FIRST EDITION

The

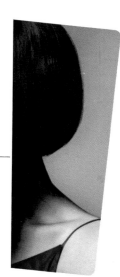

ing

∴ CENGAGE
Learning

Australia • Brazil • Japan • Korea • Mexico • Singapore • Spain • United Kingdom • United States

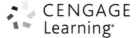

HABIA SERIES LIST

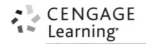

**Hairdressing & Barbering: The Foundations —
The Official Guide to Hairdressing and
Barbering VRQ at Level 2**
Martin Green

Publishing Director: Linden Harris

Commissioning Editor: Lucy Mills

Development Editor: Claire Napoli

Editorial Assistant: Lauren Darby

Production Editor: Alison Cooke

Production Controller: Eyvett Davis

Marketing Manager: Lauren Mottram

Typesetter: MPS Limited

Cover design: HCT Creative

Text design: Design Deluxe

For product information and technology assistance,
contact **emea.info@cengage.com.**

For permission to use material from this text or product,
and for permission queries,
email **emea.permissions@cengage.com.**

British Library Cataloguing-in-Publication Data
A catalogue record for this book is available from the
British Library.

ISBN: 978-1-4080-7111-3

Cengage Learning EMEA
Cheriton House, North Way, Andover, Hampshire, SP10 5BE
United Kingdom

Cengage Learning products are represented in Canada by
Nelson Education Ltd.

For your lifelong learning solutions, visit **www.cengage.co.uk**

Purchase your next print book, e-book or e-chapter at
www.cengagebrain.com

Printed in Malta by Melita Press
1 2 3 4 5 6 7 8 9 10 – 15 14 13

Contents

PART ONE Salon Skills

PART TWO Technical Skills

11 Cutting facial hair 324

13 Perming 404

12 Colouring and Lightening 348

14 Develop creativity 428

Foreword

Vocational qualifications in hairdressing have seen phenomenal success since the introduction of the NVQ Level 2 in Hairdressing in 1989, based on the standards developed by Habia.

NVQs and SVQs became the established qualification for the industry. And in time, other vocational qualifications such as the VRQ (Vocationally Related Qualification) were developed, also based on the Habia standards.

VRQs focus more on classrooms delivery, teaching and testing the underpinning knowledge required to develop skills further. This book aims to help learners achieve that underpinning knowledge.

There is no better person to guide you through it than Martin Green – one of the top hairdressing educators and writers in the UK, and author of some of the most respected and widely used textbooks in the sector, including *Begin Hairdressing & Barbering – The Official Guide for Level 1* and co-author with Leo Palladino for *Professional Hairdressing – The Official Guide to Level 3*.

Martin is passionate and enthusiastic about his industry, and has that rare skill in being able to communicate that to others, translating it into knowledge based on years of experience working in salons with clients.

The Foundations: The Official Guide to Hairdressing and Barbering Level 2 VRQ is the most up-to-date learning resource available for VRQs and reflects the changes that have taken place in the QCF.

I have no doubt it will help you achieve your qualification, and put you on the path to achieving success in your hairdressing career.

Rob Young, Habia MD

Acknowledgements

The author and publisher would like to thank the following:

For providing the cover image:

Habia

For providing images for the book:

Avlon

BaByliss PRO

Banbury Postiche Ltd

Beauty Express

Denman

Dr John Gray

E A Ellison & Co Ltd

Erik Lander

The Glove Club

Georges Hair Salon

Goldwell

HairTools Ltd

HSE

IT&LY

Jaguar

Ken Franklin

Kent

King Research, Inc.

L'Oréal Professionnel

MG Hairdressing Artisitic Team

Majestic Towels

Matador

MOSKO Hairdressing Artistic Team

MUSE

Mediscan

Media Select International

Nathan Allen

Patrick Cameron

Paul Falltrick for Matrix

Prof. Andrew Wright

Redken

REM UK Ltd

Wella

Wellcome Library

The publisher would like to thank the many copyright holders who have kindly granted us permission to reproduce material throughout this text. Every effort has been made to contact all rights holders but in the unlikely event that anything has been overlooked please contact the publisher directly and we will happily make the necessary arrangements at the earliest opportunity.

Introduction

This book provides a comprehensive course guide for anyone who wants to do a level 2 qualification, in hairdressing, barbering or in a qualification that combines both. In addition to this and because of the way it is structured, it is an excellent learning resource for people studying at all QCF credit values, whether it be award, certificate, or diploma, in a variety of different settings.

The book is written in a way so that each chapter addresses a different topic, and this enables potential students to *mix and match* the content, to suit their individual needs. For example, a student may want to do hairdressing initially, but wants to extend their skills later on to do other individual units. This allows them to progress at their own pace of learning and gain further or higher qualifications in their chosen area of work.

There are three sizes of qualification in the QCF:

- Award, between 1 and 12 credits

- Certificate, between 13 and 36 credits

- Diploma, 37 credits and above.

The structure of the QCF and the way in which qualifications are represented in it is shown in the diagram below.

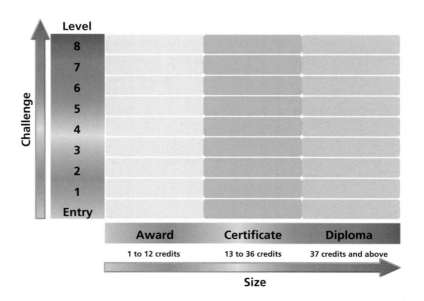

What is a Hairdressing or Barbering VRQ?

Qualifications are *littered* with abbreviations and unpronounceable words and this can all be very confusing. They often consist of a range of numbers or letters and at different types or levels, so which qualification do you choose? What credit value should it be, an award, certificate, or diploma? It is all very confusing, and when you are trying to choose, or make comparisons between one and another, you need a career councillor to help you! The good news is that you can accumulate unit credits that contribute towards a qualification.

The most important decisions that you need to make is *"what do I want to be and how am I going to get there?"*

The VRQ is a nationally recognized Vocationally Related Qualification with its content based on Habia's Hairdressing and Barbering National Occupational Standards (NOS). VRQs are known as 'preparation for work qualifications' and may take place in a simulated, although realistic, hairdressing or barbering learning environment. This could include schools, colleges, training providers, the workplace and distance learning.

Each awarding organization is required to cover the same standards in the design of their qualification. The National Occupational Standards are provided by the government-approved standards-setting body for hairdressing, beauty therapy, nails and spa therapy, Habia (Hairdressing and Beauty Therapy Industry Authority). This ensures that a future employer or training provider can be confident of the skills you will have acquired in accordance with the VRQ level you have achieved, whichever awarding organisation has accredited it. When you have successfully qualified, your diploma will bear the logo of the awarding organization you registered and qualified with, as well as the Habia logo to show that Habia approves the qualification.

The Habia website provides a list of the qualifications that can be studied. See www.habia.org.

The aim of the VRQ is to develop the skills and knowledge required when preparing to gain employment and work in the industry. Another type of vocational qualification available is the NVQ (National Vocational Qualification). The main difference between a VRQ and an NVQ is that an NVQ is a 'job ready qualification', meaning that an NVQ assessment identifies your competence and capability and readiness for work. If competent, you are said to be ready to perform your skill, meeting both the industry's, and the clients' commercial expectations. A VRQ does not assess competence', but capability and knowledge. With further experience you will become 'job ready'.

Judgment is made upon your level of practical skills and underpinning knowledge. Commercial competence requirements are less important as it is recognized that these will be achieved with experience.

Mapping Grid

VRQ Diploma (QCF) – What does it contain?

Habia i.e. The Hair and Beauty Industry Authority is the representative organization, responsible for defining the standards for our hair and beauty industry. The National Occupational Standards (NOS) that they produce are then used by awarding organizations to create the qualifications that you take part in.

All National Occupational Standards have a common structure and design. That is to say, they all follow a particular format for all vocational sectors. Each vocational qualification is made up from a number of grouped components.

Learning outcomes Each grouping or unit addresses a specific task or area of working e.g. reception. Therefore, when a staff member is asked to 'do reception' the work involves many different tasks such as; handling payments, making appointments, receiving clients and restocking products and stationery materials.

STRUCTURE and MAPPING OF UNITS The following table provides you with information relating to the names of the units addressed within this book. It also provides an indication of the individual credit value towards the qualification, an indication of the minimum Guided Learning Hours (GLH) spent on delivering the unit, and finally, where you will find this information within this book.

Unit title	Credit value	GLH	Chapter
Working in the hair industry	4	35	2
Salon reception duties	3	24	3
Display stock to promote sales in a salon	3	24	4
Promote products and services to clients in a salon	3	28	4
Follow health and safety practice in the salon	3	22	5
Client consultation for hair services	3	30	6
Shampoo and condition the hair and scalp	3	29	7
The Art of Dressing Hair	5	30	8
Plaiting and Twisting Hair	3	30	8
Styling men's hair	3	30	9
Cut women's hair	8	75	10
Cut men's hair	6	53	10
Cut facial hair	4	32	11
Colour and lighten hair	10	91	12
The Art of Colouring Hair	7	60	12
Perm and neutralise hair	7	60	13
Create an image based on a theme within the hair and beauty sector	7	60	14
Provide scalp massage services	4	33	Online in CourseMate

Units and Learning outcomes The individual units denote the smallest components of the VRQ that can be certificated. Each unit comprises a unit title and one or more objectives or **learning outcomes** and these are the smallest meaningful components within VRQ.

Unit title and Learning outcomes (example from: client consultation):

Unit title	Learning outcomes
Client consultation for hair services	Be able to consult and advise clients
	Know the characteristics of the hair

The Learning outcomes Learning outcomes are brief statements that outline what someone needs to be able to do and know. Their titles are always expressed in competency terms, e.g. 'Be able to consult and advise clients'. However, while giving you an idea of what **needs** to be done, it does not say **how** it has to be done.

These standards are comprehensive because they specify how each task is to be performed by listing; the **performance criteria**, they also cover the circumstances, i.e. the conditions or situations in which these actions must be done, which is called the **range**.

Performance criteria The performance criteria are a list of the essential actions. Although these may not be necessarily in the order in which they should be done, they do provide a definitive checklist of what needs to be done. During assessment, these performance criteria form the *'checklist'* of how a task must be done.

An example of performance criteria; showing how the task must be done:

Learning outcome	Performance criteria
Be able to consult and advise clients	**A.** Communicate in a manner that creates confidence and trust, and maintains goodwill **B.** Establish client requirements for products and services, using appropriate communication techniques **C.** Consult and complete client records **D.** Identify factors that may limit or prevent the choice of services or products **E.** Advise the client on any factors which may limit, prevent or affect their choice of service or product

Range The range statements provide a number of conditions or situations in which the learning outcomes must be performed. Quite simply, they state under what particular contexts, and on what occasions, or in which special situations, the activity must take place.

An example of range statements – identifying which situations or circumstances need to be included when doing the task:

Learning outcome	Range
	You must practically demonstrate that you have:
Be able to consult and advise clients	Provided an effective consultation for both new and regular clients
	Used questioning and observation consultation techniques and carried out tests
	Considered all influencing factors such as: Adverse hair, skin and scalp conditions, Incompatibility of previous services and products, and Lifestyle
	Dealt with suspected infections and suspected infestations

Knowledge and understanding VRQs are not just about doing though; when you do your work properly, you need to know **what** you are doing and **why** you are doing it. The terms 'theory', 'learning' and 'principles' generally refer to essential knowledge and understanding, in other words, **what you must know**.

Typical knowledge statements covering what you need to know:

Learning outcome	What you must know
Be able to consult and advise clients	**You should know:** how to communicate effectively
	You should know: the communication techniques used during client consultation
	You should know: the importance of consulting client records

At the point where a task's performance criteria and range have been covered and knowledge has been learnt and understood, the task is carried out competently and a skill has been achieved.

Ready for assessment Your competence i.e. your ability to carry out a task to a standard, is measured during **assessment**. Your ability to carry out the task, 'performance evidence', will be observed and checked against the performance criteria. Therefore, your assessor will be watching to see how you carry out your work.

Sometimes it is not possible to cover all the situations that might crop up in one performance. Therefore, in that situation, your assessor might ask you questions about what you have done and how you might apply that in different circumstances. To help you get used to this, the activities that appear throughout the book contain many types of questions that you might be asked.

Your understanding and background knowledge of work tasks is also measured through questions asked by your assessor. Sometimes you might be asked to give a personal account of what you have learned. This could take the form of writing a sequence of events that need to be done to complete the task satisfactorily. Other questions may ask you specifically about particular tasks; more often than not, these types of questions take the form of short-answer, or multi-choice type questions. Again, the activities covered within this book give plenty of examples and practice.

About the author

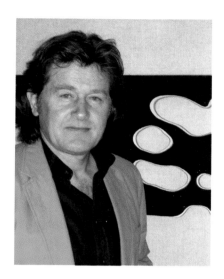

Martin Green is an experienced hairdresser and college lecturer with 40 years in the industry. During that time, he has been a consultant to Habia, where he was part of the original team that created the first NOS. He has worked for awarding organizations such as City and Guilds of London Institute (C&G) where he was a Regional Verifier for the South West, and at the Vocational Training Charitable Trust (VTCT) writing assessment materials.

Martin writes the *Official Guides to Hairdressing*. These include *Begin Hairdressing NVQ Level 1, Hairdressing and Barbering the Foundations NVQ Level 2 and Professional Hairdressing NVQ Level 3*.

Martin's energy and passion for the craft is not only demonstrated through being a practitioner, teacher and author, his enthusiasm has been unyielding, and he has keen interests in the development of e-learning and online resources too. More recently, he won a national award at *Advanced Level for Widening Participation* in education through e-learning, awarded by JISC RSC.

About the book

Throughout this textbook you will find many colourful text boxes designed to aid your learning and understanding as well as highlight key points. Here are examples and descriptions of each:

Working in hairdressing and barbering

PRACTICAL SKILLS

Learn about salon services, treatments and products

Learn how to communicate professionally in the salon with clients and colleagues

Learn about the different jobs that people do in the industry

Learn about the different training and education options that are available

Learn about the career opportunities that are available

Learn about employer rights and responsibilities

Learn about performance appraisals

Learn about transferring to other related parts of the sector

UNDERPINNING KNOWLEDGE

Conducting yourself and behaving in a professional manner

Promoting yourself in a professional way

Maintaining a professional image suitable for personal services

Taking part in self-development activities

Achieving the goals and targets that have been set

BEST PRACTICE

Suggest good working practice and help you develop your skills and awareness during your training.

HEALTH & SAFETY

Draw your attention to related health and safety information essential for each technical skill.

ACTIVITY

Feature within all chapters and provide additional tasks for you to further your understanding.

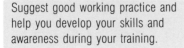
Directional arrows point you to other parts of the book that explore similar topics, in order for you to expand your learning.

CourseMate video boxes highlight some techniques which are available to view online

Tools & equipment Box

Products, tool and equipment lists help you prepare for each practical treatment and show you the tools, materials and products required.

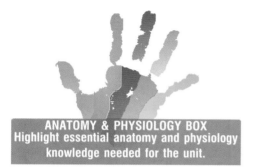

ANATOMY & PHYSIOLOGY BOX
Highlight essential anatomy and physiology knowledge needed for the unit.

TOP TIP

These share the author's experience and provide positive suggestions to improve knowledge and skills for each unit.

Knowledge Check

These boxes are designed to check your knowledge of the subject being discussed on the page. These will often include information about the current laws surrounding a topic.

SUMMARY

Summary boxes can be found at the end of each chapter and are designed to:

1 Provide a final reflection on what you have covered in the chapter.

2 Provide a clearer picture of all the essential aspects of the topic, including the tools and equipment you should be using.

3 Ensuring you have a basic understanding of the key principles.

ASSESSMENT OF KNOWLEDGE AND UNDERSTANDING

These sections provided at the end of all core chapters. You can use the questions to prepare for oral and written assessments and help test your own knowledge throughout. Seek guidance from your supervisor/assessor if there are areas you are unsure of.

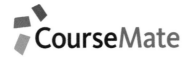

About the website

Use Hairdressing and Barbering Level 2 VRQ CourseMate alongside the *The Official Guide to Hairdressing and Barbering Level 2 VRQ 1e* textbook for a complete blended learning solution!

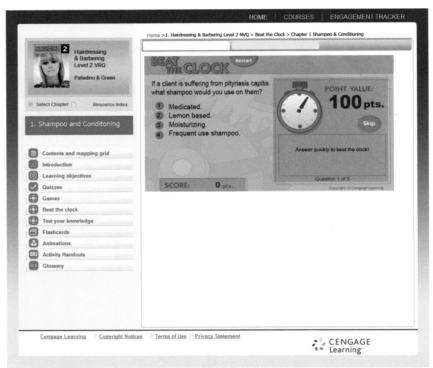

This highly interactive resource brings course concepts to life and is designed to support lecturers and students through the range of online resources which can be perfectly integrated in to the classroom to cover the guided learning hours for each unit.

For Students:

- Searchable eBook
- Step by step videos
- Interactive multiple choice quizzes

- Interactive activities and games

For Lecturers:

- Lessons plans
- PowerPoint slides
- Activity handouts

- 'Engagement Tracker' tools so students' progression and comprehension can be fully monitored

For more information please email emea.fesales@cengage.com

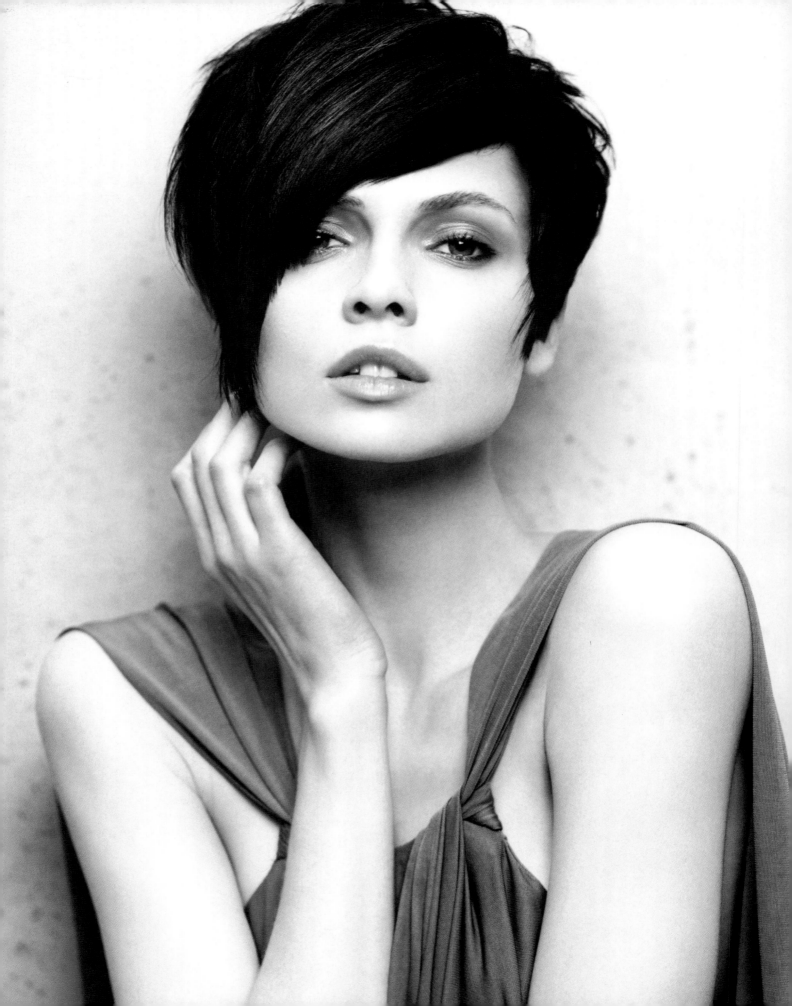

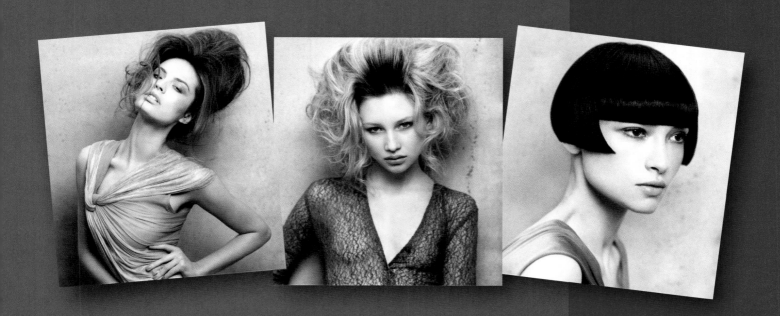

PART ONE
Salon Skills

This section provides you with some preparation for starting out, and some other, non-technical, things that could be used in a wide variety of different situations.

The first chapter looks at the tools and equipment you will be using, and gives you plenty of advice on how to look after and maintain them. The second chapter gives you more of an insight to the hair industry; the jobs that people do, along with the various routes that you could take to be a hairdresser or barber. Following this, the next three chapters have a wider application in the more general areas of work and the final chapter in this section addresses the more technical aspects of client consultation.

If you are new to hairdressing or barbering, start this book by reading this section first, as it provides the logical, and first, tiny steps into the craft.

1 Your tools and equipment box

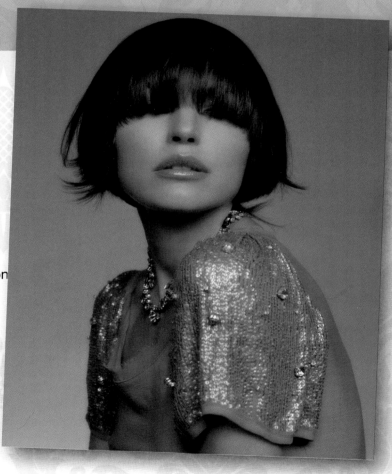

LEARNING OBJECTIVES

◆ Become familiar with the tools and equipment typically found in a college hairdressing kit

◆ Understand the uses for essential hairdressing equipment

◆ Understand how to maintain your tools and equipment to keep it in good, working condition

◆ Understand the techniques associated with each piece of cutting equipment

◆ Become familiar with the different types of cutting blocks and their uses

◆ Understand how to use and maintain modelling blocks

KEY TERMS

accessories
alkaline
back-combing/back-brushing
baselines
beta keratin
braid
clipper over comb
clippers
contact dermatitis
cornrows/corn rowing
cuticle
cutting comb

debris
Denman brush
density
diffuser
disulphide bonds
dressing
dry hair
fading (cutting reference)
freehand cutting
grade
grips and hair pins
hair extensions

knots
materials
nape
natural hair
outlines
partial colouring
perming (permanent wave)
pH balanced
pleat
porous hair
PPE (Personal Protective Equipment)

practise
radial brush
rollers
rotary massage
scalp
stylists
tapering
tension
thinning
thinning scissors
tonging
Vented brush

INTRODUCTION

The first things that you will need to get started on your college course are:

◆ This book
◆ A hairdressing kit
◆ Salon uniform

And from these items, the purchase of your college kit will be the best investment that you will ever make in the development of your career. Bearing this fact in mind, you can now get a *flavour* of what this chapter is about.

The investment made in tools for any trade is an investment for the future; it doesn't matter whether it is in carpentry or cooking, as any professional cannot work without their tools. Following on from this, the next thing to consider is the work that needs to be done; this is because having the right tools for the right job is essential.

For example, can you imagine trying to measure the height of a wall with a rolling pin, or a chef trying to peel an apple with a screwdriver? Yes, this does seem like a ridiculous analogy, but it does happen every day in hairdressing and barbering too.

Think about the following and what you would do in that situation.

Imagine that you need to comb the hair through on a long hair modelling head but you couldn't find a detangling comb. What would you do?

A Spend time looking for one?
B Try to borrow one from someone else?
C Carry on combing the modelling head with the tail comb that you have on the shelf?

Now imagine a similar situation with a client with long hair. What would you do then?

A Spend time looking for one?
B Try to borrow one from someone else?
C Carry on combing the client's long matted hair with a tail comb?

I am sure that even if you chose to comb the modelling head with your tail comb, you wouldn't dream of doing the same thing on a client. Well hopefully not!

The first thing that you need to think about is professionalism. You can't have double standards, i.e. you do one thing in one situation and something totally different in another. A true professional approaches the same procedures in the same way. That way they can standardize the results and are consistent in their approach.

Hopefully you have realized that answer C is incorrect in both situations. The reason for that is that it doesn't matter if you are practising or not, you need to put yourself in a realistic situation and therefore, in order to achieve the correct result, you have to use the correct comb. But of course, in a salon situation you can't leave a client unattended while you *forage* around for a spare detangling comb, and likewise, it would be wrong to ask someone else for their detangling comb, as they need it for their practise too.

You need to look after your tools and they need to be ready for use in the salon for all practical sessions.

Your hairdressing tools and equipment

PRACTICAL SKILLS

Know what each of your hairdressing kit items are for

How to use your tools and equipment

How to handle your modelling heads

How to maintain your modelling heads

How to maintain your tools and equipment

UNDERPINNING KNOWLEDGE

Be able to use your tools and equipment correctly

Be able to maintain your tools and equipment

Be able to prepare and use your modelling head correctly

Your hairdressing and barbering kit

This section takes you through a typical college kit item by item. For each piece of equipment, you will see:

- A picture of what it looks like.

- What the equipment is used for.

- Easy —— Hard   How hard it is to master the techniques associated with it.

- Weak —— Strong   How strong it is and therefore the care you need to take to look after it.

- Rare —— Often   How often you will be using this during your course.

- Rare —— Often   How often you will be using this after you have qualified.

- The services associated with the equipment.

- How to maintain this item.

- How to use this item.

Cutting Comb (long, parallel body, two sets of teeth)

E A Ellison & Co Ltd

Kit item use

- Sectioning and **dressing** and all cutting and barbering techniques.

- Especially useful for creating and maintaining straight base lines in longer hair.

Services involved with this item	Maintenance
◆ Cutting	✓ Remove hair and **debris** from teeth after use.
◆ Dressing out	✓ Wash in hot, soapy water and towel-dry.
◆ General combing and detangling	✓ Place in Barbicide® when not in use.
◆ Combing through setting and styling products for even application	✓ Rinse and dry after Barbicide® and before using.
◆ Some conditioning treatments	✓ Alternatively, place in UV cabinet for 15 minutes then turn over for another 15 minutes.
◆ Sectioning for colouring	✗ Do not put in back pocket as the comb will bend (it's also unhygienic!).
◆ Sectioning for **perming**	

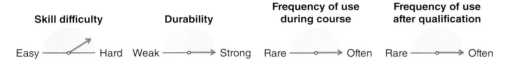

Skill difficulty	Durability	Frequency of use during course	Frequency of use after qualification
Easy ——→ Hard	Weak ——→ Strong	Rare ——→ Often	Rare ——→ Often

How is this item used? The longer **cutting comb** is a strong, durable comb that serves a multitude of purposes and you will find that you are constantly using it in many different situations. It may be more difficult to use if you have smaller hands, but is far better in maintaining accuracy for perimeter **outlines/baselines** in longer length hair.

For detangling A long backed cutting comb with two sets of teeth is useful for detangling, when a *detangling comb* is unavailable. You can comb a client's hair after shampooing and conditioning when they have been moved back to the styling unit.

◆ Take off the towel from around the client's hair.

◆ Squeeze out the excess moisture and towel-dry thoroughly.

◆ On shorter, layered hair, start at the back of the head near to the **nape** and comb through, gently removing any tangles at the point ends of the hair first and work back up the hair to nearer the root ends. Do this working up to the crown, then at the sides and backwards from the front hairline. Finally, let the natural parting fall into place and comb the hair in directions so that the hair sits properly and is ready for the next service.

◆ On longer hair lengths, start at the back of the head and separate the bulk of the hair with your fingers so that you can hold the upper bulk of the hair in one hand, while you gently comb from the point ends first and then as the tangles are removed, back up the hairshaft towards the root ends. As each section of hair is detangled, gently divide off another mesh of hair to work with in the same way. Do this all over the head, working from the back, up to the crown, into the sides then up to the natural partings. When all of the hair has been combed through, it is ready for the next service.

For sectioning The main purpose for the cutting comb is the sectioning aspect during cutting and other technical services. Sectioning is usually quite hard for any new student to master, and because of this it has been identified as fairly difficult to use.

However, when sectioning is mastered, you will find that this comb is almost as important to you as your scissors.

You will need to practise your sectioning on your modelling head for quite some time and as the hair on a 'block' is not the same as that on a client's head; once you can do it on the block you can section hair of any quantity or texture on a client's head.

Most sectioning is done to create horizontal or vertical divisions in the hair. The idea of parting the hair subdivides the main bulk; allowing you to work with and handle smaller amounts of hair that are easier to manage and will help to provide better accuracy throughout the technical service.

You can start to learn how to section on your modelling head.

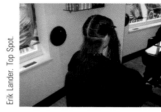 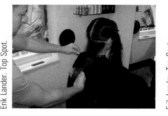 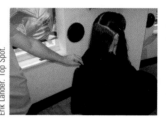

Erik Lander. Top Spot.

- Make sure that the hair is tangle free, then, using the tip, i.e. the last tooth on the coarser set of teeth, place this centrally at the back of the head; just below the crown area.

- Then, start to divide the hair downwards as if you were using the comb like a pen, making sure that you maintain contact with the **scalp**. Don't apply too much pressure, as this could hurt the client.

- As you draw the comb downwards, make sure that you use your thumb from your other hand to separate the bulk away from the comb and gather this hair into your hand.

- When you reach the lower part of the block at the nape, don't let go of the hair. Now lift it away to create a 'pony tail' to one side.

- Take the comb away from the scalp area and now with the section you are holding, place the tip again at the lower part of the hair about 2cm above the nape hairline.

- Keep the tip tooth in contact with the scalp and draw across horizontally, to a position behind the ear.

- Let the mesh you have just taken fall away from the amount of hair you are holding and you should have a clean, horizontal section that creates a straight line (parting) on the scalp.

- Secure the bulk of the hair that you are still holding into a clip on the side of the head at a point above the ear.

- You have created your first section – all other sections are created in a similar way.

For Dressing out: Go to **CHAPTER 8** for setting and dressing pp. 241–263 for more information on all the techniques associated with dressing out after setting.

BEST PRACTICE

Combs should always be clean and ready to use; make sure that all hair and debris is removed and that they have been immersed in Barbicide® for at least 30 minutes.

Cutting Comb (short, parallel body, two sets of teeth)

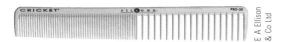

E A Ellison & Co Ltd

Kit item use

◆ Sectioning and dressing, and all cutting and barbering techniques.

For Cutting: Go to **CHAPTER 10** for cutting pp. 292–303 and **CHAPTER 11** for cutting facial hair pp. 340–343 for more information on all the techniques associated with cutting hair.

Services involved with this item	Maintenance
◆ Cutting	✓ Remove hair and debris from teeth after use.
◆ Dressing out	✓ Wash in hot, soapy water and towel-dry.
◆ Applying styling products	✓ Place in Barbicide® when not in use.
◆ Colouring	✓ Rinse and dry after Barbicide® and before using.
◆ Perming	✓ Alternatively, place in UV cabinet for 15 minutes then turn over for another 15 minutes.
	✕ Do not put in back pocket as the comb will bend (it's also unhygienic!).

Skill difficulty	Durability	Frequency of use during course	Frequency of use after qualification
Easy ——— Hard	Weak ———→ Strong	Rare ———→ Often	Rare ———→ Often

How is this item used? The shorter cutting comb is as strong and durable as its bigger *brother*, although it does lack some of the larger comb's benefits. A shorter comb is **not** suitable for detangling anything more than short hair and it doesn't provide the same advantages for helping with accuracy when cutting baselines and angles. But it is ideal for smaller hands as it is easier to control and hold between the fingers when holding sections of hair to cut.

For Sectioning See larger cutting comb as previously detailed.

Pin-tail Comb (a comb with a single row of teeth and a 10cm metal spine)

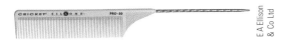

E A Ellison & Co Ltd

Kit item use

◆ Sectioning during setting and dressing-out hair.

◆ Sectioning and placing pin curls.

◆ Sectioning for heated styling equipment.

◆ Sectioning for woven highlights.

◆ Sectioning for perming.

◆ Sectioning for plaiting techniques.

Services involved with this item	Maintenance
◆ Setting and dressing ◆ Putting hair up ◆ Plaiting and twisting ◆ Colouring ◆ Highlighting ◆ Perming ◆ **Hair extensions**	✓ Remove hair and debris from teeth after use. ✓ Wash in hot, soapy water and towel-dry. ✓ Place in Barbicide® when not in use. ✓ Rinse and dry after Barbicide® and before using. ✓ Alternatively, place in UV cabinet for 15 minutes then turn over for another 15 minutes. ✗ Do not put in any pocket, as the comb is very sharp and will pierce the clothes and skin! (It's also unhygienic!).

Skill difficulty	Durability	Frequency of use during course	Frequency of use after qualification
Easy ——→ Hard	Weak ——→ Strong	Rare ——→ Often	Rare ——→ Often

How is this item used? The pin-tail comb is ideal for working with small sections or meshes of hair typical in; highlighting, perming, plaiting and hair extension services. It has a narrow, parallel, steel spine that divides the hair with greater accuracy than the plastic tail comb will and this makes it far more popular for professional hairdressers. In fact, many **stylists** who use a pin-tail comb would never use the plastic version, as it seems cumbersome (i.e. clumsy) in comparison.

Like many other tools, once you have learned the skill of handling this item and achieved the results that you want, you will wonder why you worried about it.

For Sectioning The main purpose for the pin-tail comb is precision sectioning. The narrow tip of the comb allows you to divide the hair in any direction and its rounded edge enables you to run it across the surface of the scalp without causing any discomfort.

The first and second finger on one side of the comb's back and the thumb on the other hold the comb firmly. This holding position enables the stylist to turn their hand at the wrist, with palms facing downwards; which introduces the teeth of the comb to the hair, or palms upwards; which introduces the metal spine towards the hair.

This comb twisting technique ensures for setting, styling, hair-ups and perming that:

◆ Horizontal sections can be taken easily.

◆ Hair can be divided into any mesh thickness.

◆ The sectioned hair can be combed to remove tangles.

- ◆ (For setting and perming) the roller or curler can be introduced to the ends of the hair and wound in.

- ◆ (For heat styling) the body of the tongs or straighteners can be introduced to the hair and styled.

- ◆ (For hair-ups) the weft or section of hair can be manipulated and fixed into position with **grips and hair pins**.

This comb twisting and weaving technique ensures for highlighting and **partial colouring** services that:

- ◆ Horizontal (or vertical) meshes can be divided off into workable amounts.

- ◆ The sectioned hair can be combed to remove tangles.

- ◆ The hair can be held in the other hand while the tip of the comb can lift away amounts of hair from within the width of the held section.

- ◆ The woven pieces of hair can be lifted 'off' the metal spine and placed into a foil, colour wrap, easy meche, etc.

- ◆ The colour/lightener can then be applied to the hair.

HEALTH & SAFETY

Pin-tail combs are very sharp and should never be put into your pocket as they will easily pierce through clothing and your skin!

Tail Comb (a single row of teeth within a fixed plastic body and integrated tail)

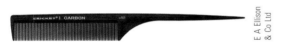

E A Ellison & Co Ltd

Kit item use

- ◆ Sectioning hair during setting and dressing-out hair.

- ◆ Sectioning and placing pin curls.

- ◆ Sectioning for heated styling equipment.

- ◆ Sectioning for plaiting techniques.

Services involved with this item	Maintenance
◆ Setting and dressing	✓ Remove hair and debris from teeth after use.
◆ Putting hair up	✓ Wash in hot, soapy water and towel-dry.
◆ Plaiting and twisting	✓ Place in Barbicide® when not in use.
◆ Perming	✓ Rinse and dry after Barbicide® and before using.
◆ Hair extensions	✓ Alternatively, place in UV cabinet for 15 minutes then turn over for another 15 minutes.
	✕ Do not put in back pocket as the comb will bend (it's also unhygienic!).
	✕ Do not put in any pocket, as the comb is relatively sharp and could cause injury.

Skill difficulty	Durability	Frequency of use during course	Frequency of use after qualification
Easy ——————— Hard	Weak ——————→ Strong	Rare ——————— Often	Rare ——————— Often

For Sectioning: Go to **CHAPTER 1** for Pin-tail Comb p. 9.

HEALTH & SAFETY

Plastic tail combs may be safer than metal pin-tail combs, but you should never put these into your pockets as it is unhygienic and will permanently bend your comb.

How is this item used? The solid-backed tail comb is not as popular or used as often as the pin-tail comb. It's not that it is any more difficult to master than the pin-tail comb and in many respects, it is more durable as the comb is made from one single injection mould.

Hairdressers, and barbers for that matter, tend to get used to a relatively small number of 'core' items that will do a large number of jobs.

This comb duplicates many of the applications that the pin-tail comb does, but it does lack the same precision and accuracy needed for sectioning;

◆ Woven highlights;

◆ Partial colouring techniques; and

◆ Some perming techniques.

Back-combing Comb (a multi-pronged comb with a single row of notched teeth)

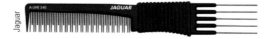

Kit item use

◆ Applying firm **back-combing** during dressing out.

◆ For lifting shape and maintaining balance during dressing out.

Services involved with this item	Maintenance
◆ Dressing out ◆ Putting hair up	✓ Remove hair and debris from teeth after use.
	✓ Wash in hot, soapy water and towel-dry.
	✓ Place in Barbicide® when not in use.
	✓ Rinse and dry after Barbicide® and before using.
	✓ Alternatively, place in UV cabinet for 15 minutes then turn over for another 15 minutes.
	✗ Do not put in back pocket as the comb will bend (it's also unhygienic!).
	✗ Do not put in any pocket, as the comb is relatively sharp and could cause injury.

Skill difficulty	Durability	Frequency of use during course	Frequency of use after qualification
Easy —— Hard	Weak —— Strong	Rare —— Often	Rare —— Often

How is this item used? The multi-pronged back-combing comb has a single row of teeth with 'notched' serrations at the lower end of each tooth near to the comb's spine. These are designed to create a very firm and solid base of back-combing into any hair type, or hair length. The other end of the comb has four fine (usually metal) prongs that are used during dressing out to provide lift and volume and maintain the hairstyle shape, without disturbing the overall effect.

Because back-combing is not as popular as back-brushing and potentially is more damaging to hair, this type of comb is hardly ever used. Admittedly, it will provide a quick, firm result, but because other combs will do a similar job, most stylists tend to leave it in their tool-pouch.

You can practise back-combing on your modelling head.

◆ Make sure that the hair is dry, brushed and tangle free.

◆ Hold the comb centrally, between the first two fingers and thumb.

◆ Starting at the upper part of the block near the crown, tilt the comb so that a single prong can be used to lift a generous, oblong section of hair away from the bulk.

◆ Hold the section vertically, away from the rest of the hair with one hand, while you smooth the remainder down with the comb.

◆ Comb through the section from the root area, up through the length to create an even **tension** throughout the section.

◆ Engage the teeth into the held section about 10–15cm away from the head and push the hair back down to the scalp area in one movement. This will immediately create a knotted mass or ball of hair at the lower end nearer to you and less knotting at the front of the section.

◆ Depending on how much back-combing you want to produce, you can repeat this action two or three times to increase the back-combed base and support.

This describes the technique of back-combing, but in a dressing out situation this is applied to any area over the head, where a 'strong base' is required for the hairstyle effect.

> **BEST PRACTICE**
>
> Handle with care. Back-combing combs are more delicate than plastic combs and the lifting spines are easily damaged.

Back-brushing Brush

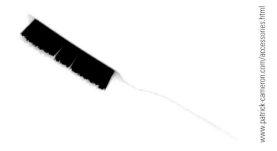

www.patrick-cameron.com/accessories.html

Kit item use

◆ Applying firm back-combing during dressing out.

◆ For lifting shape and maintaining balance during dressing out.

Services involved with this item	Maintenance
◆ Dressing out ◆ Putting hair up	✓ Remove hair and debris from the bristles after use. ✓ Wash in hot, soapy water and towel-dry. ✓ Place in UV cabinet for 15 minutes then turn over for another 15 minutes.

Skill difficulty	Durability	Frequency of use during course	Frequency of use after qualification
Easy —— Hard	Weak —— Strong	Rare —— Often	Rare —— Often

How is this item used? Back-brushing is far more popular in dressing out than back-combing. It is kinder to the hair and easier to remove from the hair (by the client, or the stylist) causing less *physical* damage, and therefore, the stylist's obvious choice for maintaining hair condition and quality.

Because the structure and support provided by back-brushing in dressing out is virtually the same as back-combing and the hair is smoothed more easily, forming a neater, desired effect, this brush should be considered as one of your main 'go to' tools.

You can practise back-brushing on your modelling head.

◆ Make sure that the hair is dry, brushed and tangle free.

◆ Hold the brush centrally, between the first two fingers and thumb.

◆ Starting at the upper part of the block near the crown, insert the tail of the brush into the hair to lift a generous, oblong section of hair away from the bulk.

◆ Hold the section vertically, away from the rest of the hair with one hand, while you smooth the remainder down with the brush.

◆ Gently brush up through the section from the root area, up through the length to create an even tension throughout the section.

◆ Engage the tips of the bristles into the held section about 10–15cm away from the head and push the hair back down to the scalp area, gently, in one movement. (This will immediately create a looser, knotted mass or ball of hair at the lower end nearer to you and no knotting at the front of the section.)

◆ Depending on how much back-brushing you want to produce, you can repeat this action two or three times to increase the back-brushed base and support.

Again, this technique can be applied to any area within a hairstyle to create lift, volume and support in the desired effect.

Detangling Comb

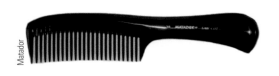
Matador

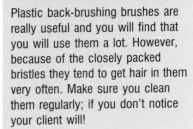

HEALTH & SAFETY

Plastic back-brushing brushes are really useful and you will find that you will use them a lot. However, because of the closely packed bristles they tend to get hair in them very often. Make sure you clean them regularly; if you don't notice your client will!

Kit item use

- Removing tangles from wet hair after shampooing and conditioning.

- Applying conditioning treatments evenly into longer hair.

Services involved with this item	Maintenance
◆ Conditioning treatments	✓ Remove hair and debris from teeth after use.
	✓ Wash in hot, soapy water and towel-dry.
	✓ Place in Barbicide® when not in use.
	✓ Rinse and dry after Barbicide® and before using.
	✓ Alternatively, place in UV cabinet for 15 minutes then turn over for another 15 minutes.
	✓ Do not put this comb in your pocket; it's unhygienic and can cause cross-infection.

Skill difficulty	Durability	Frequency of use during course	Frequency of use after qualification
Easy ——→ Hard	Weak ——→ Strong	Rare ——→ Often	Rare ——→ Often

How is this item used? For detangling you can comb a client's hair after shampooing and conditioning when they have been moved back to the styling unit.

- Take off the towel from around the client's hair.

- Squeeze out the excess moisture and towel-dry thoroughly.

- On shorter, layered hair, start at the back of the head near to the nape and comb through, gently removing any tangles at the point ends of the hair first and work back up the hair to nearer the root ends. Do this working up to the crown, then at the sides and backwards from the front hairline. Finally, let the natural parting fall into place and comb the hair in directions so that the hair sits properly and is ready for the next service.

- On longer hair lengths, start at the back of the head and separate the bulk of the hair with your fingers so that you can hold the upper bulk of the hair in one hand, while you gently comb from the point ends first and then, as the tangles are removed, back up the hairshaft towards the root ends. As each section of hair is detangled, gently divide off another mesh of hair to work with in the same way. Do this all over the head working from the back, up to the crown, into the sides then up to the natural partings. When all of the hair has been combed through, it is ready for the next service.

For conditioning treatments the comb is used in the same way as detangling, but for the purpose of spreading conditioner through the hair evenly so that all porous areas are treated.

Denman brush

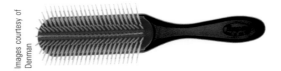

Images courtesy of Denman

Kit item use

◆ Blow-drying different hair lengths into smoother styles.

◆ Achieving small amounts of lift during blow-drying.

◆ Brushing out **dry hair** and moderate detangling before shampooing.

◆ Brushing out roller marks after setting and before dressing out.

Services involved with this item	Maintenance
◆ Blow-drying ◆ Dressing out ◆ Putting hair up ◆ Detangling and general brushing prior to many other services	✓ Remove cushioned, rubber brush head by sliding out of handle and open flat. ✓ Check rubber head for splits or damage. ✓ Remove rows of nylon bristles from rubber head and wash bristle rows, brush head and brush back in hot, soapy water and towel-dry. ✓ Place individual items in UV cabinet for 15 minutes then turn over for another 15 minutes. ✓ Reassemble the bristle rows into the brush head and fold into shape. ✓ Apply a little talc to the slotted grooves and slide back into the handle.

For blow-drying: Go to CHAPTER 8 for blow-drying techniques pp. 232–237.

For setting and dressing out hair: Go to CHAPTER 8 for brushing out hair pp. 246–247.

For general brushing and detangling: Go to CHAPTER 7 on shampooing and conditioning pp. 210–213.

Skill difficulty
Easy —— Hard

Durability
Weak —→ Strong

Frequency of use during course
Rare —→ Often

Frequency of use after qualification
Rare —→ Often

How is this item used? The **Denman brush** is the most useful brush item that a hairdresser can own. If looked after properly, it will give several years of unfailing service. It has several applications and is used as a styling item as well as for general brushing.

BEST PRACTICE

The Denman is the most versatile brush that you will own; they are very durable and comfortable for the clients too. You can make them last longer by making sure that you dry the rubber head after cleaning; this will help to prevent the rubber from splitting and perishing.

Paddle brush

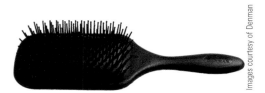

Images courtesy of Denman

Kit item use

◆ Blow-drying longer, one-length hair into smoother styles.

◆ Brushing out dry hair and moderate detangling before shampooing.

Services involved with this item	Maintenance
◆ Blow-drying ◆ Detangling and general brushing prior to many other services	✓ Remove hair and debris from teeth after use. ✓ Wash in hot, soapy water and towel-dry. ✓ Place brush in UV cabinet for 15 minutes then turn over for another 15 minutes.

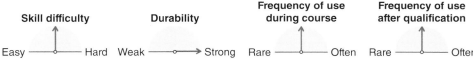

Skill difficulty Easy ——————— Hard

Durability Weak ——————→ Strong

Frequency of use during course Rare ——————— Often

Frequency of use after qualification Rare ——————— Often

How is this item used? The paddle brush is designed for longer hair; it has a cushioned, wide head, with coarser, soft tip bristles. This makes it the most comfortable brush for detangling any length hair before shampooing and general brushing for longer hair. If there is one brush that should be recommended for use by clients on their own hair or their daughter's long hair, then this is it. As a general brush, it is very easy to use and lasts a long time. As a blow-drying brush it is slightly harder to master, but the wider flatter head helps to control the hair during drying.

For blow-drying The width of the brush head makes the user place sections of their hair upon the brush before they can dry them. In many ways this removes a lot of the problems that a novice could encounter as:

◆ It makes the user place the (their) hair onto the brush head, which uses both hands and stops them from using the brush to twist the hair over the bristles.

◆ A wider brush with wider teeth is easier to hold and doesn't tangle so easily as narrower brushes.

◆ It helps the hair to dry faster than narrower, bristled brushes.

BEST PRACTICE

Paddle brushes are really suited for longer or thicker hair types; get used to using the right brush for the right job.

Vented brush

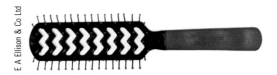

E A Ellison & Co Ltd

Kit item use

◆ Blow-drying short, medium and longer length hair.

◆ Achieving small amounts of lift during blow-drying.

◆ Brushing out roller marks after setting and before dressing out.

Services involved with this item	Maintenance
◆ Blow-drying	✓ Remove hair and debris from teeth after use.
	✓ Wash in hot, soapy water and towel-dry.
	✓ Place brush in UV cabinet for 15 minutes then turn over for another 15 minutes.

Skill difficulty	Durability	Frequency of use during course	Frequency of use after qualification
Easy — Hard	Weak — Strong	Rare — Often	Rare — Often

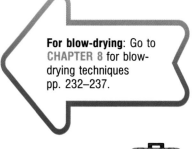

For blow-drying: Go to CHAPTER 8 for blow-drying techniques pp. 232–237.

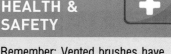

HEALTH & SAFETY

Remember: Vented brushes have very stiff bristles and this can be quite painful for clients with sensitive scalps.

How is this item used? The vented type brush is made by many manufacturers and has both advantages and disadvantages. The cheaper versions of this brush are made from one piece and have narrow, strong bristles that are 'planted' directly into its handle. The more expensive versions have a 'soft-touch' handle, which improves the grip, so has less chance of ending up on the floor. One of its disadvantages is that it can be painful for the client if the stylist has had little practice or training in using it, as it is very light in weight, and can lead to a stylist being 'heavy handed' in use.

Vented brush bristles are quite stiff and they can scratch the client's scalp during use, especially the first row of bristles, as these engage with the head first when picking up hair. Because of this, a vented brush is **not** recommended for general brushing and detangling.

The vented brush does have one main advantage over all other brushes, i.e. the speed at which it can dry hair during blow-drying; which is due to the brush's design. The brush head has a *skeletal* construction, which allows the flow of air from a blow-dryer to pass through the hair rather than being deflected off the surface of the brush head. This simple scientific benefit speeds up drying by up to a half, and in a busy salon, this has obvious attractions.

Radial brush

There are two types, and a typical radial brush set of either type will have up to five different sizes.

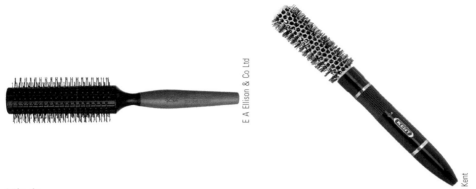

E A Ellison & Co Ltd

Kent

Kit item use

◆ Blow-drying short, medium and longer length hair.

◆ Achieving strong lift during blow-drying.

◆ Creating end curl and movement in all lengths of hair.

Services involved with this item	Maintenance
◆ Blow-drying	✓ Remove hair and debris from teeth after use.
	✓ Wash in hot, soapy water and towel-dry.
	✓ Place brush in UV cabinet for 15 minutes then turn over for another 15 minutes.

Skill difficulty	Durability	Frequency of use during course	Frequency of use after qualification
Easy ——— Hard	Weak ——→ Strong	Rare ——→ Often	Rare ——→ Often

How is this item used? The radial brush is the only tool for adding volume and curl into a blow-dried style. They are very durable and designed to be heated and cooled by a dryer; all day long and throughout the working week. Admittedly, there are different qualities and the brush set that you start with may need replacing within a few years, but a more expensive set will last you most of your hairdressing career.

There are two main types of radial brush and these are illustrated.

◆ Type 1. This type of brush has strong, plastic teeth like a 'vented' brush. This type of brush is quicker to use and dries hair more quickly than a Type 2. It is designed to be used in a similar way to a Denman or Vent brush, in that it is used by one hand while the blow-dryer is held in the other. During use, the leading edge/rows of bristles are engaged with the hair to pick up and roll it around the brush's body while it is dried into shape. This type of brush is good for providing lift and end curl.

◆ Type 2. This type of brush has softer bristles that are positioned closer together in a *'bottle brush'* design. These bristles try to prevent the hair from falling inwards, i.e. lying closer to the brush's body. Therefore, the Type 2 brush works in a way more similar to a setting roller than a blow-drying brush. This provides a much stronger root lift, volume and end curl than the Type 1. However, because the hair is more easily tangled on this type of brush, you need two hands free during the blow-dry so that you can pick up and position the ends around the brush carefully before drying into style.

Please note: You may only have one set of brushes in your college kit and you really need to master the techniques associated with both. You may need to consider purchasing additional brushes when you can afford them.

Neck brush

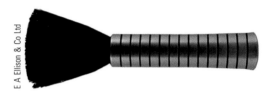

E A Ellison & Co Ltd

Kit item use

◆ Brushing wet or dry clippings away from the skin during cutting of women's or men's hair.

◆ Brushing away fragments of dry hair during clippering and beard or moustache trimming.

Services involved with this item	Maintenance
◆ Cutting women's hair ◆ Cutting men's hair ◆ Cutting beards and moustaches	✓ Wash in hot, soapy water and towel-dry. ✓ Place brush in UV cabinet for 15 minutes then turn over for another 15 minutes. ✗ Do not allow the brush to dry with bristles in a bent position, as it will shorten the brush's life dramatically.

Skill difficulty	Durability	Frequency of use during course	Frequency of use after qualification
Easy ——— Hard	Weak ——— Strong	Rare ——→ Often	Rare ——→ Often

How is this item used? Unfortunately, the longer bristle neck brush is prone to shedding hairs and becoming misshapen, particularly if they are not looked after carefully. As an alternative, you can purchase a shorter length bristled brush. These are not as comfortable for the client, but they are more durable. Remember during cutting to use the neck brush regularly, as the client is unlikely to tell you that the cut hair is irritating them. Make a point of stopping at different points during cutting to brush away (from side to side) any hair that is resting near the cutting collar or that has fallen forwards on to the client's face. This is particularly uncomfortable during cutting of men's facial hair as the fragments tend to fly all over the place and are far stiffer, and stronger, than hair cut from the upper part of the head.

Cutting collar

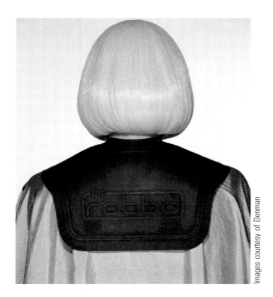

Images courtesy of Denman

Kit item use

◆ Protecting the client from clippings going down their neck during cutting services.

◆ Keeping the client comfortable during cutting services.

◆ Keeping clothes smooth under the cape or gown during cutting, providing a flatter base on which to cut, and improving cutting accuracy.

Services involved with this item	Maintenance
◆ Cutting women's hair ◆ Cutting men's hair ◆ Cutting beards and moustaches	✓ Wash in hot, soapy water and towel-dry. ✗ Do not put in direct sunlight or place on anything hot, as this will change the material's properties, causing it to distort or split.

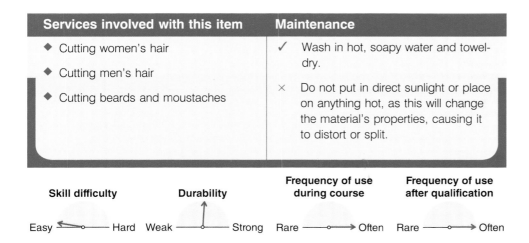

Skill difficulty	Durability	Frequency of use during course	Frequency of use after qualification
Easy ⟵○— Hard	Weak ——○— Strong	Rare —○—→ Often	Rare ——○—→ Often

How is this item used? **Note:** Cutting collars vary in price and quality dramatically; a typical college kit item will be at the entry level quality, and may not last the length of the course. The more expensive versions are made from **materials** that are more durable and have 'weighted' fronts that help to keep cumbersome clothes down. These will last for several years, providing they are maintained properly.

The cutting collar is an invaluable piece of equipment and any hairdresser or barber that doesn't use one is being unprofessional in their work. It provides **PPE** for the client and helps to maintain accuracy during the haircut by either providing a base to establish balance and do **freehand cutting** against, or by keeping clothes out of the way, which enables the stylist to see the position of the shoulders in relation to the cut length of the hairstyle.

Cutting collars keep the hair fragments out of necklines and clothes.

Water spray

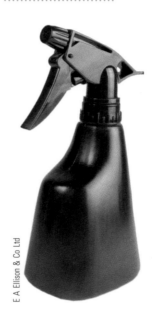

E A Ellison & Co Ltd

Kit item use Keeping hair damp during:

◆ Cutting services

◆ Rollering while setting

◆ Winding while perming

Services involved with this item	Maintenance
◆ Cutting ◆ Setting ◆ Perming	✓ Remove spray top and wash bottle and spray in hot soapy water, rinse with clean water and dry with a towel. ✓ **During use*** – rinse out stale water often and replace with fresh, clean water.

Skill difficulty	Durability	Frequency of use during course	Frequency of use after qualification
Easy ⟵——— Hard	Weak ——↑—— Strong	Rare ——→ Often	Rare ——→ Often

How is this item used? Apply a light misting to the hair during:

◆ Cutting – to provide more control when cutting dry or to stop hair from drying while you work when cutting wet.

◆ Rollering – so that all the hair being set doesn't have a chance to form an unstretched 'beta keratin' state before going under a dryer.

◆ Winding perms – to help wind sections with an even tension and to help with the correct placement of the 'hair points' around the perm rod (eliminating fish hooks).

BEST PRACTICE

Keep your water spray filled with fresh water. Stale water can smell and can even make the client's hair feel greasier.

Sectioning clips (Two types – 'crocodile' clips and flat clips)

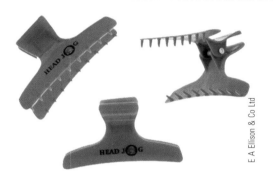

E A Ellison & Co Ltd

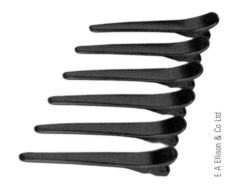

E A Ellison & Co Ltd

Kit item use

◆ Sectioning and fixing hair out of the way while you work methodically, in a variety of hairdressing services.

Services involved with this item	Maintenance
◆ Cutting	✓ Wash in hot, soapy water and towel-dry.
◆ Colouring	
◆ Lightening	✓ Place brush in UV cabinet for 15 minutes then turn over for another 15 minutes.
◆ Perming	
◆ Setting and dressing	
◆ Plaiting and twisting	
◆ Putting hair up	
◆ Conditioning treatments	
◆ Consultations	

Skill difficulty	Durability	Frequency of use during course	Frequency of use after qualification
Easy ——○—— Hard	Weak ——○—— Strong	Rare ——○—→ Often	Rare ——○—→ Often

How is this item used? It may seem that they do the same job, so you would be asking;'why have both?' Well, you will need both and as they are easily mislaid or broken, you will probably have to replace them during your course.

Each one does have advantages and disadvantages.

The 'Crocodile' clip *Good for holding bulk and weight*

◆ Advantage – Has *powerful jaws* that are great for holding large amounts of hair or dense, heavy hair out of the way.

◆ Advantage – good for holding longer hair up and out of the way.

◆ Disadvantage – the clip is quite vicious and can easily be placed too tightly and will pull or catch on the client's hair.

◆ Disadvantage – doesn't last as long as a flat clip, and the springs tend to give out quicker so it has to be thrown away.

> **BEST PRACTICE**
>
> Tip – only use this type of clip on heavy, dense or thicker, longer hair. Never use on finer; more delicate hair types.

The Flat clip *Good for delicate or precision placement and better organization of work.*

◆ Advantage – more useful on shorter or layered hair.

◆ Advantage – easier to remove and doesn't catch on the client's hair; far more comfortable to wear.

◆ Advantage – clips the hair parallel to the head so it is easier to judge balance during cutting.

◆ Advantage – does not crush or distort dry, styled hair. You should only ever use these during hair-ups, plaiting, twisting and heated styling; i.e. **tonging** and straightening, etc.

◆ Disadvantage – not as strong as the crocodile so will not hold heavy hair securely and is more prone to breaking.

> **BEST PRACTICE**
>
> Different types of flat clips do different jobs. You need to have both; the crocodile clips for large amounts of thick or heavy hair and the flat clips for precision sectioning and hair placement.

Colouring set (brush, bowl and measuring flask)

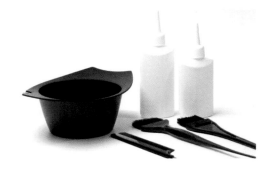

Kit item use

Services involved with this item	Maintenance
◆ Colouring ◆ Lightening ◆ Highlighting	✓ Wash items in hot, soapy water and towel-dry. ✗ Never leave colour on the brush around the top of the bristles as it will affect the next colour that you use with it. ✗ Never leave developer in the measuring flask.

Skill difficulty	Durability	Frequency of use during course	Frequency of use after qualification
Easy ———→ Hard	Easy ———→ Hard	Rare ———→ Often	Rare ———→ Often

How is this item used? The standard college kit colouring set is very durable and will last you for years. Although more manufacturers are trying to modify something in its design in the hope of selling more, the classic brush set is still the best. Newer versions may look appealing with colourful, larger bowls, wider brush tips and chamfered edges. But if you have the choice, choose a brush that is conventionally narrow like the one shown and a bowl that has a rubberized (neoprene) grip to stop it sliding about on your work trolley when you try to use it.

This type of brush provides the stylist with far greater control and accuracy in colouring or lightening:

◆ Small or narrower root areas.

◆ Woven highlights.

◆ Partial colouring techniques.

In addition to this the brushes last longer and are less prone to misshaping/bending.

For Colouring and lightening services: Go to CHAPTER 12 on colouring and lightening hair p. 348.

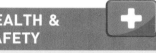

HEALTH & SAFETY

Clean your colouring brushes thoroughly; making sure that you get to the base of the bristles and removing any previously used product. If you don't you may get a very surprising colour result next time you use them!

Highlighting cap

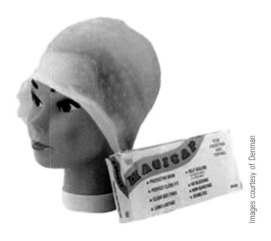

Images courtesy of Denman

Kit item use Quick applications of full head or part head, single colour highlights

Services involved with this item	Maintenance
◆ Highlighting	✓ The cap must be prepared before it can be used – all seals must be pierced before use.
	✓ After use – cap must be washed in hot, soapy water and rinsed and towel-dried well.
	✓ Talc the inside of the cap before applying to a client's head; this will help to slip on the cap more easily. Otherwise, the rubber will pull the client's hair.

Skill difficulty	Durability	Frequency of use during course	Frequency of use after qualification
Easy ——— Hard	Weak ——— Strong	Rare ——— Often	Rare ——— Often

How is this item used?
The cap highlighting method is far less popular in professional salons than other more creative options and only exists to any *real* extent in barbering and mobile work as an affordable solution to quick colour effects.

There isn't any skill required for using it and this method of highlighting has limited applications in professional hairdressing and barbering. There are particular reasons for this:

1 Specific placement of colour is very inaccurate as it is very difficult to see through the cap to the client's hair beneath.

2 The cap is totally unsuitable for thicker hair or hair over 10cm long as it is too painful for the client during the process.

3 The cap has a fixed size and can be very uncomfortable for certain clients.

4 The cap is made of rubber and the holes start to split after a couple of uses – this allows product to 'bleed' through and affect other areas of the hair, causing problems and not solving them.

5 It only allows the stylist to apply a single colour, whereas foils, easy meche, etc. facilitate multiple colour applications.

Disposable gloves (Nitrile or Vinyl)

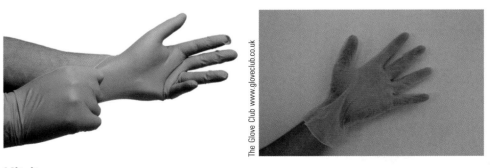

The Glove Club www.gloveclub.co.uk

Kit item use
◆ Standard PPE within the salon and must be worn in all situations where hands may come into contact with chemicals and wet working, such as shampooing.

◆ Eliminating the risk of **contact dermatitis**.

Services involved with this item	Maintenance
◆ Shampooing and conditioning ◆ Conditioning treatments ◆ Colouring – mixing and application ◆ Lightening – mixing and application ◆ Perming – application of lotion ◆ Neutralizing	✓ None – disposable gloves have very limited life and a new pair is worn for each service/treatment.

Skill difficulty	Durability	Frequency of use during course	Frequency of use after qualification
Easy ⟵—○—— Hard	Weak ——————— Strong	Rare ———○——▶ Often	Rare ————○——▶ Often

How is this item used?

There are two forms of acceptable disposable gloves, nitrile and vinyl. The choice of which one you wear is up to you, but it is an essential item of PPE for hairdressers, and they need to be worn at all times. Nitrile are a bit thicker and may last longer if they are looked after, whereas the vinyl glove does not catch on the client's hair and has more sensitivity for the hands when worn.

Step 1. Wear disposable non-latex gloves when rinsing, shampooing, colouring, lightening, etc.

Step 2. Dry your hands thoroughly with a soft cotton or paper towel.

Step 3. Moisturize after washing your hands, as well as at the start and end of each day. It's easy to miss fingertips, finger webs and wrists.

Step 4. Change gloves between clients. Make sure you don't contaminate your hands when you take them off.

Step 5. Check your skin regularly for early signs of **dermatitis**.

HEALTH & SAFETY

Don't undertake ANY hairdressing technical service that involves contact with chemicals without wearing gloves.

Plastic apron

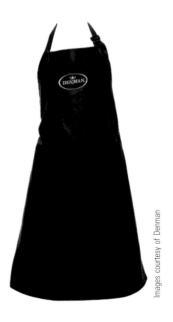

Images courtesy of Denman

Kit item use

◆ Standard PPE within the salon and must be worn for all chemical treatments or services.

Services involved with this item	Maintenance
◆ Conditioning treatments ◆ Colouring ◆ Lightening ◆ Perming ◆ Neutralizing	✓ Simply wipe over with a cloth to remove light staining. ✓ Wash in hot soapy water to remove heavier soiling, blot dry with a towel and hang up so that creases fall out.

Skill difficulty	Durability	Frequency of use during course	Frequency of use after qualification
Easy ⟵ Hard	Weak ↑ Strong	Rare → Often	Rare → Often

How is this item used? A typical hairdressing apron has adjustable neck straps to suit different heights and for extra comfort. They usually have two large front storage pockets for holding a range of hairdressing items, gloves and **accessories**. Most aprons are designed with ease of maintenance in mind so many are machine washable.

The salon apron must be worn as standard PPE for all of the above salon services.

Setting rollers (Several sizes ranging from large to very small)

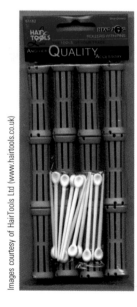

Images courtesy of HairTools Ltd (www.hairtools.co.uk)

Kit item use

◆ Wet setting – providing all hair lengths with lift, volume, movement or curl.

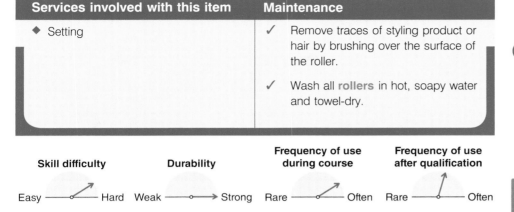

Services involved with this item	Maintenance
◆ Setting	✓ Remove traces of styling product or hair by brushing over the surface of the roller.
	✓ Wash all **rollers** in hot, soapy water and towel-dry.

For setting: Go to **CHAPTER 8** for setting hair pp. 241–244.

Skill difficulty	Durability	Frequency of use during course	Frequency of use after qualification
Easy ——→ Hard	Weak ——→ Strong	Rare ——→ Often	Rare ——→ Often

How is this item used? The skills relating to setting and dressing out are directly applicable to other aspects such as blow-drying and the use of heated styling equipment. Few students say that they enjoy setting, but it is one of those essential processes of professional hairdressing.

Setting hair, i.e. rollering, is quite difficult for any new student hairdresser to master; a lot of your training will be spent applying rollers onto your mannequin head. When you have worked out the sizing of the rollers in relation to the effect you are trying to achieve, and the placement and apportioning of hair into the roller, this skill will never be forgotten.

HEALTH & SAFETY

Setting lotions and other styling products are dried onto the rollers each time they are used. This builds up a dirty layer upon the roller making them unhygienic to use. They will need regular washing and drying before they are used.

Pins, grips and clips

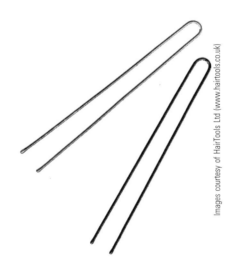

Images courtesy of HairTools Ltd (www.hairtools.co.uk)

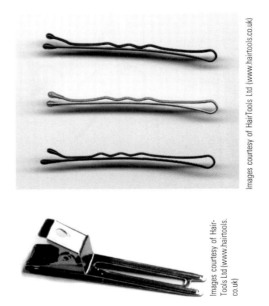

Images courtesy of HairTools Ltd (www.hairtools.co.uk)

Images courtesy of HairTools Ltd (www.hairtools.co.uk)

Kit item use

- ◆ **Pins:** Securing rollers into wet hair while setting.
- ◆ **Grips:** Securing dry hair into position for all sorts of hair dressings and hair-ups, e.g. **pleats**, plaits, **knots**, rolls, twists, folds, etc.
- ◆ **Clips:** Pin curling – a setting technique where clips often form part of the overall set hair style.

HEALTH & SAFETY

Pins, clips and grips are small fiddly items that can drop on the floor, particularly when you try to handle them. Never use a clip, pin or grip if it has been on the floor; if it can't be cleaned it must be binned.

Services involved with this item	Maintenance
◆ Setting	✓ The metal pins, grips and clips have no method for cleaning and maintaining hygiene.
	✓ Plastic pins are often used in college kits instead of metal pins. These can be washed in hot soapy water and dried with a towel before putting away.

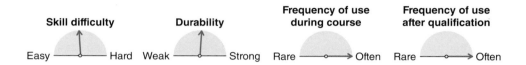

Skill difficulty	Durability	Frequency of use during course	Frequency of use after qualification
Easy ——○—— Hard	Weak ——○—— Strong	Rare ——○—→ Often	Rare ——○—→ Often

Scissors

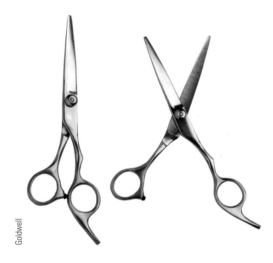

Goldwell

Kit item use

◆ All cutting services for men and women.

Services involved with this item	Maintenance
◆ Cutting women's hair ◆ Cutting men's hair ◆ Beard and moustache trimming	Good quality scissors need very little maintenance and, providing they haven't been dropped, they should last well and can be re-sharpened when the blades are dull. After use: ✓ Remove any hair fragments from around the pivot screw with a small, (electric clipper) maintenance brush. ✓ Oil the pivot screw with electric clipper oil.

(Continued)

(Continued)

✓ Wipe the blades over with any remaining clipper oil to assist the cutting action then remove any excess.

✓ Place brush in UV cabinet for 15 minutes then turn over for another 15 minutes.

✓ Keep them in a tool pouch when not in use.

✕ Do not put in any pocket, as they are very sharp and will pierce the clothes and skin it's also unhygienic!.

✕ Do not leave out on the work surface as they can easily be knocked off and get damaged.

Go to **CHAPTER 10** on cutting women's and men's hair.

Go to **CHAPTER 11** on cutting men's facial hair. See pp. 340–342 for more information.

Skill difficulty	Durability	Frequency of use during course	Frequency of use after qualification
Easy ➔ Hard	Weak ➔ Strong	Rare ➔ Often	Rare ➔ Often

How is this item used? Scissors are the most important tool that you will ever own for furthering your career. You will find by the end of your course that your standard, entry level 'college kit' scissors will not be suitable for the commercial work that you will be doing, so you need to be ready to make a further investment in your future, and be prepared to spend considerably more on them.

Scissors vary greatly in their design and quality, ranging from around £25.00 up to £500.00.

BEST PRACTICE

Never ask to borrow someone else's scissors, you may damage them accidentally and find that you have an expensive bill to pay.

BEST PRACTICE

Scissors are the best investment in your styling future, buy the best you can afford when it comes to upgrading.

Thinning scissors

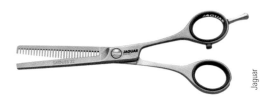

Jaguar

Kit item use

◆ **Thinning** hair

◆ **Tapering** hair

◆ Texturizing profile hair around the face and neck

Services involved with this item	Maintenance
◆ Cutting women's hair ◆ Cutting men's hair	✓ Remove any hair fragments from around the pivot screw with a small, (electric clipper) maintenance brush. ✓ Oil the pivot screw with electric clipper oil. ✓ Wipe the blades over with any remaining clipper oil to assist the cutting action then remove any excess. ✓ Place brush in UV cabinet for 15 minutes then turn over for another 15 minutes. ✓ Keep them in a tool pouch when not in use. ✗ Do not put in any pocket, as they are very sharp and will pierce the clothes and skin it's also unhygienic!. ✗ Do not leave out on the work surface as they can easily be knocked off and get damaged.

Skill difficulty
Easy ——————— Hard

Durability
Weak ——————— Strong

Frequency of use during course
Rare ——————— Often

Frequency of use after qualification
Rare ——————— Often

HEALTH & SAFETY

Thinning scissors are prone to getting dirtier than normal scissors; make sure that you keep yours clean and hygienic to use.

Blow-dryer

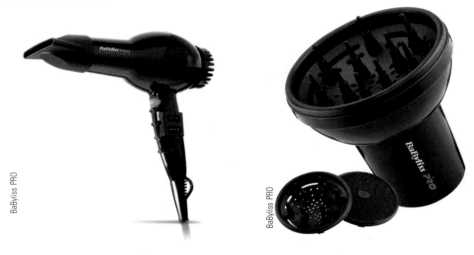

BaByliss PRO

BaByliss PRO

Kit item use Blow-drying women's or men's hair with a nozzle to produce:

- Smoother effects

- Volume

- Styles with curl or movement

Using the **diffuser** attachment for:

- Finger drying

- Spot processing/developing colour or lightener

Services involved with this item	Maintenance
- Blow-drying - Finger drying	Blow-dryers of all qualities are made from tough durable plastics. They need little maintenance, although you do need to take care when ravelling the lead around the hairdryer. ✕ If the cable is constantly coiled up, unwound and recoiled, this can, in certain instances, work the contacts in the plug loose. Always check the cable and plug before you plug the dryer into a socket. ✕ Never wash or make the dryer wet, simply wipe over the casing and leads with a dry cloth.

Skill difficulty	Durability	Frequency of use during course	Frequency of use after qualification
Easy ———— Hard	Weak ———— Strong	Rare ———→ Often	Rare ———→ Often

The blow-dryer is one of the most commonly used items of equipment in the salon. There is a huge range of models available, with a variety of power outputs, speeds and heat settings. The latest ionic dryers can even reduce the 'flyaway' effect that is produced by static electricity when hair is heated in a colder environment.

A good professional blow-dryer should:

- Have at least two speeds and two heat settings.

- Have different shaped nozzles to channel the heat onto the brush or comb.

- Have a lead long enough for it not to tangle around the chair or client.

- Be powerful enough to dry damp hair quickly (1300w–1500w).

- Have a cool shot button – to enable hot hair to be fixed (set) into shape around a brush.

- Be not too long so that it is balanced in the hand and can be held away from the client's hair during drying.

- Be light enough so that it can be manipulated easily and used for long periods without fatigue.

- Be quiet enough so that it allows natural conversation with the client.

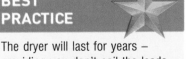

For Finger drying: Go to CHAPTER 9 on p. 276.

BEST PRACTICE

The dryer will last for years – providing you don't coil the leads around the handle as it will work the cables loose or damage the leads.

Electric clippers

Go to p. 292 for detailed information about routine maintenance and safety checks.

For Clipper techniques: Go to **CHAPTER 11** for cutting hair and cutting facial hair pp. 334–342.

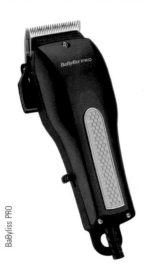

BaByliss PRO

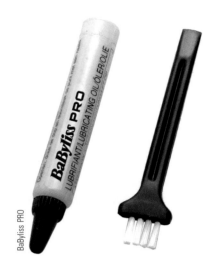

BaByliss PRO

BEST PRACTICE

Clipper blades are expensive in relation to a brand new pair of clippers. Maintain the blades regularly and make sure that you use the oil provided with them. This will prolong the clippers' life and save you money!

Kit item use

◆ Close cutting or layering with clipper **grades**

◆ Beard trimming

◆ Moustache trimming

◆ **Clipper over comb**

◆ Freehand profiling, **fading** and shaping necklines

Services involved with this item	Maintenance
◆ Cutting women's hair ◆ Cutting men's hair ◆ Beard and moustache trimming	Maintenance of **clippers** is quite involved and has serious implications for safe use and handling.

Skill difficulty
Easy ——→ Hard

Durability
Weak ——→ Strong

Frequency of use during course
Rare ——→ Often

Frequency of use after qualification
Rare ——→ Often

Straightening irons

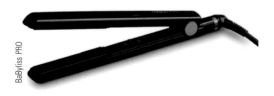

BaByliss PRO

Kit item use

◆ Smoothing and straightening hair after blow-drying.

◆ Forming wave, volume or curls on dry hair.

Services involved with this item	Maintenance
◆ Blow-drying ◆ Putting hair up ◆ Dressing out hair	Heated styling tools are made to be tough, so like blow-dryers they too are very durable. They need little maintenance; although you do need to take care when ravelling the lead around the body of the straighteners; remember to leave plenty of slack in the cable, otherwise tight coiling will shorten their life considerably. ✓ Make sure that any build-up of styling products on the surface of the hot plates is removed with a dry cloth/wipe before they are plugged in and used. ✓ Always use a heat mat or purpose built holder when they are hot or in use and leave them to cool down fully before putting away. ✗ If the cable is constantly coiled up, unwound and recoiled, this can, in certain instances, work the contacts in the plug or body of the straighteners loose. Always check the cable and plug before you plug them into a socket. ✗ Never wash or make the equipment wet, simply wipe over the plastic body and leads with a dry cloth.

For heated styling equipment: Go to CHAPTER 8 for styling hair pp.. 223–238.

BEST PRACTICE

Keep the surfaces of the hot plates clean; free from product build-up, as it will 'grab' and burn the hair next time you want to use them.

HEALTH & SAFETY

Never try to clean hot surfaces; wait until they have cooled down.

Skill difficulty	Durability	Frequency of use during course	Frequency of use after qualification
Easy ——○—— Hard	Weak ——○↗ Strong	Rare ——○→ Often	Rare ——○→ Often

Curling tongs

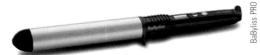

BaByliss PRO

Kit item use

◆ Forming wave, volume or curls on dry hair

Services involved with this item	Maintenance
◆ Blow-drying ◆ Putting hair up ◆ Dressing out hair	Heated styling tools need little maintenance; although you do need to take care when ravelling the lead around the body of the tongs; remember to leave plenty of slack in the cable, otherwise tight coiling will shorten their life considerably. ✓ Make sure that any build-up of styling products on the surface of the hot styling body is removed with a dry cloth wipe before they are plugged in and used. ✓ Always use a heat mat or purpose built holder when they are hot or in use and leave them to cool down fully before putting away. ✗ If the cable is constantly coiled up, unwound and recoiled, this can, in certain instances, work the contacts in the plug or body of the tongs loose. Always check the cable and plug before you plug them into a socket. ✗ Never wash or make the equipment wet; simply wipe over the plastic handle and leads with a dry cloth.

Skill difficulty: Easy —— Hard
Durability: Weak —— Strong
Frequency of use during course: Rare —— Often
Frequency of use after qualification: Rare —— Often

Modelling blocks – your new best friend

Your training mannequin head is always referred to as a modelling block. You will find during your course; or certainly the early part of it, that you will be using the modelling block every day. You will find that the skills you learn in the hours spent in training will not be wasted because each time that you use it, you are one step closer to working on real clients.

The modelling block is fairly durable but, in order for you to get the best out of it, there are things that you can do and other things that you shouldn't do. First of all and like everything else in life, they do come in a range of different qualities and types, and generally speaking, the blocks that you get in your college kit are at the cheaper end of the scale. If you do want to upgrade your block, talk to your tutor to investigate other options.

Most colleges recommend a minimum of two blocks within your college kit. One block will be used primarily for cutting and the other will be saved for setting, blow-drying, perm winding, colouring, heat styling, etc. As you can see with all these treatments and services, they do take a lot of *punishment* during your training and if you don't keep them in 'tip top' condition, you will be losing out because you won't be able to practise your skills.

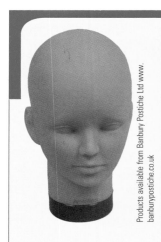

Products available from Banbury Postiche Ltd www. banburypostiche.co.uk

1. The basic ladies head form

This type of block is used with 'slip-overs'. These are pre-knotted wefts of hair that can be placed over the head form to enable you to create hair styles.

Dos and Don'ts

✓ Cutting

✓ Heat styling

✓ Setting

✓ Dressing/plaiting/twisting

✓ Hair-ups

✗ Colouring

✗ Highlighting

✗ Lightening

✗ Perming

✗ Chemical relaxers

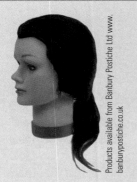

Products available from Banbury Postiche Ltd www. banburypostiche.co.uk

2. Standard modelling block

This is the general modelling head that you will find in your college kit.

100 per cent human hair 30–35cm long Medium **density**: 230–260 hairs per square cm.

The hair is chemically treated and pre-coloured to mid brown. The hair is implanted backwards around the front hairline to enable the hair to be brushed or styled back away from the facial area, smoothly and without a definite parting.

Dos and Don'ts

✓ Cutting

✓ Heat styling

✓ Setting

✓ Dressing/plaiting/twisting

✓ Hair-ups

✓ Colouring

✓ Highlighting

✓ Lightening

✓ Perming (water wind only)

✗ Chemical relaxers

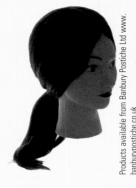

Products available from Banbury Postiche Ltd www. banburypostiche.co.uk

3. High quality modelling block

100 per cent Human hair 30–35cm long Medium density: 230–260 hairs per square cm.

This higher quality training head has a neck and shoulders and this makes it suitable for display work, precision cutting, styling and hair-ups generally associated with competition work.

Dos and Don'ts

✓ Cutting

✓ Heat styling

✓ Setting

✓ Dressing/plaiting/twisting

✓ Hair-ups

✓ Colouring

✓ Highlighting

✓ Lightening

✓ Perming

✗ Chemical relaxers

(Continued)

(Continued)

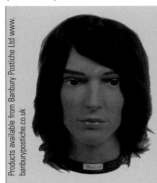

Products available from Banbury Postiche Ltd www. banburypostiche.co.uk

4. High quality male modelling block

100 per cent human hair – Large head circumference of 59cm. Forward fringe implant – 20cm long, High density 260–290 hairs per square cm.

The head circumference is larger than the standard modelling block, so there is a lot more coverage of hair over the head form, which provides a greater density and allows you to produce fringes and forward lying hair styles.

This type of block will also tolerate close clipper grades without exposing scalp/nape thin areas.

Dos and Don'ts

✓ Cutting

✓ Heat styling

✓ **Cornrows**/twists

✓ Colouring

✓ Highlighting

✓ Lightening

✓ Perming

✗ Chemical relaxers

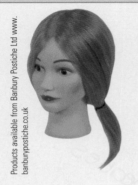

Products available from Banbury Postiche Ltd www. banburypostiche.co.uk

5. Very high quality female modelling block

100 per cent human hair – Large circumference of 59cm. Forward fringe implant – 30–35cm long. High density 260–290 hairs per square cm.

The head circumference is larger than the standard modelling block, so there is a lot more coverage of hair over the head form, which provides a greater density and allows you to produce styles with fringes or forward lying hair and hair-up finishes that are more elaborate or intricate.

Dos and Don'ts

✓ Cutting

✓ Heat styling

✓ Setting

✓ Dressing/plaiting/twisting

✓ Hair-ups

✓ Colouring

✓ Highlighting

✓ Lightening

✓ Perming

✗ Chemical relaxers

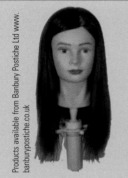

Products available from Banbury Postiche Ltd www. banburypostiche.co.uk

6. Standard quality long hair modelling block

100 per cent **Natural hair** (not necessarily human). Medium density: 230–260 hairs per square cm – 60cm long.

This type of block requires a lot of maintenance and will deteriorate quickly if the hair is NOT taken down and brushed out after EACH styling.

Dos and Don'ts

✓ Hair-ups

✓ Dressing/plaiting/twisting

✓ Cutting

✗ Heat styling

✗ Setting

✗ Colouring

✗ Highlighting

✗ Lightening

✗ Perming

✗ Chemical relaxers

(Continued)

(Continued)

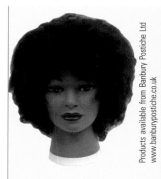

Products available from Banbury Postiche Ltd www.banburypostiche.co.uk

7. Ladies African-Caribbean modelling block

100 per cent Human hair 20cm long. Medium density: 230–260 hairs per square cm.

This type of block has very curly hair and is chemically pre-treated. It will tolerate *one chemical process but generally, these blocks are better without, and can be washed and conditioned to reactivate the curl after styling.

Dos and Don'ts

- ✓ Cutting
- ✓ Heat styling
- ✓ Setting
- ✓ Dressing/plaiting/twisting
- ✓ *Colouring
- ✓ *Highlighting
- ✓ *Lightening
- ✓ *Chemical relaxers

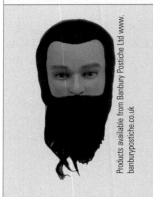

Products available from Banbury Postiche Ltd www.banburypostiche.co.uk

8. Gents head with beard and moustache

100 per cent human hair 20cm long. Medium density: 230–260 hairs per square cm.

This type of block is ideal for practising beard and moustache shaping and will tolerate reasonably close cutting without exposing scalp/nape and facial contours.

Dos and Don'ts

- ✓ Cutting
- ✓ Beard shaping
- ✓ Moustache shaping
- ✓ Heat styling
- ✓ Plaiting/twisting
- ✓ Colouring
- ✓ Highlighting
- ✓ Lightening

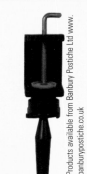

Products available from Banbury Postiche Ltd www.banburypostiche.co.uk

9. Standard clamp

All modelling blocks are packaged with a nylon/plastic adjustable clamp.

These types of clamps will enable you to affix the block to a table top or styling shelf.

Dos and Don'ts

- ✓ Make sure that you protect the surface of the shelf from scratches or dents by covering it with a towel or cloth first.
- ✕ Do not over-tighten the clamp as the screw thread area will snap off!

The table illustrates a variety of different blocks with particular uses in mind. It is advisable that if you want to specialize in longer hair work or gents barbering that you get a block fit for that purpose. For more information visit specialist retailer to the industry Banbury Postiche **http://www.banburypostiche.co.uk**.

Modelling block care and maintenance

If you want to get the most out of your block, you must look after it. Even though most blocks are made from human hair, it doesn't make them very durable. In fact, even heat styling with very hot straighteners will shorten its life and the handling properties of the block.

The main problems with handling are more to do with the way that the blocks are initially prepared and processed.

When the block manufacturers buy hair, it has to be:

✓ Cleaned

✓ Coloured

✓ Stabilized

BEST PRACTICE

ALWAYS brush out your block after styling and place a plastic bag over it to keep it tidy.

See **CHAPTER 13** on perming for more information.

Generally, the bulk hair bought for making blocks is of Asian origin and this hair is usually black. The first part of the processing is cleaning, so in the interests of hygiene, the bulk hair is washed and sterilized, and this kills off any infestations or contamination. These are strong **alkaline** chemicals and this tends to swell the hair, making it coarser in texture.

The hair is then dyed, or in some cases lightened, to produce mid-browns, golden blondes or black colour options. But the most popular colour is brown. Finally, the hair is conditioned and **pH balanced** so that the **cuticle** flattens and so that it helps with brushing and combing.

As you can see from all this chemical treatment, your block is very porous and *sensitive* to further processing. Admittedly, some blocks do seem to cope with some processes better than others and as a *rule of thumb* they cope better with colouring and lightening than they do with the chemical rearrangement of their **disulphide bonds** during perming and relaxing.

Read this before you use your block!

Process, service or treatment	What you should do	Why do I need to do this?
Shampooing	✓ Always use a mild or moisturizing shampoo with cold water. ✓ Try to get someone to hold the block in the basin so that you can run the water down through the lengths. ✓ Avoid using **rotary massage** technique, use effleurage or squeeze between your palms instead.	This will help to stop the cuticle from becoming raised, which locks the hair together making it almost impossible to detangle. This will make the hair matted, again making it difficult to detangle.
Conditioning	✓ Always use an anti-oxidant or deep moisturizing conditioner after shampooing.	This will fill damaged sites along the hairshaft and fill areas of torn or missing cuticle, helping you to detangle after use.
Detangling	✓ Always use a wide tooth comb, never use a pin-tail or cutting comb. ✓ Always start at the lower nape area first, nearer the points of the hair and remove these tangles first. Then work slower back towards the mid lengths and root area last.	The hair is going to be difficult to comb even if it hasn't been coloured or lightened, so you need to make the job easier for yourself.

(Continued)

(Continued)

Blow-drying	✓ Always dry the block off well beforehand. Squeeze excess moisture into a towel without using a rubbing action.	This will make the hair matted and lock the hair together.
	✓ Avoid overheating the hair when using flat, paddle or radial brushes as this will raise the cuticle and damage the hair further.	This will create problems for the next time you shampoo the block as the hairshaft will be swollen and the cuticle raised.
Heated styling equipment	✓ Always prep the hair first by using a heat protection.	This will extend the life of your block by helping to maintain it in a reasonable condition.
Dressing out (after setting)	✓ Setting the block in rollers doesn't create any problems but avoid back-combing during the dressing out stage.	Back-combing is potentially more damaging on any type of hair than back-brushing, so you are likely to create longer term problems and shorten the life of your block.
Plaiting – twists, cornrows, *braids*	✓ Always remove the plaits after your training session; never leave them in overnight.	When small plaits are left in for any length of time they tend to damage or distort/kink the hair and this will limit your styling options in the future.
Colouring and lightening	✓ Modelling blocks will tolerate most colouring and lightening techniques although they don't respond well to higher strength developers.	If lightening the hair to extra light blonde, it won't work; the hair will break off long before it reaches your target shade.
Styling products	✓ Avoid using any firm hold styling products on your block such as gels, hairsprays, waxes, pomades.	Blocks tend to have **porous hair** and this can make them difficult to manage after styling products have been applied.

SUMMARY

As a final reflection on what you have covered in this chapter, you should now have a clearer picture of all the essential aspects relating to the tools and equipment that you will be using. In particular, you should now have a basic understanding of the key principles of:

1 The wide variety of tools and equipment available and what they are used for.

2 How to maintain your equipment and optimize the durability (life-span) of each item.

3 How to look after and maintain your modelling heads.

And collectively, how these principles will help you to work as a true, professional hairdresser or barber.

ASSESSMENT OF KNOWLEDGE AND UNDERSTANDING

Project

There are many manufacturers of professional equipment and your kit is a small example of what is available within the craft. For this activity, look at the following brand names and find out from the Internet, the main sorts of products that they provide, what country they come from and how much their products cost.

◆ **Joewell**

◆ **Bob Tuo**

◆ **Babyliss**

◆ **Cricket**

After you have done your preliminary research, answer the following questions.

Q1.   Joewell is a manufacturer of?

Combs	☐
Brushes	☐
Clippers	☐
Scissors	☐

Q2.   Bob Tuo make cutting _____

Q3.   Babyliss make electrical equipment   True or False

Q4.   Cricket manufacture?

Scissors	☐
Rollers	☐
Brushes	☐
Combs	☐
Perm curlers	☐
Clippers	☐

Q5.   Joewell is a manufacturer in?

UK	☐
France	☐
Japan	☐
USA	☐

Q6.   Bob Tuo only manufacture products in black   True or False

Q7.   Which manufacturer produces tongs, straighteners, hair dryers, crimping irons and conical wands?

Joewell	☐
Bob Tuo	☐
Babyliss	☐
Cricket	☐

Q8.   Cricket manufacturer their products in the _____

Q9.   Joewell make metal products   True or False

2 Working in the hairdressing industry

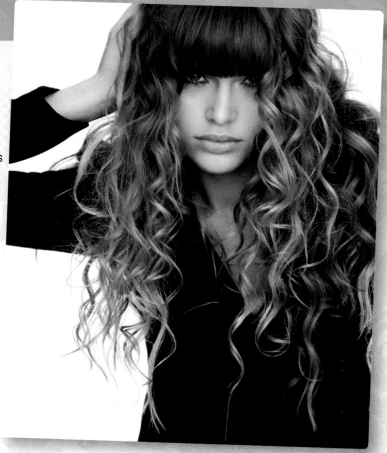

LEARNING OBJECTIVES

◆ Know the different options, timings and patterns of attendance, for full and part time courses

◆ Understand the main differences between qualification levels and how you can benefit from participation

◆ Understand the differences between employment and apprenticeships and that of college based courses

◆ Know what is expected within a salon and the basic standards that are required

◆ Know a variety of services within hairdressing and barbering and what they mean

KEY TERMS

appointment
appointment systems
appraisals
artificial colouring
awarding organization
bacteria
barrier cream
body language
body odour (BO)
C/BW
colour correction
communication

'continuing professional
    development' (CPD)
D/C
Data Protection Act
deodorants
diseases
franchised
guideline
Habia
Hair and Beauty
    Industry Authority
hair colour

Individual Learning Plan (ILP)
infections
NVQ – National Vocational
    Qualifications
Personal Development
    Plan (PDP)
PW
restyle
risk
salon policy
SWOT
sweat glands

sweat
temporary colour
Trichologist
trim
trimming
twist
VRQ – Vocationally
    Related Qualifications
W/C

Working in the hair industry; give clients a positive impression of yourself and your organization.

INTRODUCTION

There is an annual survey done in the United Kingdom on people and their work. Each year the survey looks at all the different occupations ranging from accountancy to zoo keeping, to find out how happy people are within their jobs. Over the past decade, a strong, repetitive pattern has emerged.

The findings show that the happiest groups of people are those that have contact with others. That may sound rather obvious, but when you think of the types of jobs that people do, then it isn't so simple. The vast majority of people work in some form of office environment, in administrative jobs such as data processing, payroll, insurance, local government and sales admin, to name but a few. All of these people have one thing in common; they don't get to meet anyone else other than the people they work with in the office.

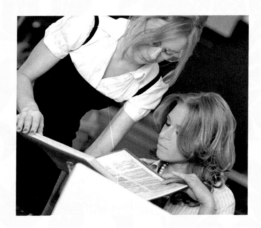

Then again, there are many who do get to work with other people, but not necessarily when they are in their best of health. This is particularly noticeable for people working in the care sector, such as those working for the NHS, or looking after the elderly in residential care, or looking after sick and the infirm in their homes. Some of the happiest people work with animals, but the drawbacks are obvious as communication can be a little limited! The winners, year after year are hairdressers.

Yes, people in hairdressing are the happiest people in their jobs and there are probably some underlying, *philanthropic* reasons for this. For many people at work, the nature of what they do has a negative impact upon their wellbeing. Many people have jobs where they spend their time in the constant support of others, or deliberately trying to 'out-do' people by selling them things that they do not want or need. All this work is tiring and tedious, and it begins to show after a while in the ways that people say they hate their job! Not so for hairdressers and barbers, as people in this industry get to meet new people and do new and exciting things every day.

Our clients rely upon us to bring a welcoming, social break in their routine, *'same old'*, busy lives. But that's not all. Our clients trust us and that is because they have built up a relationship over time. They know that what we do for them works and they are happy to pay for the services and advice that we provide.

What could be better than making a living out of making others feel good about themselves?

Working in hairdressing and barbering

PRACTICAL SKILLS

Learn about salon services, treatments and products

Learn how to communicate professionally in the salon with clients and colleagues

Learn about the different jobs that people do in the industry

Learn about the different training and education options that are available

Learn about the career opportunities that are available

Learn about employer rights and responsibilities

Learn about performance appraisals

Learn about transferring to other related parts of the sector

UNDERPINNING KNOWLEDGE

Conducting yourself and behaving in a professional manner

Promoting yourself in a professional way

Maintaining a professional image suitable for personal services

Taking part in self-development activities

Achieving the goals and targets that have been set

Learning to be a hairdresser or barber

There are many routes into the industry and many roles to fill. So how can you get started, where can you learn? If you want to consider a future in hairdressing or barbering, you have several options that you can consider, and some of these will depend on your starting point.

Young learners

We tend to think of younger learners as those that have chosen to enter the industry after leaving school. Quite often, the school leaver entrant to the craft has had some experience or links with hairdressing or barbering before. The educational system that these people have experienced has given them the *Year 10* opportunity to do work experience in industry and, historically, hairdressing has been a popular option.

Work experience has been (and still is) a big motivator for many students, as it gives them the opportunity to see what the industry has to offer and without any firm commitments. This has encouraged many young people to progress further and to approach salons and barbers to get Saturday jobs or holiday work.

Adult learners

This group of people tends to fall into two different categories:

1   As far as colleges of further education are concerned, an adult learner is some-one over the age of 19. Of course, a 19-year-old entrant may have also been in mainstream schooling, but had stayed on to do other qualifications, so their understanding of vocational futures will be similar to that of a student leaving school at 16.

2   However, the adult learner covers a wide age band and the industry tends to find that it attracts people of all ages. Many adults consider hairdressing or barbering as an alternative career and will take it up after working in another sector for years. The options available to this type of learner will often need more flexibility in attendances, so programmes held in evening classes and short courses provide popular alternatives.

College-based programmes for hairdressing and barbering

There are hundreds of further education colleges available for providing vocational qualifications in hairdressing and barbering. You will have one that is local to you, so you should be able to find out what they offer by looking at their website or by calling the hairdressing department.

TOP TIP

There are two qualification routes into hairdressing/barbering via further education colleges or private training providers:

1   NVQ – National Vocational Qualifications

2   VRQ – Vocationally Related Qualifications

And these two types of qualification are very different in their approach to entering the hairdressing and barbering industry.

TOP TIP

The NVQ route into the industry is available in:

1   College

2   Private training providers

3   Employers/employment

This educational system has been popular for entry into the industry since the mid-80s. Learners who take the NVQ route into hairdressing or barbering have to participate in a balanced programme of 'on', and 'off' the job training. In a college, this approach is delivered through work experience. That is, students attend college on a part-time or

TOP TIP

The VRQ route differs from the NVQ in that it is not really an industry-led qualification.

The content of the qualification is weighted towards full-time college attendance and provides extra, additional content beyond the craft skills, in areas such as:

1 Science

2 Business studies

3 **Communication**

4 Functional Skills

The awarding bodies providing these qualifications confirm that learners will be able to achieve a similar experience, although there is no 'set' status or industrially recognized role.

full-time basis and in addition to the time spent at college, they must participate in a minimum number of hours in a local salon doing work experience. The NVQ qualification that they are taking is recognized by the industry and will eventually qualify them as either a junior or senior stylist.

College flexibility There are advantages and disadvantages to college-based learning.

The main advantages are:

◆ Structure – With an organized programme of studies and course content.

◆ Learner support – Providing access to additional help not available from employer based training.

◆ Funding support – Providing access to government grants, benefits, bursaries and scholarships.

◆ Attendance times – Flexibility for a wide variety of learners with differing needs.

◆ Safety and security – ECM(Every Child Matters) safeguarding, equality and diversity.

The main disadvantages are:

◆ Academic year and terms – September enrolment for some colleges, inflexible to open recruitment patterns. This is not usually the case with private training providers.

◆ Costs – Course fees (over 19s), college kits and uniforms.

Courses available in hairdressing and barbering

Course level	Course content/aims	On completion, you can:
Level 1 Hairdressing and barbering	This qualification will: ◆ Develop your practical hairdressing and barbering skills to a basic level. ◆ Enable you to provide the professional image needed to work in a personal service industry. ◆ Develop team working skills necessary for working with others in a salon.	Assist in a salon and: ◆ Work on a salon reception. ◆ Have basic skills in dressing and blow-drying hair. ◆ Be able to apply **temporary colour**. ◆ Shampoo and condition hair. ◆ Display retail stock. ◆ Be able to plait and **twist** hair.

(Continued)

(*Continued*)

Course level	Course content/aims	On completion, you can:
		◆ Style men's hair. ◆ Promote products and services to clients. ◆ Provide scalp massage.
Level 2 Hairdressing and barbering	This qualification will enable you to: ◆ Cut both women's and men's hair. ◆ Style, dress and finish both women's and men's hair. ◆ Provide consultation services. ◆ Shampoo, condition and treat hair. ◆ Demonstrate good health and safety. ◆ Colour and lighten hair. ◆ Perm and neutralize hair. ◆ Promote services and products. ◆ Display stock effectively. ◆ Work on reception.	Get a job: ◆ Working at a junior stylist level as a women's hairdresser. ◆ Working at a junior stylist level as a men's barber. ◆ Working as a technician in colouring and perming. ◆ Working as a receptionist.
Level 3 Hairdressing and barbering	This qualification will enable you to: ◆ Creatively cut and **restyle** both women's and men's hair. ◆ Creatively style, dress and finish both women's and men's hair. ◆ Creatively dress long hair. ◆ Provide advanced consultation services. ◆ Creatively colour and lighten hair. ◆ Carry out **colour correction** services. ◆ Creatively perm long and short hair. ◆ Help plan promotional events. ◆ Take part in external shows, exhibitions and competitions. ◆ Monitor healthy and safe practices.	Get a job: ◆ Working at a senior stylist level as a women's hairdresser. ◆ Working at a senior stylist level as a men's barber. ◆ Working as a senior technician in creative colouring and perming. ◆ Doing bridal hair work. ◆ Helping with promotional events and the planning of shows. ◆ Working as a receptionist.

A student leaving school with less than two good grades will probably cope better on a Level 1 programme. The level of the course taken by a student is related to their ability.

Pattern of attendance The time and pattern of attendance to a college-based course will depend on the type of course applied for. Colleges provide more flexible options than they used to, and now the learner can attend as a part-time student, or as a full-time student.

Part-time courses Typically, a part-time course for hairdressing would be delivered as evening classes. This is not the fastest route into the industry, but it does provide an educational option for learners who may have other jobs or commitments in normal, day-time, hours. This is great for adult learners as they might have families to consider and therefore can rely upon other members of the family to look after children on those evenings.

Another benefit for evening classes is the modular approach that the colleges take in order to deliver the course. For example, an NVQ or VRQ is a qualification that is broken up into units. That means the qualification is completed on a unit by unit accumulation process. This approach lends itself very well to college courses, as the people involved in the planning can set out a programme over a year where different units are delivered at different times.

For example, a college may have two later evenings and choose to deliver a flexible programme where cutting occurs on one and, say, setting and dressing on another. This gives people the option to attend on two nights and cover their qualification more quickly than just attending once a week.

Prospectuses for courses are usually available around the end of the year, advertising courses for the next academic year.

Course duration

One of the main advantages of college-based learning over salon-based training is the length of the courses. Typically, a full-time college course aims to deliver a complete programme in one academic year. The table below provides a rough guide to how long these things take.

Course	Mode of delivery	Duration
Level 1 in hairdressing and barbering	Full-time	36 weeks (one academic year)
Level 1 in hairdressing and barbering	Fast track (leading on to Level 2)	12–18 weeks
Level 2 in hairdressing	Full-time	36 weeks (one academic year)
Level 2 in hairdressing	Fast track and Intensive (suitable for returners and some adult learners)	13–18 weeks
Level 2 in hairdressing	Part-time	72 weeks (two academic years)
Level 2 in barbering	Full-time	36 weeks (one academic year)
Level 2 in barbering	Fast track and Intensive (suitable for returners and some adult learners)	13–18 weeks
Level 2 in barbering	Part-time	72 weeks (two academic years)
Level 3 in hairdressing	Full-time	36 weeks (one academic year)
Level 3 in hairdressing	Part-time	72 weeks (two academic years)
Level 3 in barbering	Full-time	36 weeks (one academic year)
Level 3 in barbering	Part-time	72 weeks (two academic years)

Fast track programmes

In the attempt to provide all sorts of options for potential learners, some colleges have more creative modes of delivery. The numbers of learners considering hairdressing has grown immensely over the past ten years. So education has had to respond and one of these flexible options is the 'Fast-track' programme. This type of option is not suited to everyone, but works on an individual basis and depends very much on ability.

The majority of people that work in hairdressing are females and this has led to an unusual pattern. Most people are aware of the flexibility of working patterns and the variety of working hours that exist within the industry.

This produces two different types of people:

- Those working in salons.
- Those working from home.

Most hairdressers do not set out with the intention of working from home, although this may be an attractive option. Initially, hairdressers tend to work in salons and then, after a few years, and after developing a sizeable clientele, they consider being freelance.

This can work very well for them until they start a family. Unfortunately, their clients' hair keeps growing; it doesn't take a *pregnant pause*. So, when a stylist starts a family, the juggling of family commitments against customer needs means that something has to give! The client usually develops a new loyalty with another hairdresser and then the bond between them is broken.

Quite often a mother who has taken a minicareer break loses more than just her clients. She can lose her confidence too, particularly when she wants to reignite her career.

This is where short courses and fast track courses fit in really well. These courses are ideal for people who are returning to work and want to refresh their skills with the latest techniques.

Intensive courses – full-time

As a guideline, there are approximately 500 hours of teaching and tuition built into a college-based hairdressing and barbering course at Levels 2 and 3. When this is timetabled throughout the academic year, it generally works out at about two-and-a-half day's attendance for each term-time week.

These guided learning hours (GLH) are a notional figure that is provided to colleges, so that they can build their courses to suit the needs of their learners. And different colleges have different approaches.

Some colleges offer a three-month intensive course, and these are quite different to full-time and fast-track programmes. First, they do not suit all learners, as the pace is fast and the courses are very short. Typically, an intensive programme would be set in one college term (13 weeks) and therefore, in order to provide sufficient guided learning hours, would require the learner to attend Monday – Friday from 09:00 until 16:00. This may sound like an attractive option for many potential Level 2 students, but you have to remember that on top of an everyday attendance, there will be private study or homework to do at weekends too!

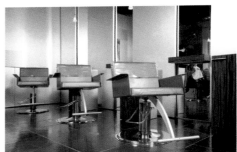

ACTIVITY

You can find out if you are suitable for Fast-tracking by contacting your local college.

ACTIVITY

Intensive courses are not that common – enquire at your local college to see if they offer this route to qualification.

Apprenticeship-based programmes for hairdressing and barbering

Apprenticeships have many distinct advantages over full-time, college delivered programmes.

Advantages of apprenticeships:

- ◆ Apprentices work in a 'commercial' salon most of their time.

- ◆ Apprentices are employed and get paid for their work while they are learning.

- ◆ Apprentices have direct contact with the salon's clients every day.

- ◆ Apprentices can only participate in NVQs as this is currently what the industry expects.

Disadvantages of apprenticeships:

- ◆ No guarantees for a job after the training.

- ◆ Training tends to be longer and is for a minimum of one year.

ACTIVITY

Many colleges offer apprenticeships as well as full and part-time courses. Contact your local college to see what options are available.

Depending upon the arrangements made by the employer, some apprentices attend a private training provider too. This can take place as a day release scheme. On day release, the apprentice attends the private training provider on a weekly or bi-weekly basis. This enables them to do class-based sessions that the salon does not want to, or cannot provide. During their planned day at the private training provider, an apprentice would typically have a morning of classroom sessions for hairdressing science and business studies, and this may be followed up in the afternoon with practical hairdressing or barbering in the private training provider's salon.

Unlike full-time students, an apprentice will get more than a qualification from an **awarding organization**. The apprenticeship itself is celebrated and this enables the apprentice to get an apprenticeship certificate as well as their NVQ diploma.

Employee rights & responsibilities All apprentices are employed within salons or barber's shops, and as their status is different to that of others in training, they need to be aware of their employee rights and also the responsibilities that they have to their employer and the employer has to them.

Brief outline of the main considerations for Employee Rights and Responsibilities (ERR)		
Contracts of employment	1	Know and understand the range of employer and employee statutory rights and responsibilities under Employment Law and that employment rights can be affected by other legislation as well. This should cover an apprentice's rights and responsibilities under the Employment Rights Act 1996, Equality Act 2010 and Health & Safety legislation, together with the responsibilities and duties of employers.
	2	Know and understand the procedures and documentation in the employee's organization which recognise and protect their relationship with their employer. Health and Safety and Equality and Diversity training must be an integral part of the apprentice's learning programme.
	3	Know and understand the range of sources of information and advice available to them on their employment rights and responsibilities. Details of Access to work and Additional Learning Support must be included in the programme.
	4	Understand the role played by the employee's occupation within their organization and industry.
	5	Have an informed view of the types of career pathways that are open to them.
	6	Know the types of representative bodies and understand their relevance to their industry and organization, and their main roles and responsibilities.
	7	Know where and how to get information and advice on their industry, occupation, training and career.

(Continued)

(Continued)

Brief outline of the main considerations for Employee Rights and Responsibilities (ERR)	
	8 Can describe and work within their organization's principles and codes of practice.
	9 Recognizes and can form a view on issues of public concern that affect their organization and industry.
Anti-discrimination	◆ Interviewees cannot be discriminated against.
	◆ Employees cannot be discriminated against on the grounds of age, disability, gender, race, religion or belief, or sexual orientation.
	◆ Men and women have the right to equal pay.
Working hours and holiday entitlements	◆ The Working Time Directive sets the number of hours that can be worked. Special provisions apply to 16 and 17-year-olds.
	◆ Employees have rights in relation to; rest periods, holidays, time off, overtime, maternity and parental leave.
Health and Safety	◆ Employers must safeguard the health and safety of employees.
	◆ Employees have a duty to their employer and fellow employees to work safely.
Data protection	◆ The **Data Protection Act** protects employees and requires for data held on file about them to be held securely, whether manual or computerized.
Issues of public concern	◆ That customers have personal and consumer rights and they are more aware of how these rights may be compromised and pursued legally.

Job descriptions For employed hairdressers and barbers, their role and the job requirements are set out in the job description. A job description is a list of the functions and roles expected within the job. The job descriptions include details of the following:

◆ Job title

◆ Work location(s)

◆ Responsibilities (to whom and for what)

◆ Job purpose

◆ Main functions (listed)

◆ Standards expected

◆ Essential requirements

◆ Desirable requirements

◆ Other special conditions

The standards expected from the job holder will often be produced in the staff handbook. They would normally include:

◆ Standards of behaviour and appearance

◆ Code of conduct

◆ Job description

◆ Grievance procedure

◆ Employee legal entitlements and responsibilities

◆ Health and safety requirements

TOP TIP

A job description is a document that should be provided to job applicants, prior to interview stage, so that the applicant may see the main remits and expectations of the job holder.

Services provided by hairdressers and barbers

There are a wide variety of services that are provided by hairdressers and barbers to their clients and this is increasing all the time. The table below looks at the main ones and an overview of what takes place. For more in-depth information on any of these services, turn to the relevant sections within this book. The service abbreviations in the table are used in **appointment** bookings which are usually written into an appointment diary or computerized **appointment systems** as a quick guide to the nature of the bookings.

Service name	Service abbreviation for appointments	What is happening in this service?
Consultation	Cons	Initially, a two-way discussion finding out the client's requirements and following this up with an examination to identify any factors that could affect the client's desired result.
Shampooing	S/S	A cleansing process that prepares the hair for further services.
Conditioning	Cond or Treat	A process (normally completed after shampooing) that will improve the look, feel, handling and physical properties of the hair.
Blow-drying	B/D	A general term for a method of drying and styling hair by using a variety of round or flat hair brushes to create directional lift and/or volume, and/or movement.
Setting	S/S	A general term for a method of positioning and fixing various sized rollers in wet or dry hair to create directional lift and/or volume, and/or movement.
Cutting Cut and Blow-dry	D/C or W/C C/BW	A collective name for a variety of techniques and methods that use scissors, thinners, shapers, razors and electric clippers to **trim**, shape, style and restyle men's and women's hair.
Colouring	Ret or FhCol R/T (root tint)	A collective name for artificially changing part, or all of a client's hair by using temporary, semi-permanent, quasi-permanent or permanent **hair colour**.
Lightening	LG	A general term that refers to a lightening process on natural hair for part or full head applications.
Highlights/Lowlights	H/L / L/L	A general term for a partial head colouring process, which may involve lightening or darkening areas of the hair to produce dual tonal or multi tonal effects.
Colour Correction	ColCor	A collective name for a variety of colouring techniques and applications which are used in order to correct an undefined number of **artificial colouring** problems or mistakes.
Perming	PW	A general term used for permanently changing the properties of hair in order to add volume, movement or curl, or alternatively, to change the direction of the natural lie of the hair.

(Continued)

(Continued)

Service name	Service abbreviation for appointments	What is happening in this service?
Relaxing	Relax	A general term used for permanently changing the properties of hair in order to reduce natural movement or curl in hair.
Hair up	H/U or P/U LHD (long hair dressing)	A collective term that covers a wide range of plaiting, curling, folding and positioning techniques, for fixing and dressing longer hair (or extended hair) into a variety of elaborate effects.
Hair Extensions	Ext	A general term that covers a wide range of systems and methods for adding artificial or natural hair to a client's existing hair, to add length, density or colour.
Beard/moustache *Trimming*	Brd Trm	A barbering service for men that cuts and styles their facial hair into a variety of managed shapes using scissors, a razor or electric clippers.
Shaving	Shv	A barbering service for men that cuts their regrown facial hair by using a 'cut-throat' razor and/or electric clippers.

Finding out more about the industry

Sources of information for hairdressing and barbering courses

Source of information	Information available	Making contact	Things to consider
College websites	◆ Course levels ◆ Qualifications available ◆ Course content ◆ Patterns of attendance ◆ Course costs ◆ Course requirements ◆ Term times ◆ Funding support ◆ Contact details	◆ Speak to members of staff first. ◆ Make appointment for interview and meeting with staff. ◆ Enrolment to courses (often online completion).	◆ Flexibility of course starts. ◆ Attendance times. ◆ Costs and funding support. ◆ Uniforms, hairdressing kits. ◆ Enrolment date. ◆ Open days/taster days.
Private training provider websites	◆ Delivery – (work/salon based training) ◆ Course levels ◆ Qualifications available ◆ Course content ◆ Patterns of attendance ◆ Course costs ◆ Course requirements ◆ Contact details	◆ Speak to members of staff first. ◆ Make appointment for interview and meeting with staff.	◆ Location of training. ◆ Employer relationships. ◆ Flexibility of course starts. ◆ Attendance times.

(Continued)

(Continued)

Source of information	Information available	Making contact	Things to consider
Connexions – career advice	◆ College-based courses ◆ Private training providers ◆ Employer-based schemes ◆ Qualifications available ◆ Career progression	◆ Careers advisory service.	◆ Young people careers advice. ◆ Links with education.
Job centre	◆ Courses available – college, private, salon-based ◆ Course levels ◆ Qualifications available ◆ Course content ◆ Career progression	◆ Call in and speak to centre staff.	◆ Location of training/ education. ◆ Links with employers.
Careers conventions and exhibitions	◆ Courses available – college, private, salon-based ◆ Course levels ◆ Qualifications available	◆ Advisors can redirect you to other sources of information.	◆ Locations for training and education.

TOP TIP

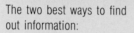

The two best ways to find out information:

1 The website.
2 Speak to someone on the phone.

The jobs that people do

The jobs that people do within hairdressing and barbering and the scope for progressing onwards in a job will depend on the size of the business they work in. There are all sorts of types of businesses, some very large and on a global scale, where many others are small independent firms.

In simple terms, there are only five types of salon business:

1 **International** – e.g. *Regis Corporation*, a very large international salon group with 13,000 locations under many branded salon names such as; Supercuts, Sassoon Salon, Regis Salons, MasterCuts and SmartStyle. The Regis Corporation owns many of the salons and the others are run as **franchised** businesses.

2 **Large** – e.g. *Headmasters*, an expanding London group with over 40 salons in different parts of the capital.

3 **Regional** – e.g. *Dimensions*, a county-wide group in the north, offering hair and beauty options along with training and education.

4 **Local** – e.g. *Philosophy*, a small company in the heart of England with a few salons.

5 **Independent** – the vast majority of salons in the UK run by employers as sole traders or partnerships, in total over 35,000 shops.

You will see from the list of examples that the way in which hairdressing services are offered is diverse and without any particular strong patterns.

However, the larger the salon the more complicated the organizational structure will be. The examples below show two very different company structures, one large and one very small.

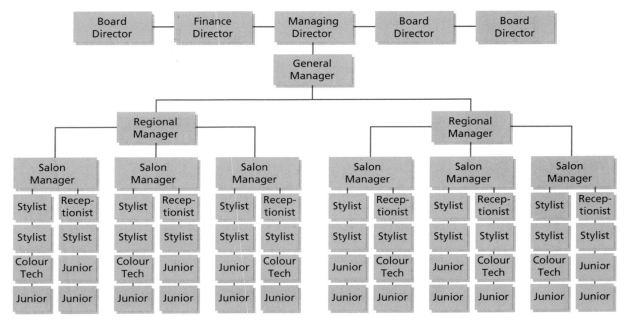

Large company structure

As you can see from both types of structure, at the bottom will be the 'junior'. The junior assists the qualified staff and carries out some parts of the service that the client has requested.

Next will be the hairdressers. They could be stylists or barbers, it will vary from salon to salon. Larger salons may have colourists, who carry out all the hair colouring in the salon, and other staff such as a receptionist. Above the hairdressers will be the manager or owner who will run the salon. Some salons, especially large ones, have more rows in their chart with different titles for the staff such as Regional Managers and General Managers as well as the Board of Directors.

As you progress within your career, gaining more experience and qualifications, you will find that your status and salary will change too. If there is a visible route for you to progress within the corporate structure, you may find that you are better off with the 'package' they can offer you. That is pension, company car, holiday entitlements, fringe benefits, etc.

Sometimes, you will find that moving to another salon is the only way that you can *geton*. Other than that, with experience *under your belt* you may be considering a business future of your own.

Small company structure

Working time expectations

Whatever you do choose to do, or whichever path you wish to take, there is one thing that you will have to think about from the start. It is not something that necessarily applies to hairdressing or specifically barbering, it is more to do with personal services industries as a whole.

Services rely upon people that are prepared to pay for them. These people are the clients. We need to remember that the client has a life and interests of their own and in order for us to count on them as one of our clients we need to provide a service that they are happy to pay for, at a time when they are able to receive it.

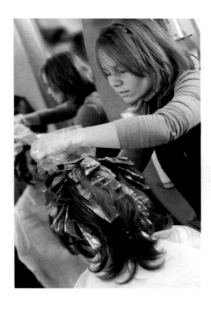

Quite simply, services industries have to be flexible in two ways:

♦ Salons need to provide a variety of services that customers want and will pay for.

♦ Salons have to provide those services at the times that the customers are available.

This could be weekends; i.e. Sundays, or even Bank Holidays (for weddings etc.), but it will definitely involve late night openings; working on into the evening.

Career opportunities in the industry

There is a wide range of job opportunities available in the hairdressing and barbering industry, the obvious ones being those in hairdressing salons and barber's shops. There are, however, lots of other opportunities for those who want more than just working in a salon and even more if you want to use your qualification and travel.

Career opportunities

Career opportunities

♦ Top hotels around the world are very *in-tune* with the needs of their customers and are experts in providing the best in personal services. So as a matter of course these destinations have lavish spas, health retreats and beauty salons, as well as catering for everyone's personal grooming and hairdressing needs.

♦ Cruising is now becoming an affordable luxury for many people's holiday preferences and all cruise liners have hair and beauty salon facilities to match the needs of their holidaymakers.

♦ Health farms and hydras offer a wide range of jobs mainly for beauty therapists, but also have opportunities for hairdressers and barbers too.

♦ Airports around the world are busier than ever before and now that many of the main ones incorporate a *one-stop-shop* approach to their provision of services, it goes without saying that along with their shopping malls, coffee shops, bars, restaurants and duty free, are barber's shops and hairdressing salons.

♦ Session stylists are another form of freelance hairdresser and there are always opportunities for the ambitious ones in film, theatre and television.

♦ Session stylists are also needed in the fashion and photographic industry. These types of fast moving jobs will definitely appeal to those who want a career at the '*cutting edge*' of fashion and innovation.

♦ The ever increasing need for health related services for the elderly, retired or infirm, includes hairdressing as a standard service. So there are always growing opportunities for hairdressers with our ageing population.

Career opportunities

◆ Field technician/sales support for a manufacturing company – a minimum four years as a hairdresser is needed, but this role provides a popular route for using your skills for a big name like L'Oreal, Wella or Goldwell.

◆ Wholesaler, wholesale supplies – another opportunity to work on the supply side of the business promoting and supporting sales in wholesale outlets, trade exhibitions and representative roles.

◆ Teaching – stylists with a minimum five years' industry experience may want to consider an educational future. With over 400 colleges of further education and a growing number of Academy and community college status schools offering vocational courses, there is always a need for people to teach hairdressing and barbering to others.

◆ Trichologist – Specialists in hair and skin dysfunctions and disorders. Literally a hair doctor providing consultation, advice and treatment for all sorts of problems.

◆ Working for an Awarding Body, e.g. City and Guilds Institute, VTCT or the Industry lead body; **Habia** – stylists with experience may want to consider working on the education side; in the development, maintenance and monitoring of standards or assessment systems.

Progressing in your career

If you want to make the most out of your decision to be a hairdresser or barber then you must find out more about these opportunities. If you want to find out more about the types of opportunities above, you should look at the following for more information:

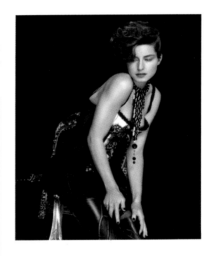

Job classifications	Source of information
Hotels	Company websites: ◆ Hilton Hotels ◆ Ramada Jarvis ◆ Marriott Hotels ◆ Intercontinental Hotels Group ◆ TAJ Hotels
Cruise liners	Company websites: ◆ Steiner Cruises
Airports	Company websites: ◆ British Airport Authorities, BAA
Session stylists/Freelancers	Website and publications: ◆ The Stage
Field technicians	Company websites: ◆ L'Oreal Professional ◆ Proctor and Gamble ◆ Schwarzkopf ◆ Unilever ◆ Goldwell

(Continued)

(Continued)

Job classifications	Source of information
Wholesaler representatives	Company websites: ◆ Sally Supplies ◆ Ellison's ◆ Salon Services Publications: ◆ *Hairdresser's Journal* ◆ *Creative Head/HeadFirst*
Teaching/Assessing	Websites: ◆ Further Education Colleges ◆ TES (Times Educational Supplement) ◆ VTCT Vocational Training Charitable Trust ◆ City and Guilds of London Institute Publications: ◆ *TES (Times Educational Supplement)*
Trichologist	Websites: ◆ Institute of Trichologists
Habia	Website: ◆ **Hair and Beauty Industry Authority**

Personal effectiveness and professionalism

Good business relies upon good service and you will need to have and demonstrate all the right attributes that are connected with promoting a professional image, while being able to deliver a quality, personal service.

The table below focuses upon the key words and phrases that professionals demonstrate in their work.

Keys to success: The characteristics of a true professional		
Good customer service	◆ Being friendly ◆ Good manners ◆ Reliable ◆ Caring ◆ Keen and enthusiastic ◆ Quick responses ◆ Putting clients first ◆ Paying attention ◆ Willing to help ◆ Being polite	◆ Put the customer at ease. ◆ Customers deserve respect and courtesy. ◆ Do what you say you will. ◆ Think about the needs of others. ◆ Provide help willingly and eagerly. ◆ Be alert and act fast. ◆ Thinking of others before yourself. ◆ Recognizing when others need assistance. ◆ Putting yourself forward first to assist. ◆ A common sign of courtesy.

(Continued)

Keys to success: The characteristics of a true professional		
Good communication skills	◆ Being confident	◆ Taking control of situations, leading others.
	◆ Positive **body language**	◆ Letting your body express your feelings in-line with what your mouth is saying.
	◆ Eye contact	◆ Demonstrates honesty and confidence.
	◆ Patience	◆ Recognizing that not everyone can respond quickly.
	◆ Self-motivated	◆ Energized into getting things done.
	◆ Enthusiastic	◆ Showing commitment and dedication.
A team player	◆ Helpful	◆ Recognizing when others need assistance.
	◆ Enjoys working with others	◆ Preferring to work collectively to a successful result or conclusion.
	◆ Listening and hearing others	◆ Responding and acting on aspects of discussion.
Being a professional	◆ Good personal hygiene	◆ Approachable and nice to be near.
	◆ Trustworthy	◆ Loyal and dependable.
	◆ Well presented	◆ Reflects the standards of the organization.
	◆ Approachable	◆ Open and willing to queries and calls.
	◆ A *walking advert*	◆ Encompasses all the attributes of the business.

Developing yourself as a professional

Being trained and educated as a stylist or barber is an important part of your professional development. However, the process of learning is not something that happens to you, it is something that you take part in.

For many this may come as rather a shock, but remember; only you can:

◆ Make the decision that you want to be a professional.

◆ Take the necessary steps in order to become that professional.

Quite simply, you are in control of your future and where you want to be. If you look again at the *Keys to success* above, re-read those statements and see which ones you need to address in order to *pass the professionals test*.

Of course, this is perfection and most of us can 'tick' some of the boxes but not all of them. It may look like a massive mountain to climb, but there is another way to think about it.

BEST PRACTICE

Some of those attributes are essential and others are ***desirable***. Having good personal hygiene is essential; but having confidence is desirable. In other words we may not have confidence now, but it's something we can continue working on in the future. Who knows, it may take years to perfect.

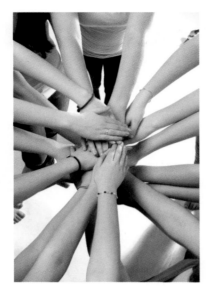

TOP TIP

The National Occupational Standards (NOS) can be obtained from the Hairdressing and Beauty Therapy Industry Authority (Habia).

Improve your personal performance

Doing well in your job really makes a difference to the whole team, as the staff in any salon situation are an integral part of the formula for success. Your work input is vital and equally as important as anyone else's in maintaining the smooth running of the business.

'**Continuing professional development' (CPD)** is the term used by professionals who continually update their skills. Working towards defined targets is standard in the world of work; without them we wouldn't know if we got things right. In employment these targets are set by others in **appraisals** or training reviews. This type of review process gives employers and educators the opportunity to look at your contribution to the team, on an individual and personal basis. It gives you the opportunity to give feedback on how work policies and targets are working in practice and affecting you while carrying out your work.

The most effective hairdressers are those who are self-motivated, keen to learn and find any opportunity to learn themselves by watching others, keeping in touch with fashions and being eager to provide assistance to fellow team members.

Your ability to meet the expected standards at work is referred to as 'personal effectiveness' and this is the result of care, interest, respect and on going training.

You should be able to:

◆ Make use of all opportunities to learn as they occur on a daily basis.

◆ Work towards the standards laid down by the Awarding Organization you are registered with.

◆ Identify your own strengths and weaknesses

◆ Work towards the targets you have been given.

◆ Self-assess your own skills and progress towards your targets.

Making use of opportunities to learn Everything that you do in the salon provides a learning opportunity. Each task that you haven't been able to carry out yourself before provides you with a target for the future. It's never a case of: 'I'll never be able to do that'. Or 'It's OK for you; you've been doing it for ages'. It's also about continual improvement. In order to learn something properly, it has to be practised, and that can mean several times in different situations before it can be done every time correctly.

Watch how others tackle difficult or complex tasks. Stand by them and offer your help; you can learn a lot more if you are able to see closely how procedures are completed. Ask questions, sometimes things are far more complex than they seem.

If you are wandering around aimlessly it is probably because you don't know what you should be doing. Just think how your colleagues will see this; they might view you as lazy or deliberately trying to avoid working as a team player. If you are unclear about what you should be doing at work, ask someone else.

Self-Appraisal Identifying your own strengths and weaknesses can sound quite daunting and particularly if you are not used to reflecting on your own progress. It needn't be; as like anything else when you are learning, there is always a hard and easier way to do things. Being able to spot your own mistakes is a starting point.

ACTIVITY

Take a piece of A4 paper and divide it into four sections in the following way:

SWOT Analysis

Strengths
I'm good at colouring.
I'm good at blow-drying.
I'm good at putting hair up.

Weaknesses
I'm not very good at cutting.
I'm not confident with clients during consultation.

Opportunities
I could take part in colour or styling competitions.
I could get noticed by doing competitions.
I could make a name for myself.

Threats
I would need to improve my cutting and client consultation because it will affect my chances of getting a job in a salon.

1   In the **Strengths** area you write down things that you are good at.

2   Then next to this in the **Weaknesses** section you write down the things that you are not so good at.

3   In the **Opportunities** section you look above at the strengths and decide what things you could capitalize upon and use them as potential opportunities.

4   Similarly, in the **Threats** area, you look above at the weaknesses and decide what things could be holding you back as a result of those weaknesses.

We all know that if we do things the right way, we gain the personal satisfaction of getting it right. Conversely, if we keep making mistakes and get it wrong more times than right, we feel wretched and that will inevitably lose the salon's clients. This low self-esteem needs to be avoided; it is negative and does nothing for our self-motivation.

One good way to start measuring your own progression is self-assessment by using a SWOT analysis. A SWOT analysis is a system for recording strengths, weaknesses, opportunities and threats. A SWOT analysis is carried out in the following way.

You can do your own SWOT analysis at any time, in fact the more often that you do it, the more you will see how you have progressed; particularly in the areas that you consider as weaknesses. Just watch them disappear.

Reviewing progress – Appraisals
The formal, periodical review process in a work setting is called an '*appraisal*'; in a college or training centre it is called a '*progress review*'. The start of a progress review or appraisal is undertaken in two ways:

◆   first, by yourself, i.e. self-appraisal (See SWOT analysis as previously detailed); and

◆   second, in conjunction with your manager on a more formal basis.

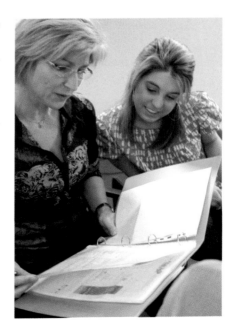

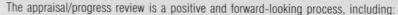

TOP TIP

The appraisal/progress review is a positive and forward-looking process, including:

◆ Positive feedback for the things that are going well.

◆ Constructive and fair criticism where there are weaknesses.

◆ Positive suggestions.

◆ Setting of specific targets.

◆ Follow-up after appraisal.

ACTIVITY

Preparing for appraisal:

◆ Think about each statement on the form.

◆ Think about the things you are good at.

◆ Think about any issues you have.

Write some notes to remind you about what you want to talk about during the meeting. These may include things that are not covered by the form. (Don't forget to take your notes with you to the meeting.)

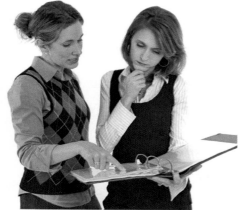

TOP TIP

The joint review process of appraisal would fulfil no purpose at all unless it looks at your current situation, your feelings and work performances. It should measure that against the mutually agreed targets and then finally, create an ongoing development plan/individual learning plan, which can be reviewed at some future date.

At the beginning of the appraisal period, the manager/tutor and the employee/student jointly discuss, develop and mutually agree the objectives and performance targets for that period. An **Individual Learning Plan (ILP)** or **Personal Development Plan (PDP)** will then be completed, outlining the expected outcomes over the next period.

During the appraisal/review period, should there be any significant changes in factors such as objectives or targets, these will be discussed and any amendments will be added to the ILP or PDP.

At the end of the review period, the results are discussed and both parties agree and sign; (at least) two copies are produced and all concerned receive a copy.

For you, the appraisal is a good way to air any problems and to make points about training needs and the future. For your supervisor/tutor, it is a good way to identify possible problems in your training and to record progress towards achieving the goals.

At the progress review meeting Refer to your appraisal form and your notes to remind yourself of what you want to say.

◆ Be positive, express yourself clearly.

◆ Ask questions.

◆ Discuss and agree your next steps with your manager/tutor.

◆ Make sure the appraisal form is filled in with details of what is agreed.

After the progress review meeting

◆ Remind your manager/tutor about how he or she agreed to help you.

◆ Make sure you keep to the agreements you made.

BEST PRACTICE

If you are having problems with any aspect of your training or your job, don't wait! You should ask for support or assistance from your tutor or manager. If you have completed the targets set out in your training before the due target date, ask for more objectives to be set. This will help to keep you more motivated by completing your training earlier and increasing your knowledge of the job, enabling you to do higher-skilled work.

Get SMART

SMART objectives **Good plans start with set objectives and well defined objectives fit the SMART principle**.

This is a common target setting system which ensures that expected outcomes are:

- ◆ **Specific** – The target(s) should be unambiguous; providing clear objectives.
- ◆ **Measurable** – Set in a context that is objective; e.g. 'Must achieve 100 per cent of sales targets'.
- ◆ **Achievable** – Within the bounds of the appraisee's capabilities.
- ◆ **Realistic** – Appropriate to the needs of the appraisee in relation to the appraisee's abilities.
- ◆ **Timed** – Set with an agreed time-line from the outset.

Improving personal appearances

Working in a salon or barber's shop puts us on display to the public from the moment we start work until the time we leave at the end of the day, so our appearance to the client is very important. The employer decides on the salon's dress code; whether it is a complete uniform or a more simple dress theme. Whichever the policy, our clothes should always reflect the image of the salon. If the salon is fashionable and trendy, then it follows that the dress policy will follow. This is an important part of how the salon or barber's shop is marketed to its clientele. In other words, if the *target* market is young and trendy, then the salon's surroundings and the people within it will reflect that particular direction. Conversely, if the target market is older and includes retired people, then the *feel* of the salon will be far more relaxed. These sorts of decisions are not made *off-the-cuff*, they are part of a much larger business plan and the staff will be an integral part of the business offering.

The effort we put into getting ready for work reflects our pride in our work and that we care about what we do. Sometimes we have to wear things that we would not wear if we had a personal choice, but professional standards and salon image must come first.

Clothes What we wear to work or college is covered in their organizational policy. Whatever the dress code it should be practical and serviceable. Clothes should be easy to clean and iron if necessary and made of suitable fabrics. They should not be tight and restrictive, which would make working harder and more tiring; they may also make you perspire and increase **body odour (BO)**.

Shoes Hairdressers and barbers should wear flat- or low-heeled shoes that enclose the feet (cover the toes). We spend most of our time on our feet so comfortable shoes will help prevent backache.

TOP TIP

Your progress review will help you to think about:

- ◆ how you feel about your job
- ◆ how your training is going
- ◆ what you would like to do in the future

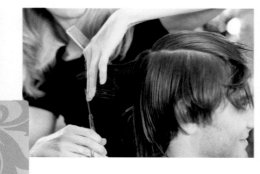

Hair As hair professionals, our hair is an advertisement for our skill in the salon. If your hair is a mess, think about how that affects your clients' confidence in you. Your hair should always look good and well styled to reflect the salon image. Your hair should always be clean, tidy and representative of the place where you work.

Make-up If you wear make-up to work, make sure that you check with your salon manager to see what is acceptable and appropriate, but as a rule of thumb, make-up should be light and fresh. It should never look like a *left over* from the night before, or some *chilling* Halloween party; we want clients to feel comfortable and not give them a fright!

Nails Hairdressers should have similar length, short, neatly manicured nails. Polish can be worn but must not be chipped or badly applied.

Jewellery Wear only a minimum of jewellery while you are working, as it is unhygienic and can harbour germs. It can also be uncomfortable for the client because it can get tangled in their hair. The policy for piercings will be down to the salon; in some situations it is actively encouraged, whereas in others, it may not be acceptable at all.

Tattoos These are similar to piercings and will depend very much on the **salon policy** and the clientele that the salon wants to encourage. It may be OK to be scantily clad and covered in body art in a salon that is eclectically different and is trying to 'carve-out' its own unique niche in the market. But it will definitely be frowned upon in a five star hotel chain in an upmarket resort.

Personal hygiene Hairdressing and barbering are personal service businesses and therefore, we must make sure we have a good standard of personal hygiene because we will be working very close to our clients. A couple of obvious things may spring to mind like BO or bad breath, but there are lots of other things to consider too.

BEST PRACTICE

Always check your appearance before you start work. Check it through the day and adjust it when necessary (but not in front of the client).

Hands and nails We must make sure our hands are very clean. Not only does it not look very good to the client if they are dirty, but it could spread germs to our clients too. Our hand are very important to us, they are the way we earn our money so need to be carefully looked after.

In hairdressing and barbering we are always working with some sort of chemicals, so disposable vinyl or nitrile gloves are essential.

By wearing them we:

◆ Protect our hands and skin from contracting dermatitis.

◆ Keep our hands and nails clean and free from unsightly staining.

◆ Demonstrate to our clients that we are professionals and take health and hygiene seriously.

Remember, we are dealing with the public every day and we need to safeguard their health as well as our own. So make sure you wash your hands before work, after using

HEALTH & SAFETY

For more information on how to avoid dermatitis, visit the HSE website at http://www.hse.gov.uk/skin/employ/dermatitis.htm.

the toilet and after coughing or sneezing; this will reduce the **risk** of spreading **infections**.

Make a point of using moisturizing creams regularly, as this will help to replace the moisture lost by the routine, daily tasks. Sometimes using **barrier cream** will also help. If the skin on your hands becomes dry, it will crack and become very sore; this may prevent you from working until it heals. Historically in hairdressing, many people suffered from a form of eczema called **dermatitis** and this was due to contact with the chemicals used in the profession. In many of those cases, the person's sensitivity to dermatitis meant that they had to give up their job. Keep your nails clean, especially underneath, and try to keep them neatly manicured and not too long.

Your body The body has **sweat glands** all over its surface and these help control our body temperature by secreting moisture out on to the surface of the skin when we are hot. This, unfortunately, provides a good breeding ground for **bacteria**, which in turn causes body odour (BO). It is essential that we have a shower or bath at least every day and use **deodorants** or antiperspirants.

Your mouth Unpleasant breath can be offensive to others and all sorts of things can cause it: smoking, things we have eaten (like onions or garlic), stomach upsets or other problems such as pieces of food that get stuck between the teeth and then decay. We tend to work very close to our clients and will be breathing very close to them, and so they will be able to smell any bad breath easily. Make sure you prevent bad breath by brushing your teeth regularly, particularly after eating, and use a mouthwash or breath freshener, or get into the habit of *flossing* regularly.

Your feet Like our hands, our feet are important because we do most of our work standing. We have looked at the sort of shoes we wear and must make sure they fit properly. We should also wash our feet regularly; some people's feet **sweat** a lot, and this can cause foot odour.

Personal wellbeing

We must look after our body and health too; it helps us work better and not put clients at risk by transferring illnesses or **diseases** to them. To work successfully as a hairdresser or barber you will need energy and stamina. So ideally, we should take regular exercise, perhaps playing sport or dancing. We should also get sufficient sleep and relaxation to help us recover from the stresses of the working day.

Good posture is a must, as we stand for long periods throughout each day. Standing properly will help prevent backache, and in the long term back problems and conditions like varicose veins. Good working posture will also reduce the risk of repetitive strain injury or upper limb disorder, caused by repetitive or overuse of muscles and tendons and nerves. When working, always stand with the back straight, your feet apart and your weight evenly distributed on your legs. Do not stand with all your weight on one of your legs and your pelvis tilted. If you stand incorrectly for long periods you will get backache and probably more serious problems with your lower back. You will also increase the risk of developing varicose veins.

The care and attention that we pay to how we present ourselves for work is very important to our future success and progression. Having a good, well balanced diet and sufficient sleep is vital to our personal health and wellbeing. We only get one life and we want to make the most of it.

BEST PRACTICE

Looking after your hands is very important. Keep them dry and use hand cream all the time, so your skin does not get dry and cracked.

BEST PRACTICE

Remember to check your hands and nails regularly for any disorders.

HEALTH & SAFETY

Make sure minor problems like verrucas, corns and athletes, foot are treated. Some disorders of the feet can make standing painful so we need to get them treated as soon as possible.

HEALTH & SAFETY

Keep your nails healthy – they should be trimmed and filed regularly.

HEALTH & SAFETY

It is often recommended that we have eight hours of sleep a day.

SUMMARY

As a final reflection on what you have covered in this chapter, you should now have a clearer picture of all the essential aspects for working in the hairdressing industry. In particular, you should now have a basic understanding of the key principles of:

1 The opportunities that are available to you within the industry.

2 How you should conduct yourself in a professional manner.

3 How you can communicate professionally with clients and colleagues.

4 How you can improve and progress within your career.

5 Identifying your own strengths and weaknesses.

6 Taking care of yourself and your wellbeing.

And collectively, how these principles will help you in the future, in your chosen career.

ASSESSMENT OF KNOWLEDGE AND UNDERSTANDING

Case Study

Job descriptions are an essential aspect of employment and in particular, the things that people are expected to do when they have a job. Without one, people wouldn't have any idea of what they should be doing. You may not have a job now, but you need to look at the roles and responsibilities that people undertake when they become a stylist. Have a look on the Internet for examples so that you can make comparisons between salons of different sizes.

Now answer the following questions:

What do you notice between the job demands of a large salon chain as opposed to a small independent?

Q1. What does ERR relate to?

    A service ☐
    A mistake ☐
    A job ☐
    A treatment ☐

Q2. BD is an abbreviation for a _____

Q3. Ext is a shortened term used in appointments

    True or False

Q4. A one year course at college is

    52 weeks ☐
    365 days ☐
    36 weeks ☐
    52 days ☐
    3 terms ☐
    10 terms ☐

Q5. Approximately, how many hours of study are there in a level 2 diploma course?

    50 ☐
    500 ☐
    150 ☐
    1500 ☐

Q6.   You don't need to be employed to be an apprentice   True or False

Q7.   An employee must have a   Contract of   ☐
                                                                          employment
                                                                     Training contract   ☐
                                                                     Day off each week   ☐
                                                                      Insurance policy   ☐

Q8.   A qualified hair doctor is called a _____

Q9.   A large company will have several salon branches   True or False

3 Reception

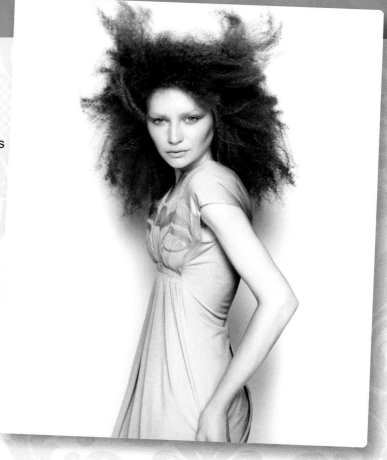

LEARNING OBJECTIVES

◆ Be able to maintain the reception and retail areas

◆ Be able to attend to enquiries

◆ Be able to make appointments

◆ Be able to calculate bills and handle payments

◆ Understand your client's legal rights in relation to consumer, and data protection

◆ Know your salon's range of products and services

KEY TERMS

BD

benefits

CBD

charge cards

cheques

Col (Rt or Fh)

confidentiality

Consumer Protection
    Act (1987)

credit card

debit cards

double bookings

effectiveness

enquiry

highlights

H/L FH or HL½H

H/L T

legal requirements

record cards

relaxer

resources

Trade Descriptions
    Act 1968

Unit topic

Salon reception duties.

INTRODUCTION

The reception is the most important area of the salon, as it is here that the client forms their first impression of the business. The area needs to be welcoming and friendly, and the décor and general appearance should reflect the overall theme and direction of the business. The feeling that clients get from this initial contact with a business provides a small *flavour* of what the clients can expect.

Throughout the day there is lots happening; with clients and visitors arriving, incoming telephone calls, stock deliveries, appointments being made and payments being taken, it's a busy place. Because there is so much to be done, the larger salon and salon chains tend to employ designated receptionists to run the reception within their salons. But more often than not, the smaller independent salons are not able to afford the additional staff salary; so in this situation, everyone needs to be able to carry out the duties.

A receptionist needs to have:

◆ A good working knowledge of the salon's services and treatments, and who within the staffing structure is capable of delivering them.

◆ Excellent communication skills.

◆ Good organizational skills.

A receptionist needs to be able to:

◆ Handle enquiries and provide accurate information to clients and staff.

◆ Make appointments for clients.

◆ Maintain the reception desk materials and stationery items.

◆ Handle different payment types and maintain the salon's record systems.

◆ Recommend retail products and support staff in retail sales.

◆ Keep the reception area tidy and inviting to all callers.

You can see from all the things listed above that the salon receptionist is key to the success of the business and their ability to meet and greet clients and visitors, make them feel welcome and attend to their needs is just a small part of a much bigger role.

The reception

PRACTICAL SKILLS

Learn how to promote a professional image

Learn how to maintain reception stationery items

Learn how to take messages for people correctly

Learn how to make appointments and record relevant information correctly

Learn about why you need to keep information private and confidential

Learn how to calculate bills for services, treatments and retail sales

Learn about different payment types used within the salon

Learn how to keep salon information, resources and money safe and secure

UNDERPINNING KNOWLEDGE

Handling enquires on the telephone and face to face

Keeping the reception and retail area tidy

Making appointments for services and treatments

Maintaining accurate client records

Handling payments at the till

TOP TIP

Sympathy is the feeling of sensing someone else's plight. Empathy is being able to put yourself in their position.

A professional salon reception

Customer service is at the heart of the hairdressing industry and it is good customer service that brings our clients back again and again. Clients want to feel that their custom is valued and that you and the rest of the staff will respond to their needs and problems with efficiency and empathy.

Making appointments requires both good literacy and numeracy skills; as well as a reasonable knowledge about the salon's services, treatments and retail product ranges.

This chapter looks at the following reception tasks:

◆ Making clients welcome and dealing with enquiries face to face.

◆ Handling enquiries.

◆ Using the phone.

◆ Handling payments for services, treatments and products.

◆ Processing card payments.

◆ Working within the laws of client **confidentiality** and consumers' rights.

Your job in reception is to receive clients and to make them feel welcome, which means greeting them properly, responding to their needs and dealing with them in a professional and friendly way.

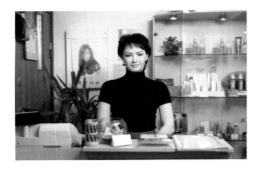

You need good communication skills for this type of work, as you will have to deal with a wide range of people who expect the best from you. You also need to know about the services you can offer so that you can explain these to clients and promote your business.

You may also be responsible for making sure that there are enough stationery items, plus accepting payments from clients and giving change. In addition, you may have to check that the money in the till is correct at the end of the day.

All this has to be done legally, so you need to know the **legal requirements** within the law and how UK laws protect the interests of our clients.

First impressions

Hairdressing is a personal service industry and if we are going to keep our clients happy, we have to provide a complete and professional service. This service is not just focused around the stylist's abilities in cutting, styling, perming or colouring. Good customer service has to be right; all the way through, from the point where clients arrive at the salon, right up to the point at where they leave. It's going to be the client's first (and last) impression of the salon.

The reception area is the hub of the salon; clients arrive, calls are received, visitors arrive, bills are paid and appointments are made. As part of your duties as the receptionist you will be responsible for:

- ◆ Making sure that the client waiting area is kept clean and tidy.
- ◆ Ensuring that magazines are regularly checked for condition and currency, and that the style books are replaced after use.
- ◆ Keeping clients happy by attending to those who have to wait so they are less likely to get angry and impatient.
- ◆ Making clients feel welcome by offering them something to drink.
- ◆ Making sure that the retail displays are regularly cleaned and refilled.
- ◆ Checking retail products for condition and visible price labels.

The retail products must look attractive; we want the clients to be encouraged to draw closer, pick them up and handle them.

ACTIVITY

Clients' interests are protected by laws. Go to www .gov.uk and find out as much information as you can about the following laws:

- ◆ Sales of Goods Act 1979
- ◆ Trade Descriptions Act 1968
- ◆ Consumer Protection Act 1987
- ◆ Data Protection Act 1998 and the information about clients which it protects.

BEST PRACTICE

Always make sure that product shelves and retail items are clean and tidy. Nobody will want to handle products that are dusty or on murky shelves!

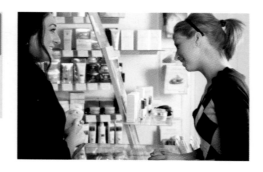

The reception area is always busy with clients arriving or wanting to pay their bill, the telephone is often ringing with clients wanting to make appointments. Therefore, the desk must be well organized. Stationery, such as memo pads, pens and payment-processing items, should be checked each morning before the salon opens, and you should make sure that there is enough to last throughout the day. The receptionist is also responsible for the till; there should be enough change and card-processing receipt rolls to last all day.

Positive body language

Watch your body language too, you can easily give clients the wrong impression if they walk in and catch you sprawling over the reception desk. Even if you're feeling tired; you can't afford to show it as it's unprofessional and it's probably your own fault anyway!

We want our clients to see us as professionals, so it's not just the way that we handle the calls on the telephone; we want to create the right impression when they walk in too. Sit up correctly, good posture shows that you are alert (and not going to cause yourself an injury). Don't sit with arms folded, it looks defensive, take a pen and be ready for work. Don't forget to smile when the clients arrive, look them in the eye and greet them properly. *'Good morning, how may I help you?'*

Reception daily checklist

✓ Desk dusted and tidied before clients arrive.

✓ Magazines are up to date and tidy.

✓ Appointment diary close to hand and ready for use.

✓ Card-payment receipt rolls and till rolls replenished and spares available.

✓ Obstructions or deliveries are moved out of the way.

✓ Stationery stocks checked and replenished.

✓ Shelves and retail products dusted and clean.

✓ Missing items or low stock levels replaced or reordered.

✓ Damaged or faulty product packaging removed and reported to the manager.

✓ Products rearranged and gaps in product lines removed from displays.

✓ Product information and pricing relevant, up to date, close at hand and easy to read.

✓ Product promotions clearly displayed, public information available and the correct product items arranged appropriately according to the current offer or promotion.

Keep stationery stocks up to date The reception desk is the first place where clients will see how organized the salon is. Even the most technologically aware salon with all the latest computerized gadgetry needs some form of desk stationery, and it is the receptionist's role to keep this well stocked. So if you are assisting, it's going to be your job to keep these things available. There is nothing worse than leaving a client unattended at the desk, while the receptionist runs off to find a pen or pencil.

Things to keep an eye on	Why do I need to do this?
Note/Memo pads	You may need to take a message for someone and rather than try to remember it, you'll need to write it down.
Pens and pencils	How will you fill in any information without them?
Client **record cards**	Client treatment records are being updated all the time and a stylist may need one during a consultation.
Skin sensitivity information cards	A client may need a skin sensitivity test 48 hours before a colouring service, they will need to know why they are having it done and what they need to do if they get any reaction to the test.
Sales receipts	Clients may want a written receipt for the services or treatments that they have had or products they have bought.
Till/Card receipt rolls	These are constantly being used and will need replacing before they run out. (Imagine if you run out of card receipt roll in the middle of a transaction – you won't be able to provide the client with written proof of purchase!)
Appointment cards	What else would you write a client's appointment on, a scrap of paper?
Price lists	What else can the client take away to keep a record of the current prices and contact information for the salon?
Product information/brochures	When products are on display the client needs to be able to take away information, either about how the products will benefit them, or about other products within a range that they might want to consider.
Cash, services and treatment summaries	A cash summary helps to record the overall sales and to show if the till receipts balance with the money in the till. A service or treatment summary may record the number of sales made for perhaps a promotion; showing the **effectiveness** of the promotion. A service or treatment summary may be kept for each stylist and be a way of calculating their commissions.

Product displays The salon's window and retail display is the focal point for passers-by and visitors to the salon. It is the most useful prompt for selling to our clients, and it's the receptionist's duty to keep an eye on the levels of stock and the overall general appearance. A receptionist needs to know about the products that the salon sells, as they are the one that the clients will ask about. They need to be aware of any current promotions and which products are suitable for certain situations or conditions.

The receptionist needs to know where the products can be found so that sold stock can be replaced, and the importance of keeping the whole area clean and inviting. Any new stock should be wiped and positioned so that it can be easily seen. Any client or visitor who is considering a purchase should be able to handle the item, read the information about it or be able to ask questions and get good advice when they need it.

Get organized

Every salon uses a tabulated system for organizing the daily work, although the way that it appears and the way in which it is completed changes from salon to salon. Some salons use the manual appointment book system; others use an electronic, computerized version. Regardless, both types do a similar job by setting out the daily, weekly and monthly work schedule. So, if the reception is the hub of the salon, then the appointment system is the most important business process within it. It provides a:

◆ Snapshot of the expected levels of business.

◆ Detailed action plan of work for staff.

◆ Minute-by-minute schedule of business activities.

◆ Record of client visits, creating a pattern of repeat business.

From this information the business can:

◆ Plan the salon **resources**, e.g. people, time, stock and equipment.

◆ Organize client records, contact details and treatment history.

◆ Prepare the till and electronic payment processes.

From this it is easy to see that the appointment system is the centre of an efficiently run business. The information it contains must be clear, accurate and up to date. However, maintaining the appointment system doesn't always guarantee the smooth running of the salon. There are late or unscheduled arrivals, staff sickness or other unexpected events, and all these situations need to be accommodated.

Attend to clients and enquiries

Communicating with clients is a fundamental and vital part of reception duties in a salon. It may well provide a new or potential client's first impression of the salon when they come in to make an appointment or an **enquiry**. Similarly, existing clients will return if they get a positive impression of the whole service, starting from the moment they walk through the door.

To make sure that clients come back to the salon time and time again, it is important to make them feel welcome when they first arrive.

Five steps to client care at reception

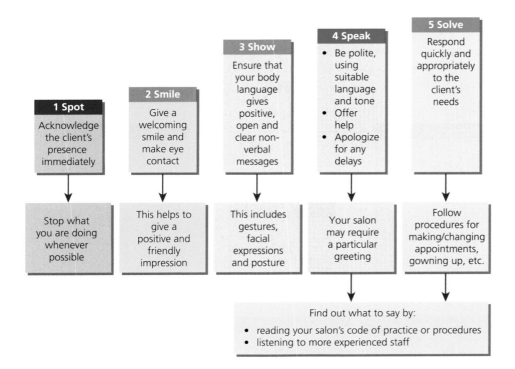

Handling enquiries

We want visitors to become clients and there are ways that we can make this happen. The first consideration is our communication skills; we want people to see us as professionals. Professional communication occurs when we handle or anticipate the needs of others in a prompt and business like manner.

We communicate in the following ways:

◆ Speech – what we say to others and the way in which we say it.

◆ Listening – hearing the requests of others properly.

◆ Writing – recording information accurately and clearly.

◆ Body language – the way we communicate our feelings and attitude to situations by posture, expression and mannerisms.

Remember, different people have differing needs, and you can help them in many ways:

◆ Clients with physical disabilities may need some help in getting through the door or assistance with a wheelchair.

◆ Clients who have a hearing impairment can usually lip read very well, so make sure that you look at them throughout a conversation; it will help them to understand you, fully.

◆ Visitors from overseas may have difficulty in making themselves understood. You can help them by using visual aids to describe a process or situation.

◆ Older clients need more time with making themselves comfortable as well as being understood, so be patient, speak clearly and ask questions to show that they understand what you mean.

◆ Don't use jargon with any visitors or clients as they won't necessarily understand the meaning of your conversation.

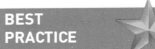

BEST PRACTICE

Be honest with clients when making appointments, you will always get found out.

On the telephone

Good telephone skills are important to give a good impression and deal with clients effectively. You will be judged by what you say, so you should be polite, cheerful and helpful from the moment you pick up the telephone to the moment you replace the receiver.

Five steps to handling calls

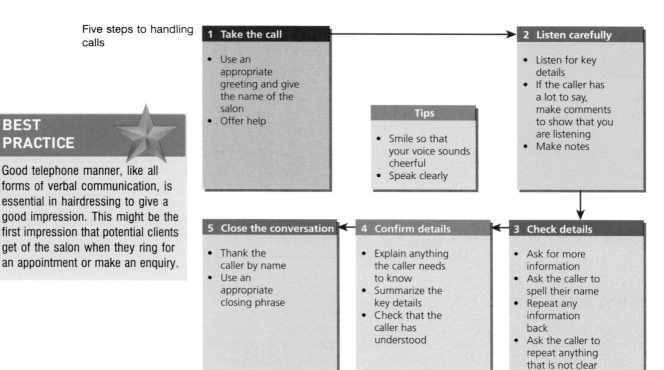

BEST PRACTICE

Good telephone manner, like all forms of verbal communication, is essential in hairdressing to give a good impression. This might be the first impression that potential clients get of the salon when they ring for an appointment or make an enquiry.

1 Take the call
- Use an appropriate greeting and give the name of the salon
- Offer help

Tips
- Smile so that your voice sounds cheerful
- Speak clearly

2 Listen carefully
- Listen for key details
- If the caller has a lot to say, make comments to show that you are listening
- Make notes

3 Check details
- Ask for more information
- Ask the caller to spell their name
- Repeat any information back
- Ask the caller to repeat anything that is not clear

4 Confirm details
- Explain anything the caller needs to know
- Summarize the key details
- Check that the caller has understood

5 Close the conversation
- Thank the caller by name
- Use an appropriate closing phrase

Smile when you answer the telephone: people will 'hear' the friendliness in your voice. At the same time, speak clearly, so that the caller can understand everything you say. After listening to the caller's request, confirm the main points back to them. This summarizes the information and ensures that all details are correct. Keep in mind the length of the call: calls cost money and waste valuable salon time.

Dos	Don'ts
✓ Always have a pen or pencil ready for taking messages or making appointments.	✗ Mumble or sigh into the telephone – it will put the caller off immediately.
✓ Answer the telephone promptly – ideally within three or four rings.	✗ Be abrupt or rude with people – give them time, be patient with people.
✓ Prepare yourself to answer – get into *character* even if you feel like you're having an off-day.	✗ Try to finish off people's sentences, listen carefully and let them speak.
✓ Be polite and cheerful – people can hear the friendliness in your voice.	✗ Tell people things that aren't true – *embellishing* the truth will get you found out.
✓ Speak clearly and slowly – calls may drop in or out of range and people could miss important information.	✗ Try to rush people on the telephone – they may not understand what you are saying and it will seem very unprofessional.

Taking messages for others

You will sometimes need to take a message on behalf of someone else. It is essential that these messages are accurately recorded and delivered promptly to the appropriate person. When taking messages, always make sure that you record the time and date, and make clear who the message is for and who it is from. Then give as much detail as you can in relation to the nature of the message:

◆ Who the message is for.

◆ Who has taken it.

◆ The date and time received.

◆ A clear description of the message content.

◆ An indication of whether a reply is necessary.

BEST PRACTICE

Always pass on a message to the person it is intended for as soon as possible.

Message:

For:	From:
	Tel Num:
Received on 　　　　Date:	Time:
Called: ☐ Called in: ☐	Needs a reply: ☐ Will call again: ☐
Message:	
Received/Taken by:	

Receiving clients – Face to face

When clients arrive at the salon, they should be attended to promptly, their appointment and time should be checked before they are directed to a seat. Always make a point of making them feel welcome; perhaps offer a magazine or a drink before informing the stylist that their client has arrived. This is important as it will avoid any unnecessary waiting or possible embarrassment when the stylist realizes (perhaps much later) that their client has actually arrived.

There will be occasions when you need to seek the assistance or advice from others. Recognizing situations when you are unable to help is not a failure – it is all part of professional communication. Some situations will require the attention of someone else; imagine scenarios when the window cleaner arrives and says 'Shall I just get on with it?'

TOP TIP

Even if our communication skills are perfect, what clients see around them has a far greater impact on their opinions than anything that we have to say.

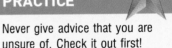

BEST PRACTICE

Never give advice that you are unsure of. Check it out first!

or requests payment, or when stock arrives and a signature is required for taking delivery and accepting the condition of the goods.

Late arrivals

On each day, at least one booked client will be late. They are not late deliberately; it's just one of those things put down to busy lives: Traffic jams, changed workloads, last-minute duties, shopping queues or just trying to fit too much into a busy day. They all have an impact on time and unfortunately, it's usually the stylist's next client.

In a situation where the client has arrived late, above all you do need to be sympathetic and understanding. The first thing to do is be sympathetic, then find out if there is still enough time to complete the service without overrunning throughout the rest of the day. If there isn't enough time left, see if one of the other stylists can help: often a bit of 'juggling' will put things back on track.

Will the client have to wait? If so tell the client immediately, let them choose between staying and waiting, or coming back a little later. Sometimes there is no other option and the appointment needs to be re-booked for some other time.

Unscheduled arrivals and 'walk-ins'

In addition to late arrivals, there is always the chance that a 'walk-in' arrives. Where possible, these new or existing clients should be accommodated in some way.

When someone arrives 'on-spec' it usually means that they have:

◆ Been recommended by other existing clients.

◆ Walked past and noticed the salon, which has interested them enough to walk in.

◆ Responded to a promotion that the salon has run in the paper or on the radio.

In any event, this is good for the salon, as it will add to the client base and increase sales.

Double bookings

Mistakes do happen. Poor communication or misunderstandings do lead to **double bookings**. The vast majority of double bookings are genuine mistakes and if they aren't handled sympathetically, it will lead to unhappy clients.

If this does happen, you need to find out if the client can be accommodated without having to wait too long. Sometimes it is easier to re-book a client for another time, but if they are unhappy about the way that they have been mishandled, the salon may lose a client and that's the last thing that the salon wants!

Ideally, try and find someone else who can help by finishing off the stylist's other client, and then at least they are able to make a start on the one that is waiting. Some businesses will smooth the situation over by offering a complimentary treatment or a scalp massage, as this will buy time while they are waiting and maintain good customer satisfaction as well.

BEST PRACTICE

Never bill a client for an amount that was not agreed.

TOP TIP

It is easier to keep a client happy than try to pacify an angry one!

Changes to booked services

There will often be occasions where a client has booked for one service, but by the time they reach the salon they have changed their mind and want something else totally different. People change their minds all the time. Don't make a fuss about this, it could be good business – a client may come in expecting a restyle, cut and finish, and go out with **highlights** too. In fact, many salons set incentives around this very activity; for example, staff performances and commissions may be targeted on 'upselling' or 'client conversions'.

Staff absences/sickness

Staff absences through sickness will always stretch the salon's resources to its limits but every salon has some sort of a contingency plan to cover in these situations.

Generally, this will involve:

◆ Checking to see if other salon staff can or have provided service to the client before.

◆ Rearranging appointments to accommodate the disruption.

◆ If all else fails – contact the client before they leave home to schedule another appointment.

BEST PRACTICE

Always introduce yourself when handling calls. People like to speak to people with whom they can associate, not strangers or machines!

Making appointments

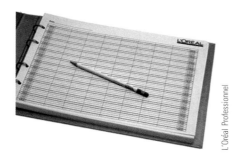

L'Oréal Professionnel

Typical appointment page/book

Know the salon's services

The appointment system is the very centre, the 'hub' of the whole salon operation. Without an appointment system the business would stop! So it is essential that appointments are made accurately and promptly, every time, whether over the telephone or in person.

Before you can make appointments, you must know the services available within the salon. Each salon provides a unique 'menu' of services. Different stylists will have different abilities and skills, and therefore offer different services and also at different levels.

You need to know the:

◆ Services and treatments available.

◆ Service and treatment timings.

◆ Costs of the services and treatments.

Making appointments needn't be difficult. It's about matching client requests with the time available. We want to help the client make the booking, while bearing in mind the time that it will take and who will be providing the service.

When clients are contacting the salon by telephone, you should always speak first saying, *'Good morning/afternoon, this is Head Masters hair salon. This is Clare speaking, how may I help you?'* This friendly and positive approach will immediately give a professional image of both the salon and yourself.

Making and confirming appointments

Each salon has its own system for making appointments but, generally speaking, accurate appointment scheduling maximizes the time available with appropriate staff members. Bearing this in mind, we should always remain ready, prompt and polite in attending to the client's requests.

Make sure when the booking is made that you record the information accurately and clearly and that you have considered all the factors:

- Date and time.
- Service required.
- Stylist required.
- The client's name.
- Client contact details.

Record the client's name clearly in the appointment system alongside the service, and check that it is booked for the correct day and time with the appropriate stylist. As a matter of customer service, it is also useful to give the client an approximate idea of service cost and length of appointment time. At the end, summarize all the information back to the client, making sure that all the details are correct.

Appointment checklist

✓ You need to know the abbreviations the salon uses for different services.

✓ You need to know the system the salon uses for making appointments.

✓ You need to ask questions to get extra information.

✓ You need good listening skills.

✓ You need to know the prices of the different treatments and services.

✓ You need to fill in appointment details.

✓ You need to know the days and hours that each stylist works.

✓ You need to know which treatments each stylist does.

✓ You need to spell clients' names correctly.

✓ You need to be able to manage times and dates.

✓ You need to know how much time the salon allows for each service.

If you're not sure, ask!

There may be situations where you are not sure. It is always better to ask someone else than to make mistakes such as:

◆ Making incorrect or inaccurate bookings.

◆ Providing inaccurate information, e.g. incorrect costings of services or products.

When unsure always ask someone for help. There is nothing worse than a stylist who is running late; particularly if this is the result of someone else's booking error. The situation will be stressful for the stylist but, more importantly, we do not want any clients waiting longer than absolutely necessary, whatever the reason.

Difficult or angry clients

There may be other situations where you have to find someone else in authority to handle the client's enquiry. If you can see by a client's face (check their expressions) that they are not happy about something, it is not your job to try and sort out their problem. Simply ask them to take a seat and then find a senior member of staff to deal with their concerns.

Service abbreviations	
Cut and blow-dry	CBD
Blow-dry	BD
Shampoo and set	S/S
Ladies' wet cut	WC
Gents' wet cut	G W/C
Gents' cut and blow-dry	G CBD
Highlights T section	H/L T
Highlights full head	H/L FH
Highlights half head	H/L½H
Retouch colour	Col rt
Full head colour	Col fh
Permanent wave	PW
Chemical **relaxer**	Relax

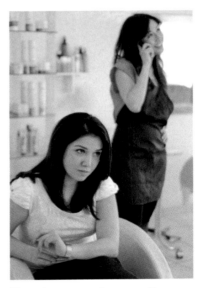

Never leave a customer waiting

No-appointment salons/barbers

Some salons and all barber's shops don't have an appointment system, they work on a walk-in basis where the staff receive the clients as they walk in from the street. This has great **benefits** from the client's point of view as they can call in, as and when it suits them. The only disadvantage of this type of system is that customers won't necessarily get the same stylist next time, so this doesn't always suit everyone.

Accurately recording appointments

When you have found out what the caller wants, you are ready to make the appointment by asking the following questions:

- ◆ 'On what day would you like the appointment?'
- ◆ 'What time do you have in mind?'
- ◆ 'What would you like to have done?'
- ◆ 'Which stylist is that with/would you like to see?'

Each time you ask one of the questions above, you are reducing the possible number of responses to a narrow range of options. This means that you are taking control of the situation and leading the conversation in a controlled professional way and eliminating unnecessary information that could lead you to making a mistake.

The four questions very quickly allow you to get to the:

- ◆ Right day in the appointment system.
- ◆ Available times for services.
- ◆ Type of service required by the client.
- ◆ The availability of their stylist to do the job.

BEST PRACTICE

Remember to take accurate information and summarize the details back to the client.

Now you have to work out if there is enough time to make the appointment for the client. This is often the most difficult part of making appointments, because some are just a single block of time, whereas others take multiple blocks.

For example, a booking for a haircut or a blow-dry is a single block appointment. The colour or perm appointment is more complex because these *straddle* other appointments to allow for the colour or perm to develop, allowing the stylist to do something else in between.

Appointment example 1

Date: *Friday 13th September*

Time	Clare	Steve
9.00		
9.15		
9.30	Taylor BD	
9.45	01 / 23 / 456	
10.00		
10.15		
10.30		

In this example we see a single block appointment made by a regular client on **Friday 13th September** at **9.30** with **Clare** for **Mrs. Taylor** for a **blow-dry**

Appointment example 2

Date: *Friday 13th September*

Time	Clare	Steve
9.00	Summers HLT	
9.15	01 / 23 / 456789	
9.30	Taylor BD	
9.45	01 / 23 / 456	
10.00	Summers CBD	
10.15	/ /	
10.30		

Here we see an additional appointment with contact details made on **Friday 13th September** at **9.00** with **Clare** for Miss **Summers** for a **highlights 'T' section**, which now straddles the Taylor appointment and is booked back with Clare to do a cut and blow-dry at **10.00**

Confirming and recording details correctly

Record the client's name clearly in the appointment system alongside the requested service, and check that it is scheduled for the correct day and time with the appropriate stylist. As a matter of customer service, it is also useful to give the client an approximate idea of service cost and length of appointment time.

At the end, summarize all the information back to the client. This will ensure that all the details are correct. If the client has come into the salon or barber's shop to make the appointment, give them an appointment card as a token of good service and as a prompt. This provides a physical copy of the appointment and another way of ensuring that all the facts are correct.

> **BEST PRACTICE**
>
> Speak clearly on the telephone, the client may have difficulty hearing you.

Handle payments from clients

All salons use some form of electronic till, some of which are computerized systems that provide detailed analysis, evaluations and reports for managing the business.

In their simplest forms, the electronic till will:

- ◆ Calculate the client's bill.

- ◆ Provide a receipt for the client.

- ◆ Provide ways to separate sales of services separately to sales of products.

- ◆ Provide readouts (during and at the end of the day) to monitor and balance sales.

- ◆ Provide a secure system for holding payments.

- ◆ Calculate VAT within sales of services and products.

The more sophisticated computer system will do **ALL** of the above and:

- ◆ Calculate stock movements and handle stock control.

- ◆ Record treatment history, contact and personal information for the salon's clients.

- ◆ Help to make appointments and identify the client's details.

- ◆ Monitor trading patterns, sales, services and treatment patterns.

- ◆ Calculate staff commissions.

- ◆ Produce management reports for budgeting and forecasting.

> **BEST PRACTICE**
>
> If the change in the till is getting low tell a relevant person immediately. Running out of change will disrupt service and give a poor impression of salon organization.

Methods of payment

Cash When taking cash from clients make sure that you follow these simple steps:

1   Carefully 'ring up' all the services and products provided to the client into the till and press 'subtotal'.

2   Inform the client of the amount to be paid.

3 Look carefully, but not suspiciously, to make sure that the money offered is legal tender (you should check that the notes are still valid, not out of date and not counterfeit, i.e. fake!).

4 Place the money tendered to you on the ledge at the top of the till drawer, so that it can be seen by the client too.

5 Press the numeric keys of the till to equal the amount tendered by the client.

6 Press the total button. The till will automatically show the amount of change to be given and the till drawer will open.

7 Take out and count back this amount into the client's hand.

8 Tear off the till receipt and don't forget to thank them as well as asking, 'Would you like to make your next appointment now?'

9 If the client disputes their change, ask how much is missing to see if you have made a mistake. It is quite simple to make a genuine mistake, but if you are in any doubt call for a senior member of staff to assist.

Payment by card

Debit Cards Arguably, the most popular form of payment in any retail location, the debit card has replaced the necessity for cash or **cheques**. A *Chip and Pin* debit card is the most secure way for clients and businesses to carry out *paperless* sales transactions.

Debit cards act as an automated cheque: the transaction process is the same as for a cheque or **credit card**, but once processed the client's bank account is automatically debited and the salon's account is electronically credited. The card-processing company applies a nominal fixed fee to the salon for each card transaction made.

Credit cards These are accepted as a method of payment at the discretion of the salon. When a card has been accepted as the method of payment, a fixed percentage of the total bill is charged by the card-processing company for the use of this facility.

Normally, a list of the salon's accepted cards should be clearly displayed on the door or front window as well as the reception desk. Clients tend to assume that payment by card will be acceptable, so failing to inform them otherwise could cause an embarrassing situation to arise. Card payments are given a 'floor limit' by the card company: payment will be honoured up to a specific amount; for large amounts, prior authorization by telephone is required. Thorough training needs to be given if staff are to understand these procedures.

Charge cards These provide another payment alternative. Many businesses now accept charge-card payments too – American Express is the main operator in this field. Charge-card payments are made in a similar way to credit or debit cards and therefore can be treated the same way. The difference is more for the card holder.

The cards are often used as business cards, for travel, accommodation and business expenses. Each month the card holder receives a statement for the purchases made on the card over the period. This statement is a request for settlement and the bill must be paid.

Processing payments by cards

Before you accept a card payment you should make sure that the card is genuine and valid. Within the salon information pack you will find a card recognition guide for each card that is permitted. The guide provides the following information:

1 **Card symbol** – This is a logo (Visa, MasterCard) which will appear at the front lower right corner of the card. On **charge cards**, i.e. American Express, the Centurion head is printed across the centre of the card.

2 **Card hologram** – The card hologram service mark is in the centre right-hand edge of the card. This service mark is etched onto a foil decal which is superimposed on the card's printed background. The service mark on the holographic service mark (e.g. Visa, which appears as a dove ascending) is visible when angled in the light. The hologram changes according to the angle from which it is viewed.

3 **Card number** – The card number will be embossed onto the surface and across the width of the card. When you use an electronic terminal, always ensure that the card number matches that which is printed on your terminal receipt.

4 **Card validity dates** – The card will show a 'valid from' date as well as an 'expires end' date. If the card is not in date it cannot be accepted.

5 **Card holder's name** – Check that the name on the card, and the title of the card holder, match the person presenting it.

Chip and pin payments

◆ Check that the terminal is in sale ready mode.

◆ Insert the card into the chip reader.

◆ Enter the amount by using the key pad (if you make a mistake you can clear the figures using the 'clear' button).

◆ Press 'enter', which will connect the terminal to the card-processing company.

◆ The customer details are automatically accessed and after a few moments, a message will prompt for 'Enter customer pin'. The customer can enter their four digit pin on the customer keypad and press 'enter'. The payment is authorized or declined automatically.

◆ Pass the receipt back to the client and retain the additional copy for the till.

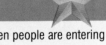

BEST PRACTICE

Look away when people are entering their pin, it is common courtesy.

Cheques There has been some controversy in recent years to the future of the cheque or at least its value as a direct payment for goods within a shop. UK banks would have preferred to remove the *Cheque Guarantee Card* and therefore the validity of cheques as a direct payment. This would encourage people to pay their regularly occurring bills by direct debit, standing order or at their local bank by the Giro banking system, or BACs payment systems. This of course is suitable for paying rent, an electricity bill or your mobile phone, but it doesn't work for paying a hairdressing bill.

Possible alternatives Many payment pilot systems are underway and future systems may incorporate NFC technology (Near Field Communication) using mobile devices featuring *Quick Tap*, and others are already using the technology in prepayment systems like the *OYSTER* cards for the London underground.

However, the banks have now retracted their request to remove cheque guarantee cards for the foreseeable future, and the historical system is still in force.

Some clients still prefer to pay their bill by cheque. Cheques must be accompanied by a cheque guarantee card. These are normally a debit card and denote a spending limit which is identified by a hologram on the back of the card. Normally this limit is set at £100.

When receiving payment by cheque follow these steps:

1 The cheque must have the correct date in the top right-hand corner.

2 The cheque must be payable to the firm or company (you may have a pre-printed stamp for this).

3 The amount in figures must match the amount written in words.

4 The client must initial any mistakes or errors made.

5 The cheque must be signed and must match the signature on the back of the cheque guarantee card.

6 The sort code and account number on the cheque must match those on the guarantee card.

7 The payment date must be within the valid **from** and **to** dates on the cheque guarantee card.

8 A cheque cannot exceed the cheque guarantee card limit.

Discrepancies Unfortunately, there will be times when discrepancies or disputes occur. They should be dealt with courteously and calmly and should avoid any unnecessary embarrassment to the client. There can be all sorts of reasons for invalid payment and these could be:

◆ Invalid currency – counterfeit notes, foreign currency.

◆ Card declined – may be out of date, or infer insufficient funds available.

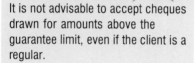

TOP TIP

A post-dated cheque, that is a cheque made out for a date later than the current day's date, is an invalid form of payment.

BEST PRACTICE

It is not advisable to accept cheques drawn for amounts above the guarantee limit, even if the client is a regular.

TOP TIP

Fraud is happening all the time, be on your guard for forged notes.

TOP TIP

If a card appears damaged, e.g. the plastic is peeling off, check closely to see that it hasn't been tampered with.

◆ Invalid cheque – figures and words don't match, post-dating, signatures don't match.

◆ Fraudulent use of card – 'hot card' warnings, or known stolen or 'cloned' cards.

Reception Security

The reception is the first part of the salon that people walk into off the street, so this area must maintain a high level of security. All monies must be kept safely locked away and products should be monitored so that they are not maliciously removed. Records relating to the business, client details, accounts books, etc. should never be left unattended. If a client were to see these things left around that would be bad enough, but if an unknown viewed them, then the salon's security measures would have been breached and personal information disclosed. In order to avoid these situations:

1 The salon reception should be manned at all times.

2 Ensure money is not kept on the premises when the salon is shut and keep cash in the till during working hours to an absolute minimum.

3 Never leave the till drawer open when it is not in use.

4 Check all notes that have been handed over in payment to avoid counterfeits.

5 Always leave the cash drawer, or at least the chassis that it fits into, open overnight: this discourages forced entries.

6 Money should be regularly transferred to the company safe or banked.

7 Never make regular visits to the bank at the same times.

8 Receipts should be given for all payments.

9 Never use the cash in the till for petty cash purchases.

10 Any other money removed for whatever reason must always be recorded.

11 Follow the salon's safety and security procedures at all times.

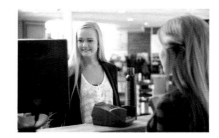

Trading safely and legally

Data Protection Act (1998)

Any organization that records information about staff or clients, whether on a card index system or a computer, must comply with the Data Protection Act 1998. The law requires people to keep information held on file about their customers safe and secure. In salons, this means that information about clients must be kept confidential and handled with the utmost professional care. All staff working within the salon have a responsibility to maintain this confidentiality at all times, even after working hours. You are not at liberty to discuss other peoples' circumstances with anyone.

DATA PROTECTION ACT 1998 – Plain-language summary of key principles

This section provides a quick overview of what the Key Principles of information-handling practice means. The Key Principles themselves are discussed below in the context of their definition in law.

◆ Data may only be used for the specific purposes for which it was collected.

◆ Data must not be disclosed to other parties without the *consent* of the individual whom it is about, unless there is legislation or other overriding legitimate reasons to share the information (e.g. the prevention or detection of crime). It is an offence for other parties to obtain this personal data without authorization.

◆ Individuals have a right of access to the information held about them, subject to certain expectations (e.g. information held for the prevention or detection of crime).

◆ Personal information may be kept for no longer than is necessary and must be kept up to date.

◆ Personal information may not be sent outside the *European Economic Area* unless the individual whom it is about has consented, or adequate protection is in place (e.g. by the use of a prescribed form of contract) to govern the transmission of the data.

◆ Subject to some exceptions for organizations that only do very simple processing, and for domestic use, all entities that process personal information must *register* with the *Information Commissioner's Office*.

◆ The departments of a company that are holding personal information are required to have adequate security measures in place. Those include technical measures (such as firewalls) and organizational measures (such as staff training).

◆ Subjects have the right to have *factually incorrect* information corrected (note: this does not extend to matters of *opinion*).

Sale of Goods Act 1979

Under the Sale of Goods Act 1979, when a salon sells something to a customer they have an agreement or contract with them.

A customer has legal rights if the goods they purchased do not conform to contract (are faulty). The Act says that to conform to contract goods should:

1 **Match their description** – by law everything that is said about the product must not be misleading – whether this is said by a sales assistant, or written on the packaging, in-store, on advertising materials or in a catalogue.

2 **Be of satisfactory quality** – this quality of goods includes:

   ◆ appearance and finish
   ◆ freedom from minor defects (such as marks or holes)
   ◆ safe to use
   ◆ in good working order
   ◆ durability

3 **Be fit for purpose** – if a customer says, or when it should be obvious to the retailer, that an item is wanted for a particular purpose, even if it is a purpose the item is not usually supplied for, and the retailer agrees the item is suitable, or

does not say it is not fit for that purpose, then it has to be reasonably fit. If there is disagreement with the customer about a particular purpose, it (the retailer) should make this clear, perhaps on the sales receipt, to protect the business against future claims.

Trades Descriptions Acts (1968/1972)

Products must not be falsely or misleadingly described in relation to their quality, fitness, price or purpose, by advertisements, orally, displays or descriptions. And since 1972 it has also been a requirement to label a product clearly, so that the buyer can see where the product was made.

Briefly, a retailer cannot:

◆ Mislead consumers by making false statements about products.

◆ Offer sale products at half price unless they have been offered at the actual price for a reasonable period.

The Consumer Protection Act (1987)

This Act follows European laws to protect the buyer in the following areas:

◆ Product liability – a customer may claim compensation for a product that doesn't reach general standards of safety.

◆ General safety requirements – it is a criminal offence to sell goods that are unsafe; traders that breach this conduct may face fines or even imprisonment.

◆ Misleading prices – misleading consumers with wrongly displayed prices is also an offence.

The Act is designed to help safeguard the consumer from products that do not reach reasonable levels of safety. Your salon will take adequate precautions in procuring, using and supplying reputable products and maintaining them so that they remain in good condition.

SUMMARY

As a final reflection on what you have covered in this chapter, you should now have a clearer picture of all the essential aspects for working in the salon reception. In particular, you should now have a basic understanding of the key principles of:

1 Meeting and greeting all the salon's clients in the appropriate way.

2 Taking messages and handling calls and enquiries.

3 Making appointments for clients.

4 Handling different payment types for the salon's services and treatments.

5 Trading safely and legally.

And collectively, how these principles will enable you to work efficiently and effectively in customer facing situations.

ASSESSMENT OF KNOWLEDGE AND UNDERSTANDING

Project

With two of your colleagues you can practise and document the different scenarios that occur in a hairdressing salon.

Let one person take the place of the client and another, the receptionist. The third acts as an observer and takes notes for the others. Take it in turns to cover the following salon situations:

1   An angry client who is not happy with their hair.

2   A client who needs assistance with buying retail products.

3   A client who wants to make several bookings for her daughter's wedding.

In your notes you need to cover how the client was handled, how, if at all, the service could be improved and what information needs to be recorded in each of the different scenarios.

Case study

A client has asked for an appointment with a stylist who no longer works at the salon. Describe your salon procedures for:

1   What you say to the client.

2   The questions you would ask.

3   The alternatives that you would offer the client.

4   What you would do if you could not deal with the situation.

Revision questions

A selection of different types of questions to check your reception knowledge.

Q1   Visa and MasterCard are both forms of _____ card.   Fill in the blank

Q2   A charge card is the same as a debit card.   True or false

Q3   Which of the following card types are debit cards?   Multi selection

Loyalty card	☐ 1
Switch card	☐ 2
American Express card	☐ 3
MasterCard	☐ 4
Maestro card	☐ 5
Store card	☐ 6

Q4   A float in the till contains 1 × £10.00 note, 2 × £5.00 notes, £20.00 in £1 coins and £5.00 in 50p coins. How much is in the float?   Multi choice

£40.00	O a
£45.00	O b
£45.50	O c
£46.00	O d

Q5   You should always take a contact number when making appointments.   True or false

Q6   Which of the following are examples of ineffective use of resources?   Multi selection

Explaining services and costs to clients on the telephone.	☐ 1
Discarding excess product after application.	☐ 2
Overrunning on appointments.	☐ 3
Turning the lights off in corridors and staff areas.	☐ 4
Washing up in the dispensary.	☐ 5
Ordering stock over the telephone.	☐ 6

Q7   _____ retail products are for maintaining hair between visits.   Fill in the blank

Q8   Which of the following procedures monitors the usage of products   Multi choice
within salons?

Stock control.	○ a
Monitoring wastage.	○ b
Retail product and display cleaning.	○ c
Stock rotation.	○ d

Q9   A job description is a document containing the employee's terms and   True or false
conditions of employment.

4 Promotion and display

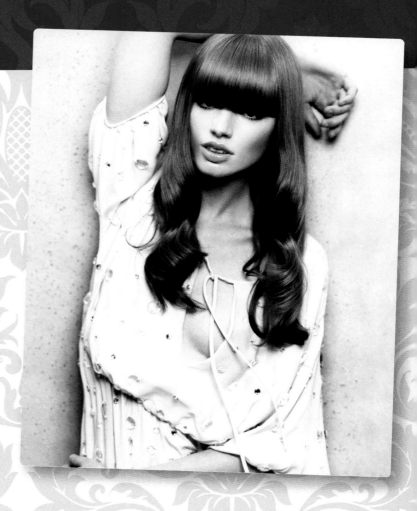

LEARNING OBJECTIVES

◆ Be able to identify additional services or products that are available

◆ Be able to inform clients about services or products

◆ Be able to promote additional services or products

◆ Understand how to promote additional services or products to customers

KEY TERMS

clarifying shampoo
dandruff
demonstrate
effective communication
features
legislation

personal presentation
Prices Act (1974)
professional advice
Resale Prices Acts (1964 and 1976)

Sale and Supply of Goods Act (1994)
salon services

Unit topic

Promote products and services to clients and display stock to promote sales in a salon.

INTRODUCTION

If you want to find out what's on at the cinema, you'll probably go online and do a quick Internet search to see what's on, when the film starts and whether there are any special deals.

Well there doesn't seem to be anything unusual in that. But did you notice that while you were looking to find what you wanted, other adverts within the cinema's website were trying to tempt you into other things as well?

◆ Visual stimulation creates *desire* and this is the basis of good selling tactics.

◆ Promotion and display is the technique or process of how that *desire* is created.

Quite simply, good selling strategies focus on things that customers either **want** or **need**.

In other words, it's easier to sell things to clients or customers when:

◆ They see things that they want.

◆ The things that they see also meet their needs.

This is where you fit in, because if the customer doesn't necessarily understand why or how those things will benefit them, then they are unlikely to buy.

Therefore, you play a vital role in the promotion of products or services by:

◆ Explaining how those products or services will benefit them.

So if we put all these things together we have a simple formula for promotion and display.

Promoting and displaying products and services

PRACTICAL SKILLS

Learn about your client's wishes, needs and requirements

Learn how to recognize opportunities to promote, recommend and sell to clients

Learn how to describe the features and benefits of products or services to your client

Learn how to promote a professional image within the salon

Learn about the legal requirements affecting the sale and supply of products and services to your client

Learn about health and safety legislation related to creating in-salon displays

Learn how to assist in the planning of salon promotions and displays

UNDERPINNING KNOWLEDGE

Communicating professionally with your client

Promoting and selling products and services to your client

Creating salon displays and promotions

Assisting others in the planning of promotional events

Features and benefits of promotion and display

Formula for success

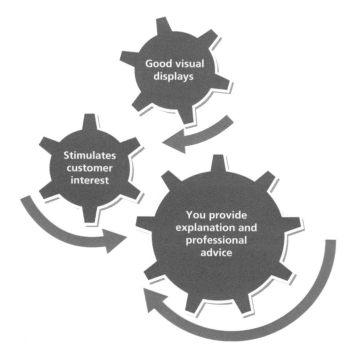

Good visual displays

Stimulates customer interest

You provide explanation and professional advice

When we think of services and products in selling or sales situations, we base our customer information upon their **features** and benefits.

Features	The qualities or characteristics of services or products

Benefits	The advantages that the clients gain from having a service or using the products

For example, suppose you recommend a client to spend £11.50 on a conditioning treatment. Why should they do this? What are the features and benefits of the service?

◆ **Features** – It re-conditions dry, damaged hair.

◆ **Benefits** – It improves the dryness and helps to smooth damaged lengths; therefore, it will improve handling, make the hair easy to manage and comb and enhance the hair further with shine and lustre.

So the client can now 'weigh up' those benefits of taking up the **professional advice** against not doing anything about the condition of their hair. Most people, when confronted with a solution to their problem, will take up the professional advice. The benefits of the products should be tailored to each client as their individual needs are different, so the benefits of the products must reflect this.

Promote a professional image in a salon

So far, we have looked in basic terms at what factors make a customer consider purchasing and we have realized that good displays, backed up with sound advice is key to the selling process. Well that's not quite everything, as you will need to be plausible too. Quite simply, you need to be seen as a professional (by the client) in order to be believable.

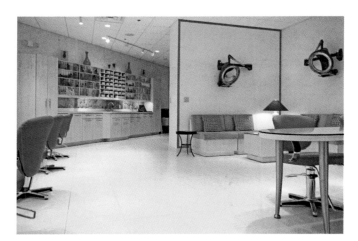

You need to reflect the same standards as those of the salon, i.e. you need to be considered a walking advert for the business. You need to present an approachable appearance to the client and be ready and willing to give help and advice. From the client's perspective, you need to have a friendly and caring attitude and be focused upon their needs. Your appearance is particularly important, paying attention to personal hygiene and tidiness, and also reflect the salon's dress code or uniform. Remember you are part of a team and therefore you play a key role in keeping up appearances for everyone's sake.

TOP TIP

Most people are embarrassed by physical contact from someone they do not know well.

Why should I bother to promote salon services and products?

You may already be thinking this and it is easier to cover this now, earlier rather than later.

You may have thought when you first considered hairdressing or barbering as a future career, that it would be an exciting opportunity to:

◆ Earn a good living.

◆ Create wonderful hair styles and effects for people.

◆ Work in a *leading edge* fashion conscious industry.

◆ Feel valued and respected for the work that you can do.

◆ Travel the world with your work.

Well you are right; you can do all of those things, but all of these things come at a price. Part of that cost relates to your own investment in your own future, and that is where you are now, learning and training to be the best. So from this you can see that your investment is measured in time and commitment, and that may seem like a big price to pay. But don't forget; others are making an investment in you as well.

◆ If you are at college, then there are course fees to be paid – so where has that money come from?

◆ If you are an apprentice in a salon, then you are receiving a wage – your employer is paying you while you learn.

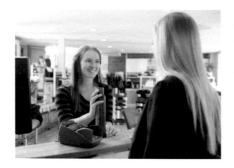

If others make an investment in you, they will expect a return on their investment; that's the way that ALL of the world works and no one can get away without repaying what they dutifully owe.

As we are already talking in terms of features and benefits, let's see who benefits from the promotion of services and products:

1   The salon benefits by increasing sales which in turn, should generate profits.

We consider a profit as the monetary value gained after say buying a product for £10.00 and selling that to a customer for £15.00. In other words, the difference between the buying cost and the final selling price generates the profit. In this case £5.00. The £5.00 is now in the till and will contribute to the business overheads, i.e. wages, rent, electricity, stock, insurances, taxes, etc.

As you can see, there needs to be lots of profitable sales in order to pay the bills. When all the bills have been paid, anything left over is the *nett profit* for the business. This money could then be spent in many ways.

2   The money could be spent in training or new products and services.

This is to your benefit as the profits generated are now reinvested in developing your skills. You will be learning new things and gaining experience in new areas of work. These are new skills that you will be able to move forward with in your future career. So who's the winner now?

You should now be able to see that you are the ultimate winner.

Cycle of success

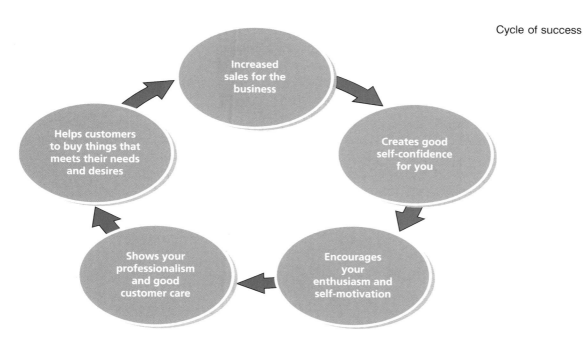

Finding opportunities to introduce services or products to clients

First and foremost you are a professional. Your role is to provide clients and prospective customers with suitable options that are *tailored* to their needs. This draws a distinct line between you and the underhand sales tactics of rogues, rascals and con-artists, who make a living out of selling people things that they don't want or need!

You are identifying a client's individual needs, so even while you are still learning, there will be many situations where you can find opportunities to recommend things to clients.

An opportunity with a client	Questions you might ask
While waiting in reception	Have you seen our new colour range Mrs XXX? I'll get you a shade chart.
During gowning	Have you noticed an increase in **dandruff** lately? I'll use one of our treatment shampoos and give you some product information about home maintenance.
When shampooing	I think that your stylist may be still finishing off. Would you like me to provide a relaxing scalp massage while the conditioner is on?
	I notice that there is some product build-up from the styling products that you are using. I suggest we use a **clarifying shampoo** and I'll mention it to the stylist so that they can recommend some alternatives for you.
While blow-drying	Does your hair tend to 'drop' very quickly Mrs XXX? I could use this mousse this time as it is designed to give root lift as well.
While their colour is developing	Can I offer you any refreshments from our café range Mrs XXX?
When they are browsing in the retail area	Can I help you with anything in particular such as styling products, home care, in-salon treatments?

Believe it or not, most additional sales in salons and barber's shops are generated through casual conversation. Typically, a discussion at the basin will start with why you are using a particular product on a client's hair. Which then leads on to the client asking, is there something that they could use to achieve the same effect, which in turn, provides an opportunity to create a sale.

All salons have price lists and manufacturers' show cards, posters or other product related materials. This provides specific, professionally produced printed information for customers, so that they can take home something about the products that the salon provides. This is also a good way of providing a talking point for staff in the salon as this often starts a discussion.

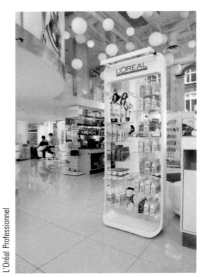

L'Oréal Professionnel

So, with all this manufacturer information being continually updated, you too will need to keep abreast of any changes and the new additions. You also need to keep up to date on all the features and benefits of newly introduced **salon services** and products. Normally, all the staff are kept informed during staff meetings, but if you were on work experience and saw recent additions that you hadn't seen before, you would need to ask the manager or your supervisor for more information.

How do you introduce products or services to clients?

Knowing when and what to say to clients is half the battle and the other half is down to your timing.

If a client feels that they are being *pushed* into a sale or being unduly hassled, they will immediately *'bring down the shutters'*, and you will be cut off quite abruptly.

First, you need to be able to provide accurate and relevant information. Make sure that you have all the correct information and are ready to answer the client's questions. There is nothing worse than running out of facts and resorting to *spouting* out rubbish, so readup on the latest product ranges and get used to using them, so you see how they work in different situations.

There is quite a difference between these two statements:

- ◆ 'I think that you should find that it works well on your type of hair' and

- ◆ 'I have tried this out in many different situations and it was particularly successful on hair similar to yours'.

Next, find the right moment to talk about your products. Choose a time when your client seems relaxed; you will find that they are far more open to being approached when they are comfortable than if they are already stressed about something. You can get an idea of the client's state of mind by the body language and mannerisms that they use.

For example, if a client arrives at the salon and they are already running late, they will be embarrassed that they have kept their stylist waiting. Their face may be 'flushed' (reddened); they may also be out of breath. They may also be talking quite quickly too. This is definitely the wrong moment to ask if they have seen this month's promotional display.

Similarly, a client who has had to wait a while for their stylist may keep checking their watch. It may indicate that they have other arrangements and be running out of time. Again, the client is preoccupied and will not be able to listen to what you have to say. The best thing that you could do in this situation is to let their stylist know and let them deal with the situation.

But at other times, when the client seems quite *chilled*, they may welcome some interaction and this is your chance.

Recognizing interest – interpreting buying signals

You need to be able to recognize the difference between genuine interest and a polite and friendly, but negative response. Just because someone responds to you in a polite or friendly way, it is not an indication of 'I want to buy that'.

Genuine interest will be expressed in at least two ways:

- ◆ The client will ask how the product will benefit them, e.g. 'Would that be suitable for my type of hair?' or, 'How does that work?'

- ◆ The client will show their interest by taking the product and holding it for closer examination, or through their positive body language.

Therefore, when you introduce or recommend the client to a new service or product, you will need to look for the signs of interest like those mentioned above.

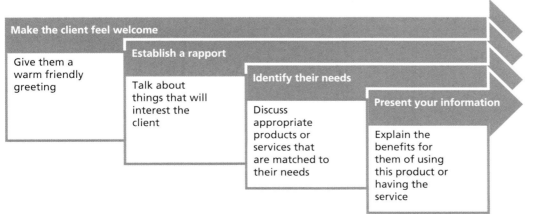

Creating the right sales environment

Make the client feel welcome

Give them a warm friendly greeting

Establish a rapport

Talk about things that will interest the client

Identify their needs

Discuss appropriate products or services that are matched to their needs

Present your information

Explain the benefits for them of using this product or having the service

Anything else could indicate a lack of interest and you should be careful how you proceed. There is little point pursuing the issue if you are receiving little or no response; even if you think it's the best product or service that they could have.

You can see from the illustration on page 101, that making them feel welcome and establishing effective, professional communication between you and the client is vital in creating the right sales environment. The relationship between stylist and client is built on quality of service, professional advice, trust, support and a listening ear. Good communication ensures productive and effective action. On the other hand, poor communication can lead to misunderstandings and mistakes.

Keeping clients informed of new services, treatments and products

In-salon promotions and product displays are the most popular way of *sending* messages to our clients. They see the promotions while they are having their hair done, and this becomes a topic of conversation between you and the client.

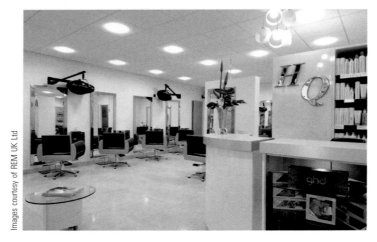

Images courtesy of REM UK Ltd

Whenever new products are introduced, the manufacturer produces a variety of point-of-sale material which provides people with professionally produced information, posters, etc. to help with the launch. The amount of support material does tend to be linked with how much the salon buys, i.e. a small independent salon that has bought an introductory deal from the supplier may only have a small amount of supporting material to use within the salon, whereas a larger salon group will bulk-buy large amounts and get more support to help promote the products.

A typical promotion will include:

◆ **Introductory discounts** – where products are available for a set period at a lower price.

◆ **Multi-buys** – typically BOGOFs – buy one get one free.

◆ **Special offers** – buy all three and get a free beach towel or bag.

In order for the promotion to work, everyone needs to be informed about the promotional plan, and any personal incentives or sales targets linked with the promotion. Each member of staff might have an individual role to play in the overall team plan. For example, the assistant may ask the client if they want to try the new conditioner on their hair at the basin. This gives the client the chance to gain their first experiences of the product.

The promotion continues at the styling position where show cards or leaflets are placed in the client's view to explain the benefits from using the product. This is reinforced by the stylist's advice and recommendations. Typically, the client would be asked if they noticed and liked the smell of the conditioner when it was applied, or if they can see and feel the difference that it has made to their hair.

Then, at the end of the service and just before the client leaves, they might be reminded again with the conditioning promotion, when they see a well put together display in reception. At this point, the receptionist may ask if the client would like to add the product to their bill so they can get the same results at home.

You can see from this example that it is really a whole-team approach and it applies whether it is a small salon or a large college.

Sensing a sale

We only have five senses and these influence our purchasing decisions. They are:

◆ What we **see**

◆ Things that we **touch**

◆ How things **smell**

◆ What we **hear**

◆ The things that we **taste**

Our five senses are the only things that can influence what we buy. So from a clever, professional approach to the mathematics of *probability and chance*, the greater the number of senses involved in the promotional event/display, then the higher chance that the client will buy. By providing professional and **effective communication** to the client, you stand a good chance of making a sale.

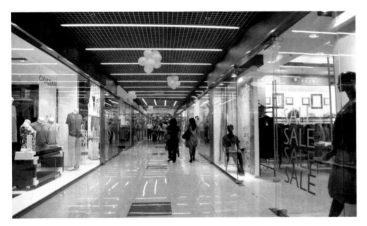

Eye-catching window displays

Closing the sale

At the point where the client has demonstrated a genuine interest, you are then able to gain their commitment by asking them if they would like to add this to their bill. Quite simply, if they have shown interest by asking about the products and then handled or removed the top to smell the product, you have stimulated their interest and initiated their desire.

With all these signals turning green, you only have to ask the question:

'Can I put it in a bag for you and leave it ready in reception for when you leave?'

TOP TIP

Genuine interest is expressed by the client wanting to know more and/or showing it by what they do.

ACTIVITY

Next time you go shopping, note how some retailers try to encourage you to use your senses. For example, what do you notice when you go into a shopping mall? Do the shops that sell toiletries or delicious pastries, open their doors so that the wonderful smells can fill the air? Is it the same for the coffee shops too? Does the smell of freshly ground coffee encourage you to start your day there?

For more information on effective communication, and different types of questions/question techniques, go to **CHAPTER 6** on Consultation, pp. 144–151.

BEST PRACTICE

Remember body zones – Do not crowd or appear over familiar with your client. Imagine how you would feel if someone came up to you and got a little too close. What would you do? Immediately back off and go onto the defensive.

When clients show no interest – what next?

Even if you have followed every step of the process, there will always be the 'odd' exception to the rule. Sometimes a client will show no interest in what you have to say about the salon's products and services, and in this event you could reflect on how you presented your pitch.

Was the information that you gave:

- ◆ Relevant – tailored to your client's needs?
- ◆ Clear – could you have been misunderstood?
- ◆ Too technical – did you overdo the 'science bit', or try to be too clever?
- ◆ Appropriate – was your timing correct, was the client relaxed?

If you didn't fall short on any of the above, you might like to look at the following sales techniques.

Key factors indicating GOOD selling techniques	Key factors indicating BAD selling techniques
◆ Listening, asking questions, showing interest.	◆ Doing all the talking.
◆ Using the client's name.	◆ Not listening, not 'hearing' unspoken thoughts, arguing.
◆ Empathy (putting yourself in the client's place), establishing a bond.	◆ Interrupting – but never letting the clients interrupt you – therefore losing an open opportunity for giving extra information.
◆ Recognizing body language (dilated pupils = 'I approve'; ear-rubbing = 'I've heard enough').	◆ Hard selling, 'spieling' (working to a script).
◆ Identifying needs; helping clients reach buying decisions.	◆ Threatening – 'You won't get it cheaper anywhere else', knocking the opposition.
◆ Knowing your products/services.	◆ Manipulating – 'Oh dear, I'll miss my sales target'.
◆ Highlighting the results or user benefits; **demonstrate** them where possible.	◆ Knowing nothing about the product.
◆ Thinking positively, talking persuasively, projecting confidence and enthusiasm.	◆ Treating 'no thanks' as personal rejection.

BEST PRACTICE

Focus on your communication skills. Excellent communicators are good listeners, they understand how to ask the clients the right questions and listen effectively to responses, building on the information given to them and then finally, helping the client to buy.

Product Displays

The importance of retail sales

Retail sales are an important part of the overall income to the business; they are a simple way of greatly increasing salon profits. Hairdressing and barbering services take up a lot of staff time in labour costs (i.e. wages) in delivering the services and, therefore, the selling of products in addition to the salon services, increases profits, without creating additional labour costs.

Salon products can be presented to the clients in two ways:

1   By **personal presentation**, recommendation and advice (covered earlier in this chapter).

2   By attractive, eye-catching displays.

The features of good salon display

There are two types of display that can be used in the hairdressing salon:

1   The '*dummy*' display.

2   The '*live*' display – from which products are sold.

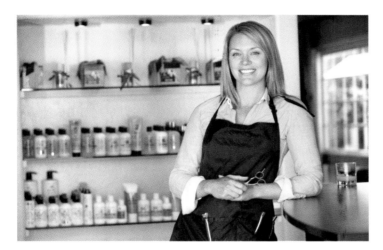

The 'dummy' display is an installation or structure that is designed, simply, to be looked at. It is created with the single objective of catching the client's attention and *informs* them of the salon's current promotions. These must be eye-catching and need to be creatively and artistically arranged, as this will stimulate interest and prompt the client to ask questions and create discussion.

They will often consist of empty product packaging or containers; this reduces the overall cost of promoting the products and creates a lighter, safer temporary structure within the salon that is easier to erect and dismantle. The dummy products are not intended to be touched or sold from, so they can be ideally situated behind glass or often create the basis for a window display.

Window displays These are essential to the advertising of a salon; services, price lists, contact information and displaying products. They can be relatively inexpensive to *dress*, particularly if they are created and maintained by the salon staff. But particular care needs to be given to the quality of window dressing, as the public are used to high quality branding and first-class advertising. Therefore, their visual expectations of any retail window space are generally high. If the standard of window dressing falls beneath the normally expected standards in industry, they *will* notice, and tell all their friends too! If that happens, it will devalue the salon and give it a poor reputation; damaging its professional standing within the local industry.

Part of the secret to creating eye-catching displays is constant change. Therefore, the display windows need to change frequently, particularly if they are to have any impact on the passing trade and stimulate them enough to stop and come in.

In-salon displays The products in an in-salon display must be attractively presented too. This type of display should encourage the client to pick products up and hold them, so therefore they need to be spaced so that they can be 'picked' (without knocking over others) and placed within easy reach. Ideally, a good display will include product testers or samples, so that clients can freely smell and touch.

Each product must be clearly priced and small signs placed beside the products or on the edge of the shelves to describe their main benefits (*Shelftalkers*).

This sort of in-salon display should always be in an area of the salon where most clients will see and walk past it – i.e. the '*main traffic routes*'. This is because a large proportion of cosmetics and hair related products are impulse buys.

Product displays should always feature in the main salon work area. The reason for this is because, when the stylist or barber uses the products, they form the topic of conversation, which helps to reinforce the benefits for using them and prompts recommendation and advice to the client. If a product display allows the customer to see, and pick from, then the sale could be *closed*, even before the client returns to reception.

TOP TIP

This is why department stores situate their perfumery concessions beside the main entrances, or right beside access points such as escalators.

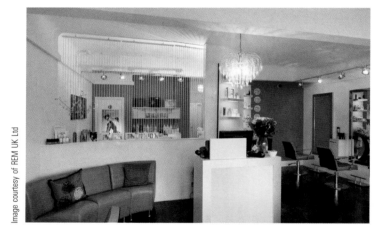

Image courtesy of REM UK Ltd

Remember products are not wallpaper! Remember that products are not decorations, bought by the salon to cheer up a dingy, dark corner; they have far more importance. Retail displays are an expensive investment for the salon, and stock waiting on the shelves to be sold is an expensive, added cost.

There are hidden benefits to the purposes of retailing (which you may not have thought about) and the promotional displays play an integral part in supporting the salon's image. If you think about it another way; the salon purchases particular ranges of products for use, and resale, that *mirror* the standards that it wants to be identified with (i.e. fits the image of the salon). Therefore, it provides the opportunity for clients to continue the salon service when they get home.

A typical in-salon promotion

In-salon display - The 'point-of-sale' promotion

Central 'island' units, open cabinet shelf displays, accessible products

'Shelftalkers' on the edge of shelves

Printed slips/cards fixed to/dangling from shelves; 'mobile' ones that bounce deliver best results

Special offers

Multi-buys, BOGOFs – buy one get one free, discounts

A good product promotion Remember: A good product promotion will:

◆ Have eye-catching displays – these are instantly informative – locate them where they'll be seen at reception or centrally in salon work areas.

◆ Be well organized/arranged – popular lines at eye level with price details – use 'price watch' stickers.

◆ Show special offers – first visit, loyalty, recommend-a-friend discounts and promotional 'tie-ins' with major local stores.

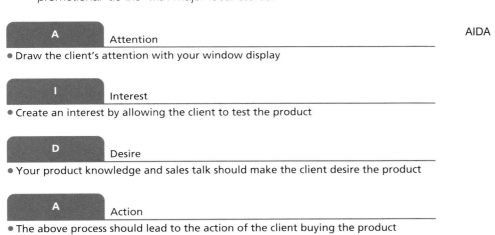

AIDA

A	Attention

● Draw the client's attention with your window display

I	Interest

● Create an interest by allowing the client to test the product

D	Desire

● Your product knowledge and sales talk should make the client desire the product

A	Action

● The above process should lead to the action of the client buying the product

Creating a salon display

Planning a display – who is it trying to attract?

The purpose of a salon display is to create customer interest by promoting the business in some way. Therefore, the main purpose of any display is to be eye-catching and attractive; it needs to make people stop and look, and that means that it has to stand out by stimulating the potential customer. This could be in a number of ways. We know that different people have different needs and we have covered this as a sales strategy, earlier in this chapter.

What we haven't really covered is the fact that different people respond to a variety of differing stimuli. Putting this in a simpler way, we could say that some people respond to promotions because of pricing, whereas others may want to be seen with the latest gadgetry; regardless of price, i.e. it's the coolest thing!

So from a display point of view, the theme can be almost anything because it works on the premise that someone, somewhere will 'buy into' that concept.

However, typical promotional strategies aim at a mass target audience and tend to reflect the following key aspects:

- ◆ Promotional offers and pricing incentives.
- ◆ Well known branding, use of logos, etc.
- ◆ Strong, bold colour themes or colour coordination.
- ◆ Key positioning and placement.

A more targeted approach will try to divide the mass target audience into *niche* groups, or in *marketing speak* segmentation. Segmentation simply means breaking down the big group, into much smaller groups of consumers who have different interests.

To give you an example of segmentation look at the following pie chart:

Segmenting the market

Numbers of people buying fruit at the supermarket each week

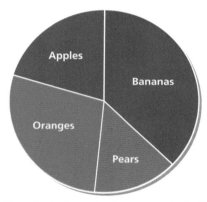

The chart above looks at people buying fruit each week. From this, we could say:

- ◆ Some people buy apples.
- ◆ Some buy pears.
- ◆ More people buy oranges.
- ◆ The largest group of people buy bananas.

We could also say that:

- ◆ Some people may be buying just one type of fruit.
- ◆ Other people could be buying two or more types of fruit.

Without going into the science and maths of statistics, the illustration tells us that some people are only interested in one thing whereas others may be interested in a number of things. Therefore, if you were selling pears, you would only be targeting your produce at a small segment of the total market.

Now with this in mind we can look at targeted promotions – i.e. attracting particular groups of people. A *niche* promotion may be attractive to only a small segment of the mass market because:

◆ It focuses on particular/specific needs.

◆ It causes emotional reactions – excitement, shock, humour, breath-taking, sympathy.

◆ It could be minimalistic, creative or artistic – working on the idea that less is more.

◆ It's exclusive – only available for a short while or to certain types/groups of people.

But even small, well planned, attractive promotions can be extremely successful and can produce very good returns and profit. Is the display to attract new customers or is it for existing clients? Will it be aimed at passers-by and be located in the salon window, or casually targeting people who are sat waiting in the reception?

Key note: *Knowing who your customers are* is the most important part of any potentially successful business plan, and good promotion and display should target the group of people that the business is trying to attract. This may seem like a simple formula for success, but even the big corporations get this one wrong.

Creating a display

The positioning of a display is vital if it is to have the most impact. Obviously, a well-designed window is the primary location for a display, particularly if it looks out onto a busy street. But the in-salon displays are equally important because they are trying to stimulate sales to the existing salon visitors. In many ways this is even better because this group of people will be around; looking at it for much longer. Therefore, there is a far greater chance of being able to *push* the promotion, particularly if everyone is well informed and asking clients if they have noticed it.

Creating the display – things to consider		
Focal point	◆ Where is it to be located? ◆ How will it catch people's eye? ◆ What is the main focus of the display?	◆ Colours ◆ Lighting ◆ Brand names ◆ Logos ◆ Prices/discounts ◆ Posters and show cards
Theming	◆ Is the promotion focused or linked to something?	◆ New products ◆ Current season ◆ Holidays

(Continued)

(*Continued*)

Creating the display – things to consider		
Schedule	◆ What is the duration of the promotion? ◆ What are the timescales involved for planning and preparation?	◆ Campaign plan ◆ Planograms ◆ Staff meetings
Constructing the display	◆ When is the best time to build it? ◆ Will you have to make the display or can the manufacturer provide it?	◆ Health and safety legislation ◆ Materials, tools and equipment ◆ Security of products ◆ Restocking, stock control
Sales support	◆ What training does the manufacturer or salon provide? ◆ What are the incentives?	◆ Product information ◆ Incentives, commissions ◆ Manufacturer's website
Customer support	◆ How do you inform the customer about the promotion?	◆ Discussion with customers ◆ Brochures, shade charts ◆ Leaflets ◆ Samples ◆ Website

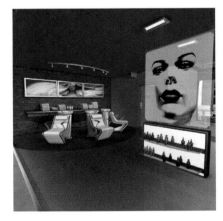

Maintaining and stocking the displays

Above all, any salon display must always be attractive and reflect the changes, or seasons, throughout the year. Therefore, they need to be changed regularly. For example, a typical promotion in summer might advertise UV hair protection, and alternatively a promotion nearer Christmas may reflect gift packs and presents.

With this in mind, the displays and the products must be checked and cleaned regularly, and in a busy salon, this will usually mean *daily*. A window display will need to be dusted, straightened and looked at from outside, just to make sure that it looks its best. The display from which products are being sold will also need to be dusted, perhaps wiped over and straightened up.

The salon display should address all the clients' needs too, it would look very 'half-hearted' if it only focused upon a small segment of the salon's clientele. It is not satisfactory to stock just a few items and expect clients to 'fit in' with the range you carry. Different ranges must be available for different client groups, i.e. fashion products for younger clients, classic styling and treatment ranges for general use, men's products for male clients and luxury products for those who can afford premium prices.

Consumer protection

Don't forget that all consumers are protected from illegal practices, misleading information, mis-selling tactics and defective products. Here is a list of legislation protecting our customers' rights.

Consumer Protection Act 1987 This Act follows European Union (EU) Directives to protect the customer from unsafe, defective services and products that do not reach safety standards. It also covers misleading price indications about goods or services available from a business. Dissatisfied clients may contact a number of organizations dealing with consumer protection for legal advice. If proven at fault the business may face legal action.

Consumer Safety Act 1978 This Act aims to reduce risk to consumers from potentially dangerous products.

Prices Act 1974 The Prices Act (1974) states that the price of products has to be displayed in order to prevent the buyer being misguided.

Trade Descriptions Act 1968 This Act prohibits the use of false descriptions of goods and services provided by a business. Products must be clearly labelled. When retailing, the information supplied both in written and verbal form must always be accurate. The supplier must not:

- Supply misleading information.
- Describe products falsely.
- Make false comparisons between past and present services.
- Offer products at what is said to be a 'reduced' price, unless they have previously been on sale at the full price quoted for a 28-day minimum.
- Make misleading price comparisons.

Resale Prices Acts 1964 and 1976 The Resale Prices Acts (1964 and 1976) tells us that the manufacturer can supply a recommended price (MRRP), but the seller is not obliged to sell at the recommended price.

Sale and Supply of Goods Act 1994 The Sale and Supply of Goods Act (1994) says that goods must be as described, of merchantable quality and fit for their intended purpose. The Act also covers the conditions under which customers can return goods.

Data Protection Act 1998 Through communication with your client it is necessary to ask clients a series of questions before the treatment/service can be finalized. Client details are recorded on the client record card. This information is confidential and should be stored in a secure area and should only be made available to persons to whom consent has been given.

Consumer Protection (Distance Selling) Regulations 2000 These Regulations are derived from a European Directive and cover the supply of goods/services made between suppliers acting in a commercial capacity and consumers. They are concerned with purchases made by telephone, fax, Internet, digital television and mail order, including catalogue shopping. Consumers must receive:

◆ Clear information on goods or services, including delivery arrangements and payment, suppliers' details and consumers' cancellation rights which should be made available in writing.

◆ The consumer also has a seven working days cool-off period where they may cancel their purchase.

Disability Discrimination Act 1995 Under the Disability Discrimination Act 1995, as a provider of goods, facilities and services your workplace has the duty to ensure that clients are not discriminated against on the grounds of disability. It is unlawful to use disability as a reason or justification to:

For more information. Go to CHAPTER 3 Reception – Trading Safely and Legally pp. 89–91.

◆ Refuse to provide a service.

◆ Provide a service to a lesser standard.

◆ Provide a service on worse terms.

◆ Fail to make reasonable adjustments to the way services are provided.

SUMMARY

As a final reflection on what you have covered in this chapter, you should now have a clearer picture of all the essential aspects for promoting and displaying products and services. In particular, you should now have a basic understanding of the key principles of:

1 Promoting a professional sales environment within the salon.

2 Introducing services and products to clients and being able to sell them based upon their features and benefits.

3 Maintaining and stocking retail and promotional displays.

4 Recognizing customer interest and being able to respond appropriately.

5 Creating promotional displays within the salon.

And collectively, how these principles will enable you to create effective, professional displays that will enhance the salon's image.

ASSESSMENT OF KNOWLEDGE AND UNDERSTANDING

Project

For this project you will need to gather information from a variety of sources.

For the following legislation find out how:

1 The Health and Safety at Work Act; and

2 The Data Protection Act,

affect the way that services can be provided to clients.

In your project pay particular attention to the aspects that would have impact on a business and the implications if this legislation were not considered.

Revision questions

A selection of different types of questions to check your sales and promotion knowledge.

Q1	Selling opportunities occur when the features and _____ of products are explained.	Fill in the blank
Q2	Business develops without promotion or advertising.	True or false
Q3	Which of the following are types of in-salon promotion?	Multi selection

Radio advertising	☐ 1
Hairdressing competitions	☐ 2
Hairdressing demonstrations	☐ 3
Point of sale material	☐ 4
Reception displays	☐ 5
Merchandising	☐ 6

Q4	PR is a term which refers to professional media handling.	True or false
Q5	What is the most cost-effective way of selling services to clients?	Multi choice

External demonstrations	O a
Internal promotions	O b
Client consultation and advice	O c
Point of sale material	O d

Q6	Merchandising is a retailing strategy.	True or false
Q7	Which of the following are laws protecting consumer purchases?	Multi selection

The Consumer Protection Act	☐ 1
COSHH	☐ 2
Trade Descriptions Act	☐ 3
RIDDOR	☐ 4
The Prices Act	☐ 5
The Data Protection Act	☐ 6

Q8	The vendor must ensure that goods they sell are of _____ quality.	Fill in the blank
Q9	When handling complaints avoid which of the following?	Multi choice

Maintaining eye contact with the client	O a
A discussion in a quieter area of the salon	O b
Telling the manager about the event	O c
Folding your arms and being defensive	O d

Q10	A prospective client forms their first impressions of salon staff in less than ten seconds.	True or false

5 Health and safety

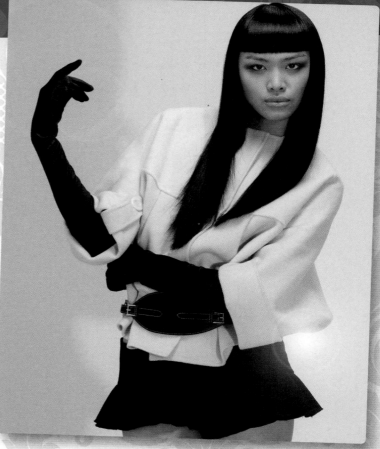

LEARNING OBJECTIVES

- Be able to identify any potential hazards within your salon

- Be able to reduce the risks to health and safety within your salon

- Know how to take action to eliminate potential hazards

- Know who you should report health and safety issues to, in situations that are beyond your normal work remit

KEY TERMS

absorption

accelerator

accident book

acute

allergy

antiseptics

autoclave

backwash

lightener

corrosive

COSHH

detergent

disinfectant

Electricity at Work
    Regulations (1989)

evacuation procedures

HASAWA

hazard

Health and Safety
    (First Aid)
    Regulation (1981)

Health and Safety
    at work Act (1974)

henna

hood dryers

hydrogen peroxide

immersed

Lightening Products

Manual Handling Operations
    Regulations (1992)

manufacturer's instructions

permanent colour/tint

personal protective
    equipment (PPE)

Personal Protective
    Equipment at Work
    Regulations (1992)

Provision and Use of Work
    Equipment Regulations
    (1998) (PUWER)

public liability insurance

RIDDOR

risk assessment

sharps

sharps box

steamer

sterile

sterilization

ultraviolet radiation

Unit topic

Follow health and safety practice in the salon.

INTRODUCTION

Stylists play a role in keeping themselves, their colleagues, clients and others safe at work, confidently managing hazards and assessing risk. Health and safety information may be given as verbal training or learners may be required to read and follow health and safety policies and procedures. It is important that this information is understood and followed, not only to maintain a safe environment, but also to protect the rights and responsibilities of both the employer and the employee.

This topic has links to many of the technical units in Level 2. Health and safety is for everyone working in the salon and it is important that you understand the responsibility that you have for yourself and others, such as colleagues and clients. The scope of the Health and Safety at Work Act 1974 covers 'all persons' whether employers, employees or self-employed. Among other things, the Act seeks to secure the health, safety and welfare of people while they work and protect other people against risks to health and safety arising from the activity of people at work.

The ways in which you and your work colleagues go about daily duties have a direct effect upon the general health and safety of everyone within the workplace. Poor hygiene or preparation, not thinking of others or clearing up properly and not noticing potential hazards can all have a disastrous impact on the safety and well-being of others. At Level 2, you should be able to identify hazards and reduce any risks within the salon/barber's shop.

This chapter looks at the types of hazard that you might find in your work and how you should go about eliminating them during you daily routine duties.

Health and safety at work

PRACTICAL SKILLS

Learn the skills required for working safely in the salon

Learn as much as possible about the job you are doing and how to do it safely

Make sure you listen to any instructions you are given

Make sure you follow written instructions and procedures

Learn how to report accidents and incidents verbally

Learn how to report accidents and incidents on forms

UNDERPINNING KNOWLEDGE

Finding the information you need

Reading health and safety documents

Listening to instructions and training

Following written instructions and procedures

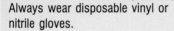

BEST PRACTICE

Always wear disposable vinyl or nitrile gloves.

ACTIVITY

If you would like to find out more about hairdressing health and safety or the relevant legislation covered in the (HASAWA) Health and Safety at Work Act (1974) go online to the Health and Safety Executive HSE website http://www.hse.gov.uk/hairdressing/index.htm to find out more about things associated with hairdressing and barbering.

HEALTH & SAFETY

Health and safety information is everywhere and you will have posters and signs where you are explaining a range of things, like how to find and use fire equipment, where you should go if there were an emergency and even how to handle the products safely.

HEALTH & SAFETY

Up to 70 per cent of hairdressers suffer from work-related skin damage such as dermatitis at some point during their career – most cases are preventable.

Hazards and risk

Almost anything may be a **hazard**, but may or may not become a **risk**. For example:

◆ A trailing electric cable from a blow-dryer is a hazard if it is trailing across a busy route through the salon, as there is a high risk of someone tripping over it, but if it lies along a wall or next to the workstation, out of the way, the risk is much less.

◆ **Hydrogen peroxide** can be a chemical hazard and may present a high risk. However, if it is kept in a properly designed **COSHH** cabinet and handled by properly trained and equipped people, the risk is much less than if it is left about for anyone to use.

◆ A failed light bulb is a hazard. If it is just one of many in a room it presents very little risk, but if it is the only light on a stairwell, it is a very high risk. Changing the bulb may be a high risk, if it is up high, or if the power has been left on, or a low risk if it is in a table lamp which has been unplugged.

ACTIVITY

Health and safety checklist: Tick the skills you feel confident about now and review again later on.

Skills for working safely in the salon	Now	Later
Finding the information you need		
Reading health and safety documents		
Listening to instructions and training		
Following written instructions and procedures		
Reporting accidents and incidents verbally		
Reporting accidents and incidents on forms		

Acting responsibly

You share a responsibility with your work colleagues for the safety of all the people within the salon (clients, visitors and staff) so you need to be aware of the types of hazards that could exist. Knowing what to do and who to approach in different situations is particularly important. In a team situation, where a group of people work together, you need to know who can and does what.

Let's look at a few examples:

You see this happening	What needs to be done?	Who needs to be involved?
Hair clippings have been left on the floor after the stylist has finished cutting.	The clippings need to be swept up immediately.	You can do this yourself.
A client waiting in reception spills their drink on the shelf.	The spillage needs to be mopped up immediately with a cloth or a towel.	You can do this yourself, but you might need to let the receptionist know.
A box of stock is delivered and is left on the reception desk.	The stock needs to be checked against the delivery note and removed from the reception desk.	The receptionist needs to be told, but you could put it down behind the desk so that it is out of the way.
A stylist 'nicks' their finger while cutting their client's hair.	The stylist needs a plaster from the first aid box.	You could get them a plaster, but remember, an incident has occurred and it needs to be recorded.
A client faints while they are having their hair shampooed.	You need to call for assistance immediately.	The first-aider needs to be called immediately and the incident needs to be recorded in the accident book.

These things could happen at any time and you may be the only one that sees it, so your swift action may make all the difference. Quite simply, you have two things to consider:

◆ You see what happens and are able to deal with the situation yourself.

◆ You see what happens and know that you need to inform someone else.

You may be keen to help out but you need to know what it is that you are dealing with.

Look at it this way; you see that the floor is wet from a spillage:

◆ What liquid has been spilt on the floor?

◆ How do you know if this is something that you can deal with?

◆ What action do you need to take about it?

In this type of situation you need to be able to assess the problem. Do you know what the liquid is? If you do, you may be able to mop it up yourself. Is it a simple spillage like water, or something more hazardous like a chemical?

If it is water, then you know that this is something that you could do yourself, but if it is a chemical it has to be handled in a certain way with the right protective equipment. The action you now take depends on the hazard. You will be either clearing the spillage yourself, or blocking the area, as a temporary measure, say with a chair, so that others are made aware of the hazard too, while you inform someone else.

Being able to spot things is one thing but having the ability to assess the potential risk and the common sense to see how this could impact on other people is quite another. Think again about the following in terms of **identifying hazards** and **reducing the risk**.

Reducing risks to health and safety

People are exposed to all kinds of hazardous substances at work. These can include chemicals that people make or work with directly, and also dust, fumes and bacteria which can be present in the workplace. Exposure can happen by breathing them in, contact with the skin, splashing them into the eyes or swallowing them. If exposure is not prevented or properly controlled, it can cause serious illness, including cancer, asthma, dermatitis and sometimes even death.

Health and safety law requires employers to control the risk of workers or trainees to the exposure of hazards in the workplace and this is done through the process of **risk assessment**. Risk assessment can cover all sorts of areas, but there are known risks that apply in our industry, that provide specific areas for scrutiny.

The health and safety laws are designed to protect you, the clients and your colleagues. So your personal health and safety and safe methods of work are absolutely essential. The table below explains how you can help reduce some common risks to health and safety within the working environment for everyone's benefit.

Hazard	Risk	Action to take
Spilled water or hair clippings left on floor.	◆ Someone may slip. ◆ This affects everyone. ◆ If not dealt with immediately, there is a **high** level of this risk occurring.	◆ Mop the water up, or sweep the area and put the clippings in the bin.
Equipment or furniture left in a corridor or blocking an emergency exit.	◆ People may not be able to get out in an emergency. ◆ This affects everyone. ◆ There is a **high** level of this risk occurring if people needed to get out.	◆ Speak to a senior member of staff immediately, see if this is something that you could help to remove.

(Continued)

(Continued)

Hazard	Risk	Action to take
Broken, worn or faulty equipment.	◆ May cause electric shock. ◆ This affects the next person who uses it. ◆ If not dealt with immediately, there is a **high** level of this risk occurring.	◆ If it is a small, portable item, remove it from the work area. Put a note on the equipment and tell a senior member of staff immediately.
Chemicals leaking through their packaging in a storage area.	◆ Could be toxic or **corrosive** to anyone touching it without protective wear. ◆ This affects everyone. ◆ If not dealt with immediately, there is a **high** level of this risk occurring.	◆ Do you know what the chemical is, e.g. perm solution, hydrogen peroxide? Put on your vinyl/nitrile gloves and mop it up. ◆ If you don't know what the chemical is, don't touch it. Tell a senior member of staff immediately.
A damaged, loose floor tile.	◆ Someone may trip. ◆ This affects everyone. ◆ If not dealt with immediately, there is a **high** level of this risk occurring.	◆ Remove any broken or loose, flapping pieces and tape down the edges. ◆ Tell a senior member of staff immediately.
Heavy boxes of stock left after delivery in the reception.	◆ Someone may injure themselves trying to move it. ◆ This affects anyone trying to move it. ◆ If someone tries to move it, there is a **high** level of this risk occurring.	◆ Tell a senior member of staff immediately. These items will need to be moved with help or assistance, e.g. a trolley or sack truck, or possibly more than one person.

The **Health and Safety at Work Act 1974** is the main, overarching legislation, made by parliament, relating to business premises, under which all other regulations exist. Although the Act contains many individual regulations the responsibility for maintaining these falls upon you and your employer.

TOP TIP

Always read the manufacturer's instructions before using their equipment or products.

Employer/employee duties

Employers have a legal duty under the **HASAWA** to ensure that:

◆ The premises are safe to work within.

◆ All equipment and salon systems are safe to use.

◆ Employees have access to **personal protective equipment**.

◆ Relevant health and safety information is provided for everyone.

◆ Adequate training is provided and that health and safety systems are appropriately reviewed and updated.

Employees have a duty to:

◆ Follow appropriate systems of work laid down for their safety.

◆ Make proper use of equipment provided for their safety.

◆ Cooperate with their employer on health and safety matters.

- Inform the employer if they identify hazardous activities/situations.

- Take care to ensure that their activities do not put others at risk.

Both the employer(s) and employees have a joint responsibility for:

- The safety of the working environment.

- Taking reasonable care of themselves or others who may be affected by their working practices and must support their employer in fulfilling their obligations in the compliance of current health and safety requirements.

HEALTH & SAFETY

Employers must display the health and safety law poster; the poster must be displayed where your employees can easily read it. The poster outlines British health and safety laws and includes a straightforward list that tells employees what they and their employers need to do.

Salon health and safety policy

Policies are written to ensure that hairdressers and salon employers work together to a common set of standards. Many policies and codes of practice are written and required by law.

All salons require their employees to follow basic rules, such as following **manufacturer's instructions**. If these simple rules are neglected, a treatment will go wrong at some point and the salon's reputation will be lost forever.

There are three levels of health and safety good practice that must be followed:

- **The law** – This is created through Acts of Parliament and enforced and regulated by HSE and local authorities.

- **Codes of practice** – This is professional practice accepted by an industrial sector, created by an industry representative organization, or recognized body.

- **Employer's policies** – These are introduced by the employer at a *local* level as an accepted method for carrying out work (within the employer's organization).

If an employer has more than five employees then they must provide a written health and safety policy for their staff to follow. But even smaller businesses will have their own rules and procedures for how things must be done. By law, a salon has to display:

- Health and safety information poster – showing employees what they must know.

- Fire **evacuation procedures** – explaining the organization's fire evacuation procedures.

Managing health and safety

In addition to the things that must be displayed by law, an employer will, as part of maintaining the business policy:

- Make assessments of all work processes to identify risks and hazards to health.

- Provide regular and appropriate training as and when necessary, to keep staff updated on safety issues.

- Maintain records for accidents or injuries where first aid treatment was necessary.

- Monitor and evaluate the health and safety arrangements on a regular basis.

◆ Provide written health and safety information to the staff.

◆ Update their own knowledge to keep abreast of health and safety developments.

◆ Provide employers' liability insurance cover for employees while at work.

Public liability insurance This is different to employers' liability insurance. It covers an employer for claims made against the salon by members of the public or other businesses, but not for claims by employees. While **public liability insurance** is generally voluntary, employers' liability insurance is compulsory.

An example of when public liability insurance is necessary If you can imagine that; a client reacts to a **permanent colour** service and is harmed in some way. The client will then take legal action against the salon and the potential costs could financially ruin someone for life, if they have not got sufficient insurance cover.

Health and safety legal regulations affecting you in the salon

The Health and Safety at Work Act 1974 is the legal framework covering a range of regulations that affects; the ways in which health and safety is managed within the workplace and the ways in which you must work.

Under HASAWA the employer must provide:

◆ **Premises** – that are safe to work in.

◆ **Systems** – that are safe to operate and use.

◆ **Safe storage** – for things that people need and use within their work.

◆ **Routes for access and egress** – that are safe at all times when the premises are in use.

◆ **Training** – for people so they know how to work safely.

The following text looks at individual aspects of the law in reference to specific, relevant regulations.

COSHH – Control of Substances Hazardous to Health Regulations (2002)

The COSHH Regulations has specific requirements for the storage, handling and use of the everyday products used in a hairdressing salon. This law requires the employer to control the exposure of workers to hazardous substances within the workplace. Many of the things we use in hairdressing are harmless, but there are some things that could be hazardous if they are not used or handled in the correct way.

TOP TIP

What is employers' liability insurance?

Employers are responsible for the health and safety of their employees while they are at work. If employees are injured at work, they may be entitled to claim compensation. The Employers' Liability (Compulsory Insurance) Act 1969 ensures that there is a minimum level of insurance cover against any such claims.

In general, COSHH covers many substances that are hazardous to health and these substances can take many forms:

- chemicals
- products containing chemicals
- fumes
- dusts
- vapours

So in order for the employer to calculate the risks associated with exposing people to these products, the employer carries out a COSHH risk assessment. The employer will not know what is in the products or which substances provide a potential risk, so part of the assessment would include obtaining the Safety Data Sheets for each product from its manufacturer. These data sheets cover all the chemical ingredients and provide an overall hazard rating.

COSHH and hairdressing related issues

The specific aspects of COSHH that affect hairdressers

- Frequent contact with water and shampoo can irritate the skin, leading to **dermatitis**.
- Some hairdressing and cleaning products can cause **dermatitis** and **skin allergies**.
- Some dusty products like *persulphates* (found in powder **lightening products**) and **henna** (a vegetable dye compound made from ground Lawsonia leaves) can cause **asthma**.
- Some hairsprays can make **asthma** worse.

The simple things you can do to prevent dermatitis and asthma

- Keep the workplace well ventilated.
- Wear disposable non-latex gloves for shampooing, colouring and lightening.
- Dry your hands thoroughly after washing with a soft towel.
- Moisturize your hands as often as possible.
- Change your gloves between clients.
- Check your skin regularly for early signs of skin problems.

HEALTH & SAFETY

The main signs and symptoms of dermatitis are:
- Dryness
- Redness
- Itching
- Flaking/Scaling
- Cracking/Blistering
- Pain

What is dermatitis?

Dermatitis is not 'catching' – it cannot be passed from one person to another. It can develop at any time, or not at all – everyone is different.

There are two types of contact dermatitis: **irritant contact dermatitis** and **allergic contact dermatitis**.

◆ **Irritant contact dermatitis** – This can flare up after a few contacts with strong chemicals like lightening products. More commonly, it develops gradually through frequent wet working or working with milder chemicals like shampoo.

◆ **Allergic contact dermatitis** – This can develop quickly after only a few contacts with substances like shampoos or colours. Sometimes it can take months or even years for the **allergy** to develop. Once you are allergic, you are allergic for life and this could happen at any time, even if you have had no problems previously in your career.

With allergic contact dermatitis, the things you can become allergic to at work might well also be things you use at home – like your shampoo or your household cleaners.

So if you become allergic to something in the salon it could well affect all aspects of your life.

BEST PRACTICE

Health and safety laws are being continually reviewed and updated. Make sure you are aware of the latest information and look at the health and safety posters within your salon.

ACTIVITY

Tick who is responsible for the following:

Duties	Who is responsible?	
	Employee	**Employer**
Drawing up a health and safety policy statement.		
Not interfering with or misusing anything provided for health, safety and welfare.		
Ensuring articles and substances are moved, stored and used safely.		
Assessing the risks to your health and safety.		
Co-operating with employer on health and safety.		
Setting up emergency procedures.		
Providing health surveillance as appropriate.		
Taking reasonable care of own health and safety as well as that of work colleagues.		
Providing adequate first-aid facilities.		
Using equipment correctly in accordance with training or instructions.		
Discussing or reporting any health and safety problems in the workplace.		

HEALTH & SAFETY

Employers have a responsibility to ensure the health, safety and welfare of the people within the workplace. All people at work have a duty and responsibility not to harm themselves or others through the work they do.

Personal Protective Equipment at Work Regulations (1992)

The **Personal Protective Equipment at Work Regulations (1992)** states that:

Every employer shall ensure that suitable personal protective equipment is provided to his employees who may be exposed to a risk to their health or safety while at work except where and to the extent that such risk has been adequately controlled by other means which are equally or more effective.

Quite simply, you are required to wear the appropriate protective equipment during chemical treatments. Protective non-latex disposable gloves and aprons are the normal requirement for avoiding contact with chemicals.

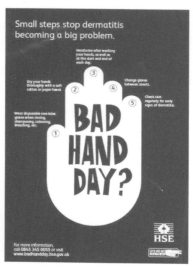

Contains public sector information published by the Health and Safety Executive and licensed under the Open Government Licence v1.0

HEALTH & SAFETY

Messages for hairdressers from the Health and Safety Executive (HSE):
- Up to 70 per cent of hairdressers suffer some form of skin damage.
- Dermatitis is caused by contact with chemicals present in hairdressing products and prolonged contact with water.
- Dermatitis causes personal suffering.
- Dermatitis is unsightly and unpleasant.
- Dermatitis is bad for your career as well as your skin.
- You can prevent it – look after your hands by wearing non-latex gloves, drying hands thoroughly and using moisturizers regularly; also take regular 'glove breaks', don't spend all day washing hair, alternate duties (e.g. cut hair instead) and change gloves between clients.

Manual Handling Operations Regulations (1992)

Lifting and moving things around the workplace can cause Musculoskeletal Disorders (MSD). This term relates to any injury, damage, or disorder of the joints or other tissues in the upper/lower limbs or the back. So correct manual handling is essential in order to prevent injury or longer term disorders. The **Manual Handling Operations Regulations (1992)** require employers to take preventative steps to avoid these injuries from occurring.

Obviously, there are far greater risks to MSD in other industries such as construction, warehousing, even the care sector, and for these areas, there is a lot of mechanical support and machinery for moving things about. This doesn't mean that hairdressing and barbering are exempt; there will always be occasions when people need to move things; e.g. deliveries, furniture, stock control would be typical, everyday situations.

HEALTH & SAFETY

The HSE advice about lifting: If manual lifting is the only option then there are a number of things that can be done to reduce the risk, including:
- Making the load smaller or lighter and easier to lift.
- Breaking up large consignments into more manageable loads.
- Modifying the workstation to reduce carrying distances, twisting movements, or the lifting of things from floor level or from above shoulder height.
- Improving the environment – e.g. better lighting, flooring or air temperature can sometimes make manual handling easier and safer.
- Ensuring the person doing the lifting has been trained to lift as safely as possible.

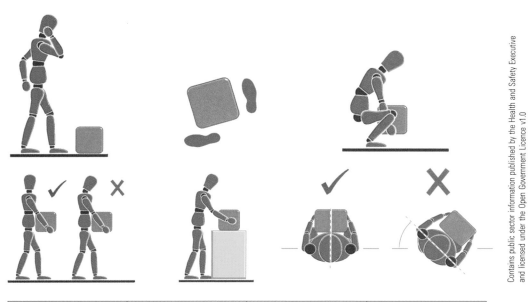

Contains public sector information published by the Health and Safety Executive and licensed under the Open Government Licence v1.0

| 1. Think about the lift. Where is the load going to? Do you need help? Is there a handling aid e.g.sack-truck available? | 2. Adopt a stable position with your feet apart and one leg slightly forward to help with balance. | 3. Bend the knees keeping the back straight. Lean slightly forward over the load to get a good grip. | 4. Lift smoothly and avoid twisting the back or leaning sideways. |

Electricity at Work Regulations 1989

The **Electricity at Work Regulations 1989** gives us safety information about electricity in the workplace. Electricity can kill. Although deaths from electric shocks are very rare in hairdressing salons, even a non-fatal shock can cause severe and permanent injury. An electric shock from faulty or damaged electrical equipment may lead to a fall (e.g. down a stairwell).

Those using electricity may not be the only ones at risk. Poor electrical installations and faulty electrical appliances can lead to fires which can also result in death or injury to others.

The law requires employers to maintain electrical equipment in a safe condition and to have them checked at reasonable intervals by a competent person.

Portable appliance testing – PAT testing

Portable appliance testing (PAT) is the term used to describe the examination of electrical appliances and equipment to ensure they are safe to use. Items are tested periodically and a written record shows: an itemized list of the equipment, date of test and who tested it.

Most electrical safety defects can be found by visual examination, but some types of defect can only be found by testing. There isn't any set timescale for re-testing of portable electrical equipment. But, the law requires that the testing should reflect the amount of usage that the appliance gets. For example, a kettle in the staff room will get more use than a pair of crimping irons, so the re-testing of the kettle should reflect this.

Get into the habit of looking for loose cables and plugs on tongs, straighteners and hair dryers before plugging them in for use. If you think that a piece of electrical equipment is faulty or damaged, tell your supervisor immediately. Make sure that no one else tries to use it.

RIDDOR – Reporting of Injuries, Diseases and Dangerous Occurrences Regulations (1995)

Under the **RIDDOR** employers must provide an online report (available through the HSE website) for any serious accidents or work related diseases. In the event of the accident causing death, then the employer must telephone the Incident Contact Centre directly.

Contact dermatitis is listed as an occupational hazard for hairdressing and barbering and is therefore a notifiable occupational health hazard under RIDDOR.

Types of reportable injury/disease	
◆ Deaths ◆ Major injuries	◆ In cases of death or major injuries, employers must notify the enforcing authority immediately.
◆ Over-seven-day injuries	◆ Cases where employees are absent from work for more than seven days – must be notified within ten days of the incident occurring using the appropriate online form.
◆ Occupational health hazard (e.g. dermatitis)	◆ Cases of disease should be reported (using the online form) as soon as a doctor notifies the employer that their employee suffers from a reportable work-related disease.

Reportable major injuries

Reportable major injuries are
◆ Fracture, other than to fingers, thumbs and toes.
◆ Amputation.
◆ Dislocation of the shoulder, hip, knee or spine.
◆ Loss of sight (temporary or permanent).
◆ Chemical or hot metal burn to the eye or any penetrating injury to the eye.
◆ Injury resulting from an electric shock or electrical burn leading to unconsciousness, or requiring resuscitation or admittance to hospital for more than 24 hours.
◆ Any other injury leading to hypothermia, heat-induced illness or unconsciousness, or requiring resuscitation or admittance to hospital for more than 24 hours.
◆ Unconsciousness caused by asphyxia or exposure to a harmful substance or biological agent.
◆ **Acute** illness requiring medical treatment, or loss of consciousness arising from **absorption** of any substance by inhalation, ingestion or through the skin.
◆ Acute illness requiring medical treatment where there is reason to believe that this resulted from exposure to a biological agent or its toxins or infected material.

Provision and Use of Work Equipment Regulations 1998

The **Provision and Use of Work Equipment Regulations 1998 (PUWER)** require risks to people's health and safety, from equipment that they use at work, to be prevented or controlled. This refers to any equipment which is used by an employee at work, to be safe to use. For example, electrical items such as clippers, hand dryers, **hood dryers, steamers** and colour **accelerators**. Similarly, if employees provide their own equipment, it is also covered by PUWER and the employer will need to make sure it complies with the law.

PUWER requires that equipment provided for use at work is:

◆ Suitable for the intended use.

◆ Safe for use, maintained in a safe condition and, in certain circumstances, inspected to ensure this remains the case.

◆ Used only by people who have received adequate information, instruction and training; and accompanied by suitable safety measures, e.g. protective devices, markings, warnings.

Preventing infection and diseases

Avoiding cross-infestation and cross-infection

Part of maintaining a safe place to work is preventing infection from spreading. Poor hygiene is usually the invisible enemy of any professional business. Infection and disease can occur by two methods within the salon/barber's shop:

◆ Externally – where visitors to the salon bring in disease which then cross-infects other people within the salon.

◆ Internally – which will also cross-infect other people but is the result of poor hygiene and cleanliness by people working in the salon.

A warm, humid salon can offer a perfect home for disease-carrying bacteria. If they can find food in the form of dust and dirt, they may reproduce rapidly. Good ventilation, however, provides a circulating air current that will help to prevent their growth. This is why it is important to keep the salon clean, dry and well aired at all times. This includes clothing, work areas, tools and all equipment.

Good ventilation is part of the solution, but in a professional salon, this is not enough, so the salon's staff use other methods to keep their tools and equipment safe. How would you feel if on a visit to the salon you saw that a stylist had used a brush on someone else's hair and was now about to use the same brush on yours?

Sterilizing tools and equipment

There are three main methods for sterilizing tools and equipment:

◆ Heat – e.g. using an **autoclave**.

◆ Radiation – e.g. using a UV cabinet.

◆ Chemical – e.g. using Barbicide®.

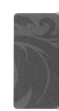

Heat The autoclave provides a very efficient way of sterilizing using heat. It is particularly good for metal tools (although the high temperatures are not suitable for plastics such as brushes and combs). Items placed in the autoclave take around 20 minutes to sterilize. (Check with manufacturers' instructions for variations.)

Autoclave

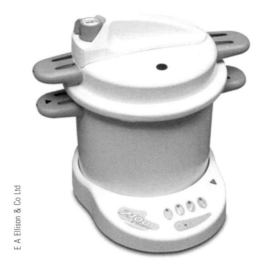

E A Ellison & Co Ltd

UV Cabinet An ultraviolet (UV) cabinet is used in a salon to sterilize tools such as brushes, combs and metal items such as scissors or clipper blades. The cabinet uses **ultraviolet radiation** which sterilizes the items, preventing bacterial growth. The UV light is emitted from a single source and it will only sterilize on the side which is exposed to the UV rays. In order to sterilize tools and equipment more effectively, the items should be washed and dried beforehand and then turned after 15–20 minutes in the cabinet to expose both sides of the items to the UV rays.

UV cabinet

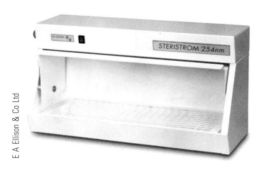

E A Ellison & Co Ltd

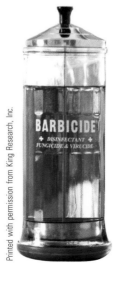

Printed with permission from King Research, Inc.

Chemicals Chemicals are the most widely used method for disinfecting tools and equipment. In hairdressing and barbering Barbicide® is the most commonly used product for hygienically preparing combs for use in between clients, and overnight. Barbicide® is contained in a jar, it is a transparent, blue coloured liquid that appears darker in colour when stronger and more concentrated, and lighter when weaker in strength. The product is prepared by dissolving with water (following the manufacturer's instructions) and will provide an effective **disinfectant** for a certain amount of time. Over time it will lose its ability to keep tools hygienically clean, so the liquid must be replaced with new Barbicide®.

Chemical	Products and equipment
◆ **Sterilization** will kill 100 per cent of germs and bacteria.	◆ Autoclaves will sterilize metal tools and equipment using heat.
◆ **Disinfectants** will kill up to 95 per cent of germs and bacteria.	◆ Barbicide® will disinfect combs when left in for one–to–two hours.
◆ **Antiseptics** will kill up to 50–60 per cent of germs and bacteria.	◆ Found in cleaning sprays will help to keep work surfaces hygienic.

TOP TIP

It is worth noting that Barbicide® is not a true sterilizing agent, it is a disinfectant.

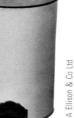

HEALTH & SAFETY

Sterilization means that it will kill 100 per cent of germs and bacteria, whereas disinfectants have a 95 per cent ability to kill germs.

Disposal of waste items

General salon waste Every day items of salon waste should be placed in a 'closed top' bin fitted with a suitably resistant polyethylene bin liner. When the bin is full, the liner can be sealed using a wire tie and placed ready for refuse collection. If for any reason the bin liner punctures, put the damaged liner and waste inside a second bin liner. Wash out the inside of the bin itself with hot water and **detergent**.

Being environmentally aware requires us to be more responsible in the ways in which we dispose of our waste items. Take care to separate the following from hair clippings and other general salon waste:

◆ Place paper, cardboard, cans, glass bottles and plastic waste into recycling.

◆ Rinse chemical hairdressing products down the drain with copious amounts of running water.

Disposal of sharp items Used razor blades and similar items (**sharps**) should be placed into a safe container (**sharps box**). When the container is full, it can be disposed of safely. This type of salon waste should be kept away from general salon waste as your local authority may provide special arrangements.

Preparing work areas

It is important you develop an awareness of health and safety risks and that you are always aware of any risks in any situation. Quite simply, a tidy salon is easier to clean so get into the habit of clearing up your work as you go.

Floors These should be kept clean at all times. This means that they will need regular mopping, sweeping or vacuuming. When working areas are damp-mopped during normal working hours, make sure that adequate warning signs are provided close to the wet areas.

Salon chairs and work surfaces Professional salon equipment is made of material that is easily cleaned. It should be washed regularly with hot water and detergent. After they have dried, the seats can be made hygienically clean by wiping over with an anti-bacterial spray.

All surfaces within the salon, including the reception, staff and stock preparation areas, should be washed down at least once each day. Most salons now use easily maintained wipe-clean surfaces, usually some form of plastic laminate. They can be cleaned with

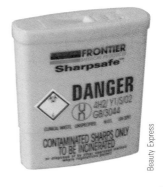

E A Ellison & Co Ltd

Beauty Express

TOP TIP

Contact your local council office's environmental health department for more information.

hot water and detergent, and after the surfaces are dry they can be wiped over with anti-bacterial spray which will not smear.

Mirrors Glass mirrors should be cleaned every morning before clients arrive. Never try to style a client's hair while they sit in front of a murky, dusty or smeary mirror. Glass surfaces should be cleaned and polished using either hot water and detergent or a spirit-based lotion that evaporates quickly without smearing.

Towels and gowns Each client must have a fresh, clean towel and gown. These should be washed on a suitable (washing machine) wash programme at 60°C to remove any hair products, dirt or staining and to prevent the spread of infection by killing any bacteria. Fabric conditioners should be used to make sure the towels feel soft and smell fresh.

Styling tools Most pieces of salon equipment, such as combs, brushes and curlers, are made from plastics. These materials are relatively easy to keep hygienically safe, if they are used and cleaned properly.

Combs should be washed daily. When not in use they should be **immersed** into Barbicide® solution. When they are needed they can be rinsed and dried and are then ready for use. If any styling tools are accidentally dropped on the floor, do not use them until they have been cleaned properly. Don't put contaminated items onto work surfaces as they could spread infection and disease.

Handle non-plastic items, such as scissors and clipper blades, with care. When they need cleaning, they can be placed into a UV cabinet or autoclave. Remember, these items are made of special steels and should not be put into disinfectants like Barbicide®. These fluids contain chemicals that will corrode and damage the precision-made cutting surfaces.

Electric clippers get a lot of use throughout the day and will require checks for cleanliness, safety and efficiency before every use. Hair gets trapped between the blades, which reduces their cutting performance, and the constant vibration may loosen the cutting edges forcing the bottom blade out of alignment. This is potentially very dangerous as the upper blade may extend beyond the lower one and cut someone the next time that they are used.

Posture for you and the client

Good posture is a must: as hair professionals, we have to stand for long periods. Correct posture by standing properly will help prevent backache, and, in the long term, back problems and other conditions like varicose veins.

Always stand with the back straight, your feet apart and your weight evenly distributed on both legs. Do not stand with all your weight on one of your legs and your pelvis tilted. If you stand like this for long periods you will get backache and possibly more serious problems with your lower back; you will also increase the risk of developing varicose veins.

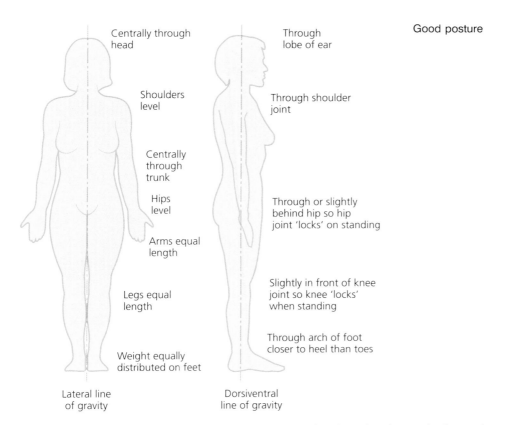

Good posture

Centrally through head

Shoulders level

Centrally through trunk

Hips level

Arms equal length

Legs equal length

Weight equally distributed on feet

Lateral line of gravity

Through lobe of ear

Through shoulder joint

Through or slightly behind hip so hip joint 'locks' on standing

Slightly in front of knee joint so knee 'locks' when standing

Through arch of foot closer to heel than toes

Dorsiventral line of gravity

Remember your client's posture too. The ways that people relax often has a detrimental effect on their personal health too. Clients need to sit in the styling seat properly; if their backs are not 'flat' against the back of the chair, then they can get lower back pain, and this can be even worse as if they have their legs crossed. Your client needs to sit with their feet on the foot rest, as if they are sat cross-legged it will alter their seated posture and the position of their head; which will make your job even harder.

Professional salon chairs have some form of height adjustment and this is particularly important for you. You need to make sure that you have a good all round access to your client, and this means above them as well as each side. During styling, you will need to be cutting over the top of their head, or winding perming curlers or placing rollers. Whatever the service, you need to make sure that you can reach without stretching or lifting your arms above horizontal, as this will cause you to tire quickly and make your shoulders ache. It is normal during a service to need to make adjustments to the seat height at least once in order to reach properly. Therefore, make sure that the chair controls/height pump is easily accessible to you and not under the client's feet.

Remember to be careful and considerate at the basin too. Most modern **backwashes** have a tilt mechanism that allows the basin to be gently inclined or 'dipped' down, as this design feature accommodates for people's different heights. If a client sits back and the basin hasn't been adjusted properly for them, then a lot of their weight can be carried by their neck. This is a dangerous sitting position, as the client may 'pass-out' because of affecting/reducing the blood supply to the brain, or get a neck injury from supporting the weight of their body.

Get your working position ready

Always remember to get organized before the client arrives; making a point of getting the record card to give you an indication of the things that you will need. Make sure

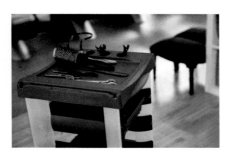

that you have everything to hand, get the equipment you need and check that it is ready for use. Look at the electrical equipment, checking the leads and the plug. If there are any signs of damage or looseness of cables, ravel up the lead, remove it from the work area and mark it for later maintenance.

Get all the rollers, rods, curlers, combs, brushes, pins, clips and grips that you need. Get a trolley ready, as when you start you don't want to be running around trying to find things that you have forgotten. Once you start on your client, you need to be staying with them for the duration. It looks unprofessional to be 'popping' off to get something else and it will be you who will feel *'the fool'* if you keep disappearing. Remember, professionals are always well organized and ready to provide a service.

Personal conduct

Remember, the salon or barber's shop is a professional environment and you are on show. The way that you react to others and the respect that you show will be apparent not only by what you say, but how you say it. Treat others with a mutual professional respect – regardless of what you think or would like to say.

Always conduct your work in a safe, professional manner; never fool around, as this could put others at risk by your actions or negligence.

- ◆ Do not rush or run around the salon.

- ◆ Follow the manufacturer's instructions always.

- ◆ Prepare and clean salon equipment before the clients arrive.

- ◆ Always use equipment for its intended purpose.

- ◆ Help prepare equipment or work areas for others.

- ◆ Keep the backwash area and basins clean and uncluttered.

- ◆ Replenish stock before it runs out.

- ◆ Behave professionally and sensibly.

- ◆ Do not endanger others in their work.

- ◆ Be responsible, spot hazards and take appropriate action to avoid injury to others.

- ◆ Remember that the client deserves respect, politeness and courtesy at all times.

Fire Action Notice

Fire Action

ON DISCOVERING A FIRE:

1. **Sound** the alarm
2. **Dial** 999 to call the fire brigade
3. **Tackle** the fire with the appliances provided if it is safe to do so

ON HEARING THE ALARM:

1. Leave the building by the nearest exit
2. Close all the doors behind you
3. Report to the assembly point in the car park

Do not take risks
Do not stop to collect belongings
Do not return to the building until authorized to do so
Do not use the lifts

Emergency procedures

HEALTH &
SAFETY

In particular, hairdressers may need to deal with electrical fires.

It is essential that all hairdressers can protect themselves and others from danger. To do this, they must be able to locate, read and understand health and safety signs in their working environment. For example, in the event of fire, delayed action could result in death. Each workplace is different and hairdressers should know exactly where the locations of the fire extinguishers are in their salon and how to use them correctly, without hesitation. To do this they will need to interpret the symbols, colours and written instructions on fire extinguishers and safety notices.

Fire safety

Under the *Fire Precautions Act 1971* – all premises must have a fire risk assessment and if five or more people work on the premises, the assessment must be in writing.

There must also be a fire and evacuation procedure for the business and there should be a fire drill at least once a year. The evacuation route must be kept clear of obstructions at all times and during working hours the fire doors must remain unlocked. The escape route must be easily identifiable, with clearly visible signs. In buildings with fire certificates, emergency lighting must be installed. These lighting systems automatically illuminate the escape route in the event of a power failure and are operated by an independent battery back-up.

In the event of fire breaking out the main consideration is to get everybody out:

◆ Raising the alarm – Anyone discovering a fire must immediately raise the alarm by operating the nearest alarm. Staff and customers must be warned, and the premises must be evacuated.

◆ On hearing the alarm – All people must exit the building via the designated fire exits and proceed to the designated assembly point. Doors should be closed on exiting the building and designated staff may assist the less able.

◆ Assembly point(s) – Everyone must remain at the assembly point, away from danger while awaiting further instruction.

◆ Call the fire brigade – After exiting the building, call the emergency services. Dial 999, ask the operator for the fire service, and give your telephone/mobile number. Wait for the transfer to the fire service and then tell them your name and the address of the premises that are on fire. Do this even if you believe that someone else has already phoned.

Fire extinguishers

◆ Fire extinguisher labels and wall signs give you important safety information.

◆ The wall sign tells you what you should and should not use the fire extinguisher for.

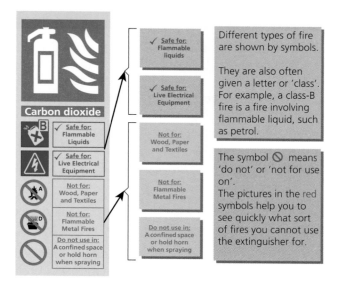

Different types of fire are shown by symbols.

They are also often given a letter or 'class'. For example, a class-B fire is a fire involving flammable liquid, such as petrol.

The symbol ⊘ means 'do not' or 'not for use on'. The pictures in the red symbols help you to see quickly what sort of fires you cannot use the extinguisher for.

◆ The extinguisher label gives information about what type of extinguisher it is, how to use it and when to use it.

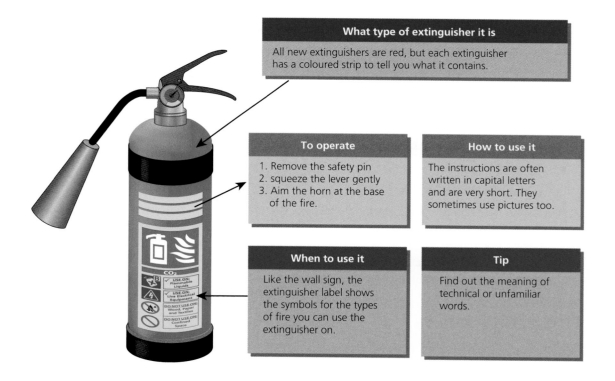

What type of extinguisher it is

All new extinguishers are red, but each extinguisher has a coloured strip to tell you what it contains.

To operate

1. Remove the safety pin
2. squeeze the lever gently
3. Aim the horn at the base of the fire.

How to use it

The instructions are often written in capital letters and are very short. They sometimes use pictures too.

When to use it

Like the wall sign, the extinguisher label shows the symbols for the types of fire you can use the extinguisher on.

Tip

Find out the meaning of technical or unfamiliar words.

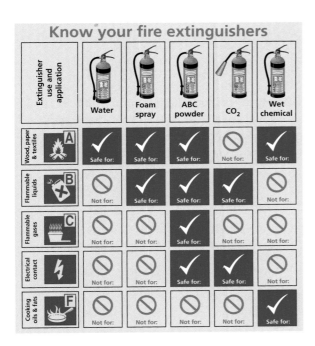

Know your fire extinguishers

Water filled Identified by: **Red label** Suitable for: **Type A fires** – Wood, Paper and Textiles		
Foam filled Identified by: **Clear label** Suitable for: **Type A and B fires** – Wood, Paper, Textiles and Flammable liquids		
ABC Dry Powder filled Identified by: **Blue label** Suitable for: **Type A, B, C and Electrical fires** – Wood, Paper, Textiles and Flammable liquids/ gases or Electrical		
CO₂ filled Identified by: **Black label** Suitable for: **Type B and Electrical fires** – Flammable liquids and electrical		
Wet Chemical filled Identified by: **Yellow label** Suitable for: **Type A and F fires** – Wood, Paper, Textiles and Cooking oils and fats		

Fire safety training

It is essential for staff to know the following fire procedures:

- Fire prevention.
- Raising the alarm.
- Evacuation during a fire.
- Assembly points following evacuation.

Training must be given to new members of staff during their induction period and this training must be regularly updated for all staff. Fire drills must be held at regular intervals.

Fire blankets

A fire blanket is made of a fire resistant material. They are useful for smothering a small fire such as wrapping around a person whose clothing is burning. They will put out flames by starving the fire of oxygen, so they should not be flapped about as this will fan the flames; they should be in close contact with the fire in order to work.

Sand

A small bucket of sand is useful for soaking up liquids which could be a source for a fire, such as cooking oil or fats.

First aid

Accidents The Health and Safety (First Aid) Regulations 1981 tell us that the employer is responsible for ensuring that employees receive immediate attention if they are taken ill or are injured at work. Accidents and illness can happen at any time and first aid can save lives and prevent minor injuries from becoming major ones.

An employer is expected to have:

◆ Completed a first-aid needs assessment.

◆ Ensured that there is either an appointed person to take charge of first-aid arrangements, or there are appropriate numbers of suitably trained first-aiders.

◆ Ensured there are adequate facilities and a suitably stocked first-aid box.

◆ Provided information about the first-aid arrangements.

What is a first-aider?

A first-aider is someone who has undertaken training and has a qualification that HSE approves. This means that they must hold a valid certificate of competence in either:

◆ First-aid at work, issued by a training organization approved by HSE; or

◆ Emergency first-aid at work, issued by a training organization approved by HSE or a recognized Awarding Body of Ofqual/Scottish Qualifications Authority.

What is an appointed person?

If an employer's first-aid needs assessment indicates that a first-aider is unnecessary, the minimum requirement is to appoint a person to take charge of first-aid arrangements. The roles of this appointed person include looking after the first-aid equipment and facilities and calling the ambulance services when required. They can also provide emergency cover, within their abilities, where a first-aider is absent due to unforeseen circumstances.

First-aid box – What should a first-aid box in the workplace contain?

There is no set requirement so the contents will depend upon the employer's assessment of first-aid needs. As a guide, where work activities involve low hazards, such as hairdressing and barbering, a minimum stock of first-aid items might be:

◆ A leaflet giving general guidance on first-aid (e.g. HSE's leaflet: *Basic advice on first-aid at work*).

◆ 20 individually wrapped **sterile** plasters (assorted sizes), appropriate to the type of work (you can provide hypoallergenic plasters, if necessary).

- Two sterile eye pads.

- Four individually wrapped triangular bandages, preferably sterile.

- Six safety pins.

- Two large, individually wrapped, sterile, unmedicated wound dressings.

- Six medium-sized, individually wrapped, sterile, unmedicated wound dressings.

- Antiseptic cream.

- Medical wipes.

- Sterile water.

- Cotton wool.

- A pair of disposable non-latex gloves.

Recording incidents – What information should be recorded?

As an indication of good practice, an employer will provide the appointed person with a book in which to record incidents that require some attention. The incident record book is not the same as the *statutory* **accident book**, although these two systems could be combined into one recording system. This would help the employer in assessing needs, as a combined system will highlight recurring patterns and help with monitoring the first aid needs.

Useful information to record includes:

- The date, time and place of the incident.

- The name and job of the injured or ill person.

- Details of the injury/illness and what first-aid was given.

- Details about what happened to the person immediately afterwards (e.g. went back to work, went home, went to hospital).

- The name and signature of the first-aider or person dealing with the incident.

Incident report/salon accident

The first-aider or staff member responsible for handling the incident at the time should fill in the report. As a measure of good practice, the record should be completed as soon as possible after the incident.

Accident record

ACCIDENT RECORD

1 About the person who had the accident

Name_____

Address_____

_____Postcode _____

Occupation_____

2 About you, the person filling in this record

If you did not have the accident, write your address and occupation.

Name_____

Address_____

_____Postcode _____

Occupation_____

3 About the accident. Continue on the back of this form if you need to

Say when it happened.　　　　Date_____ /_____ /_____ Time_____

Say where it happened. State which room or place._____

_____

Say how the accident happened. Give the cause if you can._____

_____

_____

_____

_____

If the person who had the accident suffered an injury, say what it was._____

_____

Please sign and date the record.

Signature_____ Date_____ /_____ /_____

4 For the employer only

Complete this box if the accident is reportable under the Reporting of Injuries, Diseases and Dangerous Occurrences Regulations 1995 (RIDDOR)

How was it reported?_____

Date reported_____ /_____ /_____Signature_____

SUMMARY

As a final reflection on what you have covered in this chapter, you should now have a clearer picture of all the essential aspects for working safely within the salon. In particular, you should now have a basic understanding of the key principles of:

1   The laws affecting you and your health and safety at work.

2   How working with good posture prevents injury and fatigue.

3   Identifying hazards and risks to health and safety and being able to take appropriate action in order to reduce the impact of those risks to other people within the salon.

4   Preventing the spread of infection and diseases to other people within the salon.

5   Maintaining the salon's fixtures, fittings and equipment, and hygienically preparing the tools and equipment ready for use.

6   How to respond in the event of an emergency.

And collectively, how these principles will enable you to work confidently, but safely at all times.

ASSESSMENT OF KNOWLEDGE AND UNDERSTANDING

Project

For this project you will need to use the information from the salon's risk assessments and the COSHH salon information booklet.

For each of the following:

1   One cold wave perming lotion.

2   One tube of permanent colour.

3   One powder lightening product.

find out:

1   The chemical composition.

2   How it is used safely.

3   How it should be stored safely.

4   How it is handled.

5   Any other special conditions that apply to it.

Revision questions

A selection of different types of questions to check your health and safety knowledge. (Also see Appendix 2.)

Q1	A _____ is something with potential to cause harm.	Fill in the blank
Q2	Risk assessment is a process of evaluation to develop safe working practices.	True or false
Q3	Which of the following are environmental hazards (select all that apply)?	Multi selection

Boxes of stock left in the reception area	☐ 1
Stock upon shelves in the store room	☐ 2
Wet or slippery floors	☐ 3
Shampoo backwash positions	☐ 4
Salon workstations	☐ 5
Trailing flexes from electrical equipment	☐ 6

Q4   First-aid boxes should contain paracetamol tablets.   True or false

Q5   Which of the following regulations relates to the safe handling of chemicals?   Multi choice

PPE	O a
RIDDOR	O b
COSHH	O c
OSRPA	O d

Q6   All salons must have a written health and safety policy.   True or false

Q7   Which of the following records must a salon keep up to date by law?   Multi selection

Telephone book	☐ 1
Accident book	☐ 2
Appointment book	☐ 3
Electrical equipment annual test records	☐ 4
Health and safety at work checklist	☐ 5
Fire drill records	☐ 6

Q8   The _____ regulations require employers to provide adequate equipment and facilities in case of an accident occurring.   Fill in the blank

Q9   What colour is the label on a dry powder filled fire extinguisher?   Multi choice

Red	O a
Cream	O b
Black	O c
Blue	O d

Q10   A dry powder filled fire extinguisher can be used on all classes of fire.   True or false

6 Consultation

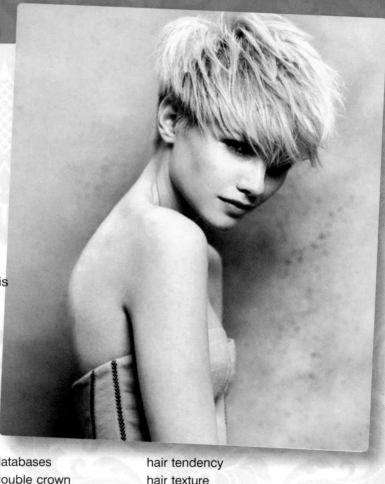

LEARNING OBJECTIVES

◆ Be able to identify what clients want

◆ Be able to analyse the hair, skin, and scalp

◆ Be able to advise clients and agree services and products

◆ Understand the salon's services, products and prices

◆ Know how to perform hair, skin and scalp analysis

◆ Know how to perform tests prior to services and treatments

◆ Be able to record information relating to the client's consultation

KEY TERMS

acids
acid conditioner
acid mantle
acne
alopecia
alopecia areata
alopecia totalis
alpha keratin
ammonium
   thioglycolate
anagen
apocrine glands
arrector pili muscle
ash/ashen

astringent
baldness
capillary
catagen
chemical reaction
cicatricial alopecia
clip-on hair extensions
colour test
contagious
contra-indication
cortex
cowlick
customer care/client
   care

databases
double crown
elasticity test
epidermis
eumelanin
facial shapes
follicle
folliculitis
fragilitas crinium
furunculosis
germinal matrix
hair bulb
hair growth patterns
hair shaft

hair tendency
hair texture
head lice
herpes simplex
impetigo
incompatibility test
inflammation
influencing factors
long facial shape
male pattern alopecia
Male Pattern Baldness
   (MPB)
medulla
melanin

monilethrix
nape whorl
organic
oval facial shape
oxidation
papilla
parasite
pediculosis capitis
pH
pH levels
pheomelanin
pigments

porosity
quasi-permanent (colour)
referral (colour)
ringworm
round facial shape
scabies
sebaceous cyst
sebaceous gland
seborrhea
sebum
semi-permanent colours

shape, proportion and balance
skin test
split ends
square facial shape
straightening
strand test
subcutaneous fatty layer
subcutaneous tissue
surface conditioners
sycosis
telogen

tensile strength test
terminal hair
tinea capitis
tone
toner/toning
traction alopecia
triangular facial shape
trichorrhexis nodosa
trichosiderin
virus
wefts
widow's peak

Unit topic

Client consultation for hair services.

INTRODUCTION

We want clients to be satisfied with what we do and we want the services and treatments that we perform to turn out as we expected.

This is a simple formula where everyone wins. If our clients are satisfied with what we do for them then they will be happy to return. Therefore, client consultation is the first and most important service within the salon or barber's shop. When done accurately and professionally, it enables you to do all the other creative things well. If done badly, or missed out completely, then a disaster is guaranteed to occur.

How can we do what our clients want unless we have a clear plan that will achieve the desired result? We cannot, so we must allow enough time to, find out if there are any reasons that will stop us from achieving the final effect.

Consultation always takes place at the beginning of the client's booked appointment. During this time, the client will sit at the styling unit while we:

◆ Talk to them about the things that they would like.

◆ Use visual aids to help decide on a suitable course of action.

◆ Look at their hair and scalp to see if there are any service contra-indications or style limiting factors.

◆ Carry out any necessary tests.

◆ Tell them how their desired result can be achieved.

◆ Provide advice about how they can manage their own hair.

◆ Recommend the right products, tools and equipment that they need to use.

◆ Agree with them about an appropriate course of action.

◆ Create or update the client's record for future reference.

Communicating with your clients

PRACTICAL SKILLS

Learn to speak clearly in the correct manner using the right tone of voice

Learn how to avoid confusion when speaking to your client

Learn to listen to your client's requests

Learn to respond willingly to your client's requests

Learn how to be polite and considerate to your client

Learn how to anticipate your client's needs

Learn how to behave in a professional manner

UNDERPINNING KNOWLEDGE

Speaking clearly and correctly

Explaining in simple language without using 'jargon' or hairdressing technical language

Listening carefully to your client

Responding in an appropriate manner

Being discrete and confidential at all times

Showing positive body language

Professional conduct and communication

Hairdressing and barbering are personal services that depend upon the relationships that we create with our clients. If the relationship is established upon a professional *footing,* then there will be mutual respect, good customer service and an on going, client loyalty. This client loyalty is essential if we are going to get returning customers, gain new clients and build up a good reputation for the future.

When you communicate with your clients, you will need to:

◆ Speak clearly in the correct manner using the right tone of voice.

◆ Avoid confusion with clients, don't use 'jargon' or hairdressing technical language.

◆ Listen and respond appropriately and willingly to their requests.

◆ Be polite, friendly and considerate; try to anticipate your client's needs.

◆ Be discrete and confidential; especially when handling information about the salon's clients.

◆ Show a positive body language.

◆ Behave like a professional.

Speaking clearly

It is important that you are clear with what you say and not misunderstood by the client. During consultation, you need to take the lead; you will be asking the client questions and trying to find enough information to make the right decisions about the course of action you need to take. You will be finding out what the client wants and then looking for anything that will affect or limit your client's expectations. You will be getting the client to agree with the various possible options and then carry out the task.

You must always treat your clients with the utmost respect and that means that you need to be polite. People can detect our innermost feelings by the way that we speak. If you use a harsh or off hand tone, your client will know and you will have lost your chance to create a good impression. You always need to create a good first impression, as this is the basic rule for professional communication and customer loyalty in any business area.

TOP TIP

You don't get a second chance to create a good first impression.

Asking questions to find out what the client wants

◆ You need to ask the right sorts of questions to get the information that you need.

◆ You need to ask the questions in a way that your client understands.

◆ You need to listen to your client's answers and act on what you hear.

The main types of question are open questions and closed questions.

Open questions These are good ways to start conversations as they prompt the client to describe things or give more in-depth information. These types of questions start with 'who', 'what', 'when', 'why', 'where' and 'how'.

Examples:

◆ How do you normally style your hair?

◆ What colours do you prefer?

◆ When is it easier for you to come in to the salon?

Closed questions These are useful for a quick 'yes' or 'no' response and are a quick way to cover different aspects of conversation.

Examples:

◆ Have you had permanent colour on your hair before?

◆ Would you like me to do it for you in your lunch hour today?

Are you against moving the parting from the centre?

By using a combination of both open and closed questions, you will be able to:

◆ Identify any limitations or **influencing factors** that affect your styling options, e.g. '*So, you have tried to wear your hair on that side before and it kept falling back?*'

◆ Help your client by making sure that they understand what you are saying/doing, e.g. '*OK, would you like me to style it that way today, so that you can see how it looks?*'

◆ Allow your client enough time to consider your suggestions without them feeling rushed or pressurized, e.g. '*There are a variety of options that you could have. For instance, if we …*'

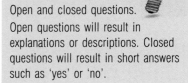

◆ Prompt your client to give you as much information as possible, e.g. 'I can see how we can improve this colour, but what was the hair like before you applied this yesterday?'

◆ Listen, hear and understand the client's requests and needs, e.g. 'Yes, Mrs Tyler, I can now see why you would prefer curl, rather than wave'.

◆ Confirm what you hear by summarizing each point before moving on to the next aspect of the consultation, e.g. 'OK, so you would like to go shorter; but do you mean, still beneath the shoulders or actually cut above; just beneath your ears?'

Avoid confusing the client

Another simple mistake made by many hairdressers is using the wrong words with clients. To us, as hairdressers these words actually mean something.

For example, think about these questions:

◆ 'OK, Mrs Clark, you would like it layered all over?'

◆ 'Will you be having a toner after you have your hair lightened?'

◆ 'I think that with a natural base 5 you wouldn't want to darken the effect by more than two levels. What do you think?'

You might think that all of these questions are normal, everyday situations.

Well they are, but you need to remember that your knowledge of the terms; layering, **toners**, bases and levels, is not necessarily the same as your client's understanding of the same words. Just because you see a faint nod of the head or hear the word 'yes,' it does not mean that your client has understood.

We tend to use jargon every day in our working lives with our fellow work colleagues and that is fine. In fact, using special technical terms is a shorter way of explaining specific things with the people we work with.

Example:

◆ 'Can you pass me the 20 vol peroxide and a colouring bowl please?'

◆ 'Who's seen the grade 4s and the neck brush?'

As you can see, to any client who had been sitting in the salon at the time that these requests were made, it would not mean a thing. However, to the stylists it was something that was urgently needed, so that they could do their job.

You must avoid confusing your clients, as if you do not you could be heading for a disaster! If you believe that the client understands, just because they give a very short acknowledgement and that's only because they didn't want to be embarrassed (by seeming ignorant or stupid), then look out when they really feel upset with what you have done!

Sometimes it is hard to judge whether we are *taking people along* with what we are saying and that is why we stop at different points to confirm what we hear and to make sure that both parties understand.

Confirm and reach an agreement at different points during the consultation Don't wait to the end of your examination and discussion to try and weigh up all the things that you have found, get into the habit of confirming and

summarizing what you think you understand, or want to recommend to the client, at many different points during your consultation. This way you will be making sure that you have covered all the necessary information and also making sure that the client has a clear understanding of what is going to happen during the service.

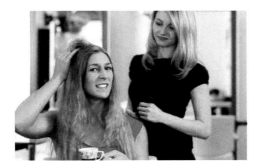

Only after you have both agreed a course of action can you take things to the next stage. When you have covered everything in your consultation, you need to summarize the points back to the client.

You could say:

'So, Mrs Jack, we've talked about the time and cost of your cut and blow-dry. Let me just run through what we are going to do. We will take 4cm off the length of the hair and introduce some layers to give it more texture and movement, then I'll finish it off with a smooth blow-dry look and apply some of that serum I was telling you about. Is that correct?'

Whatever your summary is, you must ask a question at the end of it. Unless you have the client's expressed wishes before you start then you have not given them the opportunity to accept or decline your plans. In other words, they have not agreed the services or products and they have every right to dispute this at the end!

Special situations

Some services also need additional preparation or special conditions before they can be carried out. For example, your salon may do hairpieces for hair-up work; some salons may do added **clip-on hair extensions**; others may offer the complete bonded extensions systems. In any of these cases, it would be unlikely that all the necessary materials to do all of these services will be in stock. Therefore, you need to be able to tell your client exactly when those items will be available, the differences, benefits and pitfalls, how long it will take, how they will look after them and how much it will cost.

You will also need to check to see if a deposit is needed. Often in situations where there is a large investment of salon time or stylist's time, then other preparations need to be arranged in advance and it would be normal practice to take a deposit.

There are other special situations too. You may wish to offer a colouring service to a new client, but you know that you will have to conduct your skin test first. Therefore, you will need to tell the client what they can expect and what you need to know should there be any adverse, contra-indications. All this needs to be pointed out, well in advance.

Listen and respond to clients appropriately

There are all sorts of ways to provide and demonstrate good customer service and one of those ways is the way in which we respond to the requests of others.

BEST PRACTICE

You must finish your consultation as a series of questions.

'So you would like it more like this?'

'You only want me to trim the overall length?'

'So, have I got this right …?'

This way you will be looking for confirmation and have a total agreement before you start.

Every client is different and therefore needs treating on an individual basis; each one has specific hair needs that only apply to them. True, many of those clients may come in for a similar look or colour, but when hairdressers start treating them as *all the same*, then things will go wrong and the professional link is broken.

Listening (as well as talking) is an essential skill for hairdressers, and knowing when to **stop talking and start listening** is the only way that you will be able to satisfy your client's expectations. You cannot respond appropriately to your client unless you have understood their particular needs.

So give time for your clients to answer your questions, listen to what they say and then base your reply on what you have heard.

Look at these two examples:

◆ *'I can see that your colour has faded quite a lot Mrs Ford, do you wash it a lot or go swimming frequently?'*

◆ *'I can see that your colour has faded quite a lot Mrs Ford. Do you wash it quite a lot? Do you go swimming frequently?'*

Two statements containing the same words, but one sentence rushes through to try to ask two different questions, while the other has two different sentences. *If the client answers 'yes' to the first question above, what is she admitting to?* Is it that she washes it a lot, or that she goes swimming a lot? The response 'yes' in this situation will have a very big impact, depending on what she means.

If you now think about the same situation but in a scenario where this client has come back to complain, one response will indicate that the client could be at fault; the other will indicate that the stylist who did the colour could have made a mistake!

Look for your client's visual responses
Your client's facial expressions will reflect their mood and how they are feeling. Therefore, you need to be able to understand these expressions and react to them appropriately. A confused client is one thing, but an angry one is quite another.

An angry client needs to be handled carefully and sensitively. A client who is 'bright red' in the face with narrowed eyes is quite daunting for any staff member to handle. Nevertheless, usually once the client has had a chance to put their grievances over, then their fierce expression relaxes.

For that reason, a client with a complaint should be given:

◆ Time

◆ Attention

◆ Patience (and above all)

◆ Courtesy

From the salon's point of view, it would be unrealistic to think that we can satisfy all of the clients, all of the time. In business it just doesn't work like that (well not all of the time), as unexpected things will happen, or sometimes clients have to wait. Generally speaking, the typical situations when clients feel unhappy or are angry about something are usually, easily resolved.

If you have kept a client waiting through no real fault of your own, simply say. *'I'm sorry for keeping you waiting; can I take you through now so we can start your consultation?'*

If a client arrives at the salon and appears to be angry, lead them to a quieter part of the salon so that they can be allowed to make their point without the embarrassment of 'causing a fuss' in front of other people. Always avoid being drawn into an angry exchange. Let your client state their feelings and make their point, as long as you do not interrupt them you will find that their tone of voice will soon change.

An angry outburst is a natural and human response to frustration and stress, and like a *boiling kettle* when the switch turns off, the turbulence and steam soon subsides. Do not make things worse by trying to argue or shout back, you will make things worse. You will find that in 99 cases out of 100 a simple; *'I'm sorry you feel that way'* will be enough to defuse the situation and allow some progress to be made.

Confusion is the real weakness in client consultation and you need to make sure that both you and the client have the *same* understandings. If you find that your particular line of questioning is not producing any answers that you can go forwards with, then you will need to revise your questions until you both have some commonality. Do not forget; a client who lacks confidence is unlikely to tell you that they do not understand something. Put yourself in their position, how many times have you misunderstood something, but felt unable to tackle it at the time that you should have? People never want to feel embarrassed in front of someone else, so you have to watch for other signs that say: *'I do not understand'*.

Recognizing and reading different facial expressions is something that improves with experience. You need to make sure that you look for your client's facial expression and react quickly to what you see. When you see hesitation, go back over what you have said or, even better, try to put your point across, or question, in another way. A client who misunderstands a point that you are making during consultation, may later turn into an angry one after the service has been provided.

Be polite, friendly and considerate

Customers by definition are paying for their services and good customer service will ensure that the customer is satisfied with the results. There is one common element that features in all good services and that essential component is simply, politeness.

Being polite and friendly is a prerequisite in any personal service industry, in other words it is *the expected* part, a sort of professional code of conduct. It is the way in which we communicate and is judged by the tone of our voice and the manner in which we speak. We want clients to recommend our services to other friends and colleagues; that is how business will grow. Having a polite and friendly manner with clients is demonstrated in many ways, simply by using words that show gratitude and thought:

Examples:

◆ *'Please come this way and I will show you to the basin'.*

◆ *'Thank you for waiting, so how may I help you?'*

◆ *'May I get you something to drink, perhaps a coffee or do you prefer tea?'*

On the other hand being considerate means that we make sure that our clients are comfortable and that we give them time to describe their ideas and consider our advice. Many people will bring pictures from magazines or the Internet, which will give an impression of what they have in mind. But often the client feels embarrassed to take it out of their handbag when they get to the salon, so why not ask. *'Is there anything that you have seen or brought with you?'*

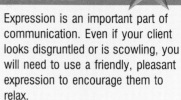

BEST PRACTICE

Expression is an important part of communication. Even if your client looks disgruntled or is scowling, you will need to use a friendly, pleasant expression to encourage them to relax.

TOP TIP

Do not use technical terms as clients will not understand you.

Guide your client through the consultation process Take control of the situation; it is essential that you guide the client throughout the service. Your professionalism is immediately evident when the client realizes that you are going to conduct the consultation. The client sums everything up (rightly or wrongly) in a few moments and you will not be able to satisfy the client fully unless you are in charge of this situation. You will have to *take your client's hand* and guide them through the whole process in order to exceed their expectations.

Big no nos – The negative exchange

◆ *Do not rush clients into making swift decisions*: you need to take them with you every step along the way. If they do feel rushed or that you are 'pushy', you will be *putting them off* from the start. That is a difficult position to be in, as you will be creating a tension during the service that would be uncomfortable for anyone.

◆ *Do not push clients into the Consultation Cul-de-sac*: by the manner of saying; '*You can only do that, or this,*' or '*I would not choose that because …*' This type of negative discussion is going nowhere. Pressurizing clients by minimizing their options is very unprofessional and clearly shows to your clients that you have not considered them at all.

Be discrete and confidential

Discretion is the safeguard to the professional code of practice. Do not forget – It is not just how we say things that matters; politeness and courtesy is one thing but what we say has an even bigger impact.

You can offend your clients very easily – even when they are not in the salon! How on earth does that work then? How can you offend people when they are not even in the salon?

Gossip is the main reason for losing customers, not poor hairdressing skills. Your clients will give you a second chance to get things right. Particularly if you have tried out something new and it has not worked. True, your client may not be very happy; but at least they will tell you and that gives you a second chance to get it right. On the other hand, if you show that you are indiscrete, by '*bad mouthing*' somebody, you will run the risk of that person finding out!

In a world that can spread rumours at the *speed of light* through social networking, texting and blogs, bad news travels fast and gossip travels even faster. The bad news is that, *once the jack is out of the box you can't get it back in*. It will always find its target and the target will find out the source. Never be drawn into a conversation in work, or college, or when out socializing about clients and their life events.

Hairdressing and barbering are professional personal services and that means that the clients rely upon our professional discretion to remain loyal to them and in return, they will continue to provide us with an income. Break that bond and you lose the money. Moreover, it gets worse! If you have been indiscrete about someone, do you think that they will keep quiet about it? *Well would you?*

If your clients spread rumours about your lack of professionalism, then you might as well choose another career.

The things discussed or overheard about a client within a salon must remain there. It is not your business and not for you to repeat; even if you think you know *half of the story*.

TOP TIP

Being 'pushy' or trying to rush clients into making a decision or choice is very unprofessional and poor customer service.

TOP TIP

Trust is hard to earn. Gaining a customer's trust and loyalty takes time. Once you have earned this, the bond remains fragile, so handle with care.

BEST PRACTICE

During consultation with your client, take enough time to find out what they want.

It's not just what you could say about clients that could get you into trouble, it's what you write down (or forget to write down) too. The law protects your client's confidentiality.

Give positive body language

The most difficult aspect of a consultation with a client is recognizing and understanding the things that we see, not just what they have said. Non-verbal communication (or body language) is reading between the lines. Your ability to understand situations based upon what has *been* said or *not* said, is important. There will be times when your client will look in a certain way, or say something that makes you stop to think. When this happens, your ability to read the situation, i.e. your sensitivity in picking this up and responding appropriately, will have a huge impact on what happens next.

Maintaining positive body language Remember, your body language is the unspoken way of letting others know what you really mean and think!

When speaking to clients, try to maintain eye-to-eye contact; this lets them know that you are paying attention. Sometimes it is easier to speak to people with your eyes at the same level too, so perhaps sit next to them while you discuss their needs, rather than looking down on them. It can be quite intimidating for the client when your eye level is above theirs and especially if you are standing above them and you appear to be *talking down* to them.

Always smile while you are speaking. This puts the client at ease and makes them feel welcome. This is particularly helpful and comforting to them as they may be feeling shy, timid or unsure of themselves; it may even be their first visit to the salon and everything may be feeling very new or uncomfortable for them.

Distances between people can be unpleasant too The spaces that people naturally keep between them produces a private, proximity area that we feel comfortable with as long as others keep out. This area or zone is something that we are happy to share with others providing we know them well, such as a member of our family, a boyfriend or girlfriend.

Therefore, you should never move in too close to a client as this could be very off-putting or even threatening. Our *'comfort zone'*, i.e. the personal space all around our bodies is extremely private, when people move into this space uninvited, there is an immediate feeling to pull back sharply.

We express ourselves with body language through posture and gestures. Here is a list of some typical mannerisms:

1   Slouching instead of sitting properly always looks unprofessional.

2   Folded or crossed arms can often represent a closed mind or being defensive.

3   Talking with open palms pointing forwards showing someone that 'you have nothing to hide' indicates openness or honesty.

4   Scratching behind the ear or the back of the neck indicates uncertainty.

5   Inspecting fingernails can indicate boredom or vanity.

6   Talking with your hand in front of your mouth may make the listener think you lack confidence or that you are dishonest.

ACTIVITY

You can try this out for yourself with a colleague; try putting your hand up in front of their face about 30cm away, see how quickly they jerk back.

Behave like a professional

Always dress and behave professionally within the salon – you will not believe how much effect your appearance has on what your client thinks about you. When we meet someone for the first time, it is human nature to rush into making our first impression of what we see. This judgement, rightly or wrongly, is a lasting impression and in a professional setting, it has to be the right one. The client assumes your professionalism by:

◆ The way that you dress, in what you wear and how you wear it.

◆ Your appearance, i.e. your tidiness, cleanliness and your hair.

◆ The way you behave and relate to other members of staff.

This is why different jobs have different dress codes. Your salon will have its own dress code or uniform along with the expected standards of behaviour.

BEST PRACTICE

It is human psychology to make quick judgements about things that we see and people that we meet. We normally make our first impressions within ten seconds of meeting someone. Make sure that your client's first impression is a good one!

Visual aids

Pictures

A picture will show many more aspects of a hairstyle than trying to find the words to describe it. It is hard enough for a hairdresser to try to explain an effect, so what chance does a client have? Details such as mood, texture, finish and quality are all very difficult to put into words. The features that we can see in a picture will cut through technical jargon and create a focus for you and the client to discuss and make your decisions.

Pictures are an immensely important visual aid and another form of language that hairdressers understand very well. Many hairdressers are *visual* learners and they have a better understanding of **shape, proportion and balance**, which enables them to look at a two-dimensional picture and devise a plan of how they will carry it out on a 'real' three-dimensional head. As a stylist, you are trained in looking into pictures to see more than just an overall image. You see things like how volume is distributed, where hair needs to be shaped in a certain way and how colour can have an impact on an overall effect. However, you cannot expect the client to see these technical aspects too, so beware when pictures are used to express a feeling or a mood instead of a hairstyle. You need to make sure that you are looking at and seeing the same things within the image.

For the client, pictures provide:

◆ Features and aspects of a hairstyle such as colour, shape, texture – that they cannot put into words in any other way.

◆ A clear vision of what they are aiming for.

◆ A theme or mood that they would like to express.*

For the stylist they provide a clear plan that:

◆ Will start a discussion about suitability, lifestyle, manageability, contra-indications, etc.

◆ Enables the client to consider options and alternatives.

◆ Forms the basis for agreement.

◆ Provides a course of action for the service.

*Be warned – when your client uses a picture that expresses a mood or feeling, it may be the atmosphere that the picture creates and not the hairstyle.

Colour charts

Colour charts are extremely useful for hairdressers. We rely on them every day. However, they are not always the best visual aid for the client. To you the colour chart is a tabular system for organizing colours.

Either in:

◆ Rows or columns – that go from lighter through to darker shades.

◆ Groups – where colours sit together in *families* such as red **tones**, golden tones, **ashen tones**.

Colour charts are exciting and stimulating for the client but that is as far as it goes. Clients have very little ability for visualizing an effect on them, but that is why they rely upon your opinions and recommendations.

Remember colour charts tend to have very small samples of coloured **wefts** called swatches, and when they are together they can often mislead the client unless you spread the swatch out so that it shows more of its colour features.

So do not forget – there will be very little value in using charts unless you can help the client to see the:

◆ Amount of colour that you will applying to the hair.

◆ Position and placement of colours, i.e. one colour against another.

◆ Bright contrast or subtle harmony of the colour against their skin tone.

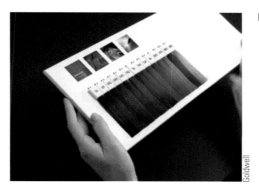

Using colour swatches on a shade chart

Goldwell

TOP TIP

Remember: A colour chart is useful to show tones and hues, but don't expect your client to be able to visualize an all over effect from a small sample.

Analyze the Hair, Skin and Scalp

In its simplest form, there are two basic parts to client consultation:

◆ You discuss your client's requirements.

◆ You see if there are any reasons why you cannot fulfil their requests.

In the earlier part of this chapter, you looked at the ways in which you communicate professionally with the client. Now you look for things that will influence what you do next.

The analysis of the client's hair takes the form of a visual inspection, so you will need to brush and separate the hair in several directions and in different areas over the head. This visual assessment will help you to find any hair features, contra-indications or aspects that will either limit or change the range of options available to your client.

You are looking for anything that could affect your styling options:

◆ **Hair texture**

◆ Hair length

◆ **Hair growth patterns**

◆ **Hair tendency**

◆ Hair density

◆ Hair condition

◆ Hair colour

◆ Hair or scalp problems

◆ **Facial shapes**

◆ Hair and skin tests

◆ Lifestyle.

Things to consider during consultation

Consultation – things to consider:	What does it mean, how will it affect the styling options?
Hair texture 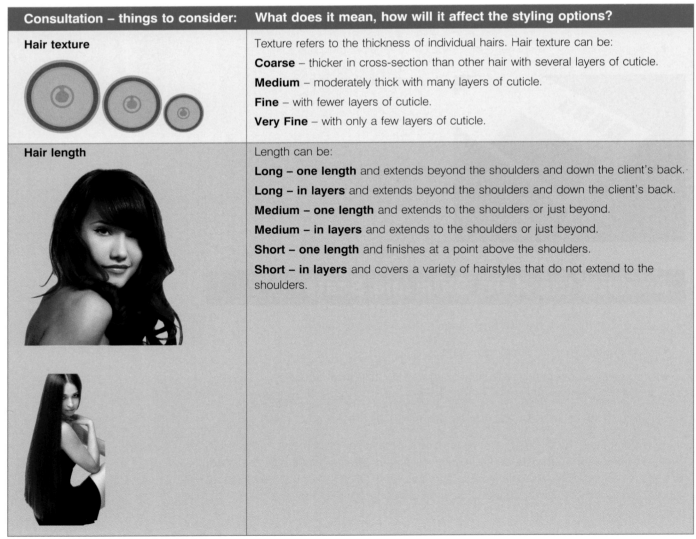	Texture refers to the thickness of individual hairs. Hair texture can be: **Coarse** – thicker in cross-section than other hair with several layers of cuticle. **Medium** – moderately thick with many layers of cuticle. **Fine** – with fewer layers of cuticle. **Very Fine** – with only a few layers of cuticle.
Hair length	Length can be: **Long – one length** and extends beyond the shoulders and down the client's back. **Long – in layers** and extends beyond the shoulders and down the client's back. **Medium – one length** and extends to the shoulders or just beyond. **Medium – in layers** and extends to the shoulders or just beyond. **Short – one length** and finishes at a point above the shoulders. **Short – in layers** and covers a variety of hairstyles that do not extend to the shoulders.

(Continued)

(Continued)

Consultation – things to consider:	What does it mean, how will it affect the styling options?
Hair growth patterns 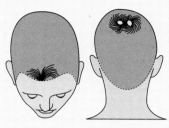 (a) (b) 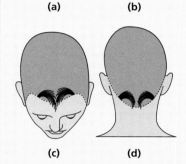 (c) (d)	These are growth directions and shapes created by the hair and will influence the way that hair can be cut and worn by the client: **Cowlick** (a) A strong, upward directional growth pattern that affects the front hairline and creates problems for fringe directions and the 'lie' of the hair. **Double crown** (b) An unusual growth feature where two crowns exist instead of one, which affects the hair over the top of the head and the lie of the hair over the rear parting and back of the head. **Widow's peak** (c) This growth pattern appears at the centre of the front hairline. The hair grows upward and forward, forming a strong peak. Similarly, to the 'cowlick' this pattern creates problems for fringes and the lie of the hair. **Nape whorl** (d) This appears as a 'sideways' growth pattern at either or both sides of the nape. It can make the hair difficult to cut into a straight neckline or close cut graduated layers. (This will often form a V-shape.) **Male Pattern Baldness** – A hereditary condition passed from father to son, where a progressive thinning occurs around the crown, at the top of the head, or at the sides of the front hairline.
Hair tendency 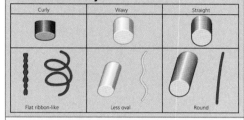	This refers to the natural fall of the hair: The amount of movement within hair is relevant to the shape of the hair **follicle** and the shape of the hair in cross-section growing from it. **Straight hair** – completely circular in cross-section. **Wavy hair** – very slightly oval in cross-section. **Curly hair** – slightly flattened in cross-section.
Hair density	The amount and distribution of hair growing from the scalp will affect the things that you can do: **Thick** – lots of hair growing closely together produces a very thick effect that takes longer to style and dry. **Medium** – a moderate amount that would give an even coverage and would be easy to style. **Thin – or thinning**, usually accompanied with finer or very fine hair types. The distribution of hair over the scalp may be the same as medium hair but will have poorer coverage and will often show the scalp through when styling; it could also be related to male pattern baldness or some other form of **alopecia**.
Hair condition	The condition of the hair will affect the manageability and durability of a hairstyle. Conditions can be: **Porous hair** – it has damaged or missing cuticles and will be rough to the touch, it will absorb moisture or chemicals too easily, take longer to dry and won't hold a style very well. **Damaged hair** – it will have damaged or broken cuticles or **cortex**, will lack moisture and need conditioning treatments, it will be weaker and more delicate than hair in normal condition and it will not hold a style very well. **Dry hair** – it will lack moisture and need conditioning treatments to improve the manageability and protect it.

(Continued)

(Continued)

Consultation – things to consider:	What does it mean, how will it affect the styling options?
	Normal hair – it has the correct balance of strength, moisture and flexibility. It will hold a style better than other conditions and will need care to maintain the condition.
	Greasy/oily – the overproduction of natural oil **sebum**, which will travel from the surface of the scalp along the **hair shaft**. This adds weight to the hair, making it look dull, lank and difficult to style.
Hair colour	Hair colour can be either:
	Natural colour – which is a result of the naturally occurring **pigments** that are produced in the living part of the hair. The pigments are collectively called **melanin** and are made up from:
	Pheomelanin – a yellow or golden pigment.
	Eumelanin – a brown or ashen pigment.
	Trichosiderin – a very rare red pigment (found in natural redheads).
	Artificial colour – which is the result of either adding chemicals that deposit semi, quasi, or permanent hair colour to the hair or by removing the natural pigments to produce lightened effects.
	Skin tone – the client's skin tone of fair, medium, olive and dark will affect the colour selection and colour suitability during consultation.
Hair or scalp problems	**Contra-indications** – There is a wide variety of hair and scalp diseases or dysfunctions that affect or limit your client's styling options.
	Go to **Hair and scalp diseases, conditions and defects** on page 169
Facial shapes	Different facial shapes suit different styles:
	Oval face shape suits any hairstyle.
	Round faces need height to reduce the width of the face. A centre parting can also help to reduce width.
	Long faces are improved with short, wider hairstyles.
	Square faces need round shapes with texture onto the face to soften them. Longer lengths beyond the jawline improve the balance and proportion.
	Triangular faces can often benefit from hair around the jawline to reduce the narrowness of the chin. These facial shapes will often suit short, 'head hugging' layered styles with soft, textured edges.

(Continued)

(Continued)

Consultation – things to consider:	What does it mean, how will it affect the styling options?
Hair and skin tests 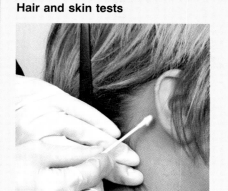	There is a wide variety of hair and skin tests that you need to perform before styling, in order to help you make decisions for courses of action.
Lifestyle	Your client's lifestyle will have a huge impact upon the ways in which they can manage their hair: **Working** clients want practical and manageable styles for their jobs. **Nurses, doctors** and people in the **services** – like the **police, army, navy, air force** – may require styles which keep the hair off the face, or they may have to wear hats or helmets. **Sporty, athletic** people need hairstyles that are easy to manage and are not in the way. People who **meet and greet** others or represent their companies in **sales or services** have to keep up a **professional** image. Younger **children** need simpler styles that are easy to maintain in the mornings, before going to school.

The structure of hair

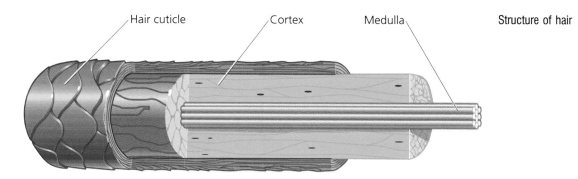

Hair cuticle   Cortex   Medulla   Structure of hair

In the image above we can see a cross-section, cut through the hair lengthways. Here we see that hair contains different areas or zones.

Hair is made from a hardened protein called keratin. This protein can be found in your fingernails and toenails and is made up from amino **acids** and polypeptide bonds. Two amino acids are connected together by a peptide to form a polypeptide chain. These polypeptide chains make up the inner structure of the cortex and look like long, spring-like structures that give the hair its strength. These polypeptides are supported by cross linkages.

Hair is made up of protein and moisture. There are 21 Amino Acids in hair protein and they account for round about 80 per cent of the weight of the hair. Moisture is in the remaining part of the hair, apart from about 15 per cent of Fatty Acids.

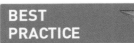

BEST PRACTICE

Give your clients time to consider your suggestions and advice.

Polypeptide chains

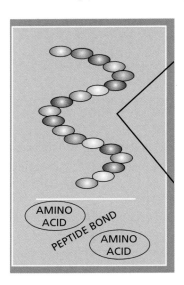

There are three different types of cross-links found in hair:

Bond/cross-link within the hair polypeptide structure	Type of bond	Relevance to hair
Disulphide bond	**Permanent** – very strong bond and can only be broken by chemicals.	The disulphide bonds are *broken during the perming* process and *reformed* (in new positions on the poly-peptide chains) *during neutralizing* to permanently re-arrange the wave or curl formation of the hair.
Salt bond	**Temporary** – weak bond broken down during shampooing.	Has no relevance to hairdressing services.
Hydrogen bond	**Temporary** – weak bond broken down during shampooing.	The hydrogen bonds are *broken during the sham-pooing process* and *reformed* (in new positions on the polypeptide chains) *when the hair is stretched and dried into style.*

Go to **Alpha and Beta keratin** on the following page.

Alpha and beta keratin

Hair that has been shampooed and left to dry naturally is known as **alpha keratin**, or in its alpha keratin state. When you shampoo hair and then dry it into style, stretching it with a brush, it is called beta keratin. This will go back to alpha keratin when the hair is moistened, perhaps by moisture in the air such as a 'steamy' bathroom.

This is the principle of heated styling and the reason why hair stays in a blow-dried or set position.

Alpha and Beta Keratin	
Before hair is shampooed, the hydrogen bonds hold the poly-peptide chains close together. Hair in this natural unstretched state is called **alpha keratin.**	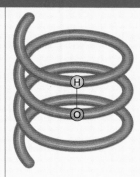 Alpha keratin: dry hair unstretched Alpha keratin
After shampooing, many of the hydrogen bonds are broken. This allows the hair to be stretched around a roller or brush.	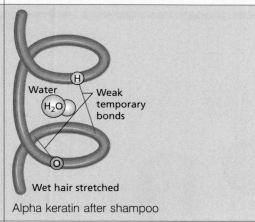 Wet hair stretched Alpha keratin after shampoo
During styling the hair is stretched, dried and allowed to cool into the new shape. The hair is now in a **beta keratin** state. Here we can see that the hydrogen bonds are reformed in new positions on the polypeptide chains.	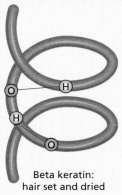 Beta keratin: hair set and dried Beta keratin

The hair will stay in this new (beta keratin) shape until the hair is made wet or it absorbs moisture from the atmosphere. (You will notice how both sets and blow-dries drop very quickly in wet, misty or foggy weather.)

BEST PRACTICE

When styling hair the hair must be: Dried fully and allowed to cool before brushing and styling.

◆ If the hair is still warm, some of the new shape may be lost during brushing/finishing.

◆ Styling and finishing products will help to protect the hair from humidity and prolong the life of the styling.

Different hair types

Hair type	Appearance	Properties
Asian hair hair types (ROUND SHAPED)	A round shape in cross-section producing straighter hair tendency.	◆ Normally have up to 12 layers of cuticle. ◆ It is usually coarser in texture and often resistant to chemicals.
Caucasian hair hair types (OVAL SHAPED)	More oval in cross-section producing a wavy hair tendency.	◆ Normally have up to eight or nine layers of cuticle. ◆ It is usually medium, or fine to medium in texture and generally quite susceptible (easy) to processing chemically.
African Caribbean hair hair types (KIDNEY SHAPED)	Is 'kidney-shaped' in cross-section producing a curly or frizzier tendency.	◆ No more than five layers of cuticle. ◆ It is usually finer in texture and delicate or fragile in chemical processing or heat styling.

Cross section of hair

CORTEX
Contains natural
colour pigments

CUTICLE
Can be many
layers thick

MEDULLA
Not always
present

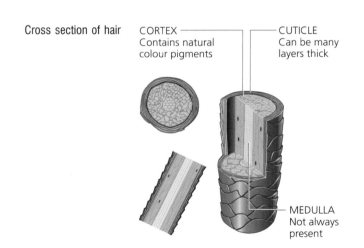

The cuticle

The cuticle is the outer layer of colourless cells that form the protective surface of the hair.

The properties of the cuticle:

◆ Regulates the chemicals entering and damaging the hair and protects the hair from excessive heat and drying.

◆ Cells overlap like tiles on a roof with the free edges pointing towards the tips of the hair.

◆ Has layers that affect the hair texture. Hair with fewer layers of cuticle is finer than coarser hair types, which have several layers.

◆ In good condition is tightly closed and resists the entry of moisture; say when shampooing, or hairdressing chemicals when colouring or perming.

◆ In poor condition will be dry or porous and have damaged or missing cuticle layers, this allows moisture and chemicals to saturate and overload the hair.

◆ In good condition will allow the hair to dry more quickly than damaged porous hair, because porous hair absorbs moisture and will take longer to dry.

◆ Temporary colours coat the cuticles, making the hair look a different colour.

◆ **Semi-permanent colours** coat the outside and penetrate to some of the lower layers to make the hair look a different colour.

◆ **Surface conditioners** coat the cuticle to add moisture, shine and increase the hair's flexibility.

The cortex

The cortex is the middle and largest layer. It is made up of long 'rope-like' fibres twisted together.

The properties of the cortex:

◆ Forms the largest part or area of the hair.

◆ All permanent hairdressing chemical processes take place within the cortex.

◆ Hair strength is directly related to the condition of the cortex.

◆ Hair elasticity is directly proportional to the condition of the cortex.

◆ Naturally occurring colour pigments (pheomelanin and eumelanin) are scattered throughout the cortex to give hair its natural colour appearance.

◆ Artificial colours such as **quasi-permanent** and permanent colours are deposited within it during chemical processing to create a new and different appearance.

◆ Condition and quality of the hair is related to the condition of the cortex.

◆ Penetrating conditioning treatments help to 'lock-in' moisture in order to improve the condition or rebuild the cortex structure.

The medulla

The **medulla** is the central, inner part of the hair.

The properties of the medulla:

◆ Only exists in medium to coarser hair types.

◆ Is often intermittent in different parts throughout the length.

◆ Is not involved in hairdressing services, chemical processes or treatments.

Maintaining healthy hair

Good conditioned hair has a direct link to healthy bodies. A healthy, balanced diet of fruit, minerals, protein and carbs, along with regular exercise, provides our bodies with a regular supply of nutrients that are carried around the body in the blood **capillary** network to the dermal **papilla**. A physiological conversion of these nutrients takes place and keratin is produced.

If our clients can get the first part of this successful formula correct, then we have a duty of care to maintain their hair condition and to be careful in the services and treatments that we provide for them.

We can complete the formula for success by providing our clients with the following information:

◆ Good advice on how they can maintain their own hair.

◆ Recommending the professional products that they should be using to achieve the correct results.

◆ Explaining how they can protect their hair before using heated styling tools and equipment.

Hair in good condition will dry quite quickly without excessive heating and the surface moisture on the cuticle will evaporate quickly. However, overheating hair, i.e. using a dryer with a high temperature, removes moisture and fatty acids from within the hair and will reduce elasticity, leaving it in a brittle and poor condition. Damaged hair is more porous than healthy hair and does not hold a style very well.

Hair is hygroscopic; that means that it will absorb water in the form of moisture from the surrounding air. The amount of water it absorbs depends on how porous the hair is; dry, damaged hair with missing cuticle, will absorb more than hair in good condition. Hair in good condition naturally contains a certain amount of 'locked-in' moisture.

Moisture and 'fatty' acids in hair will:

◆ Enable it to stretch and return, giving it good elasticity.

◆ Provide shine; one of the key indicators of good condition.

◆ Make the hair flexible enabling it to hold a style for longer.

Therefore, from the table on the previous page we see that moisture and fatty acid levels within the hair are essential for maintaining good condition. We can see the effect of this moisture by the shine that we associate with great-looking hair. 'Bad hair' denotes poor condition and a lack of shine due to the unevenness of the hair's surface, i.e. the cuticle. A roughened cuticle surface is an indicator of either physical or chemical damage.

From a **customer care** point of view the health and the condition of your client's hair is a main consideration for your consultation. Whatever you have planned for the service, you should be 'building-in' some useful advice and at least making some recommendations for conditioning treatments.

Features of hair in good condition

Features of hair in good condition	
◆ **Shine and lustre**	Locked in moisture will help the hair to look healthier and give it shine.
◆ **Smooth outer cuticle surface**	A smooth cuticle surface will help to protect the inner structure of the hair and resist the absorption of water and chemicals.
◆ **Strength and resistance**	Stronger hair is more resistant to the damaging effects of: heated styling, harsh brushing and combing, and damaging UV rays in sunlight.
◆ **Good elasticity**	Healthy hair is flexible hair and hair that is constantly being styled needs good elasticity to maintain its hold.

Features of hair in poor condition	
◆ **Raised or open cuticle**	Roughened, open cuticle scales make the hair porous allowing water and chemicals to saturate the hair.
◆ **Damaged torn hair shaft/Split ends**	Damaged, broken hair leaves the inner cortex exposed, which reduces strength and increases the risk of split ends.
◆ **Low strength and resistance**	Weakened hair will not be able to hold a style very well. It will easily break during styling and the damage will cause other longer term problems.
◆ **Over-elastic/stretchy**	Stretchy hair is weak hair and easily snaps. (This is even more noticeable when the hair is wet during combing and styling.)
◆ **Dry, porous lengths or ends**	Dry, porous hair is more delicate and will require a lot more care and conditioning maintenance than normal hair.

Reasons for damaged hair	
Physical hair damage	Rough treatment; incorrect usage of brushes, combs and other styling tools.
	Overheating the hair during blow-drying or from using excessively hot styling equipment such as straighteners, tongs, wands, etc.
Chemical hair damage	Lack of attention during the timing of colouring, lightening or perming services.
	Incorrect strengths used of hydrogen peroxide during colouring and lightening services.
	Negligent/incompetent service causing over-lightening and over-processed hair.
	Incorrect strengths of perming lotions (too strong for hair type/condition).
	Frequency of salon or home colouring, lightening or perming services – excessive, unnecessary use of chemicals upon the hair.
	Incorrect selection, application and/or timing of home colouring kits – causing damaged, over porous hair that will have less ability to hold colour in the future.
Environmental hair damage	Ultra Violet (UV) radiation from too much exposure to sunshine – raises areas of cuticle, exposing the inner hair and pigments to the effects of lightening, making the hair porous and damaged.
	Mineral (airborne) pollutants (more evident in busy, large urban areas) – affecting the **porosity** of hair due to frequency of washing and the strengths of shampoos needed to cleanse the hair.
	Chemicals in swimming pools (chlorine) – the alkaline solution changes the properties of the hair by swelling the hair shaft and often causing a discoloured 'green' effect on blonde hair with natural bases 9, 8, 7 and 6.

TOP TIP

It is far easier to keep good-conditioned hair in good condition than it is to try to correct hair in bad condition.

The structure of skin

Skin is the largest organ of the body: if it were stretched out flat, it would cover an area of over two square metres (21 square feet). It provides a tough, flexible covering and has many important features:

Basic functions of the skin

Protection	The skin protects the body from potentially harmful substances and conditions. ◆ The natural **pH** 5.5 (slightly acidic) property of skin helps to prevent the growth of harmful bacteria. ◆ The skin is a physical barrier that prevents the absorption of many substances.
Heat regulation	The temperature of the body is controlled by heat loss through the skin and by sweating.
Excretion	Waste products such as water and salt are removed from the body by excretion through the surface of the skin.
Sensitivity	The nervous system within the skin provides the feelings of touch, pressure, pain and temperature.
Warning	Intolerances to things such as plants, minerals or animals can be seen by a swelling, reddening, or irritation.

The skin is made up from many layers but the main ones are the **epidermis**, dermis and subcutis.

Basic structure of skin

Epidermis

The epidermis is the outermost layer of skin.

It has five layers:

1   **Horny layer** – Top layer, made of many flattened cells, cells shed continuously.

2   **Clear layer** – three to four layers thick, only found on palms of hands and soles of feet, acts as a protector against friction.

3   **Granular layer** – two to four layers thick, cells here begin to die and flatten, middle layer of epidermis.

4   **Prickle cell layer** – 10–20 cells thick, spines connect to other cells, sits on top of basal layer, cells here start to produce keratin and harden, melanin is produced in this layer.

5   **Basal cell layer** – Single layer of column-shaped cells, deepest layer of the epidermis, continually produces new cells which are pushed up to form next layer.

(Continued)

(Continued)

Basic structure of skin

Epidermis

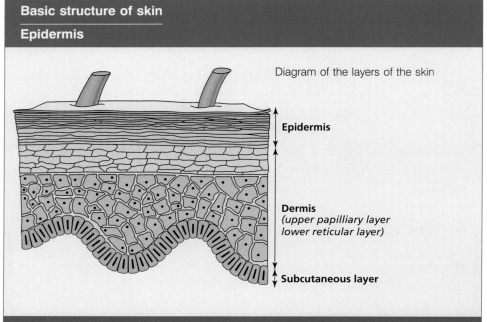

Diagram of the layers of the skin

Epidermis

Dermis
*(upper papilliary layer
lower reticular layer)*

Subcutaneous layer

Dermis

The dermis contains many structures.

It consists of two layers:

1   **Papillary layer** – is a wavy layer of tissue. It contains many blood and lymph vessels, which feed the epidermis to allow for cell reproduction and remove waste. It contains many nerve endings, which allow you to feel sensations. It joins the epidermis to the dermis.

2   **Reticular layer** – a dense, fibrous tissue. It is beneath the papillary layer. It contains the main components of the dermis:

  ◆   collagen tissue

  ◆   elastin tissue

  ◆   reticulin tissue.

It protects and repairs injured tissue.

Subcutis

The **subcutaneous fatty layer** lies below the dermis. It is also known as the subcutis.

It is composed of loose cell tissue and contains stores of fat.

The base of the hair follicle is situated just above this area, or sometimes in it. **Subcutaneous tissue** gives roundness to the body and fills the space between the dermis and muscles.

The hair follicle

The hair follicle

Hair grows from a thin, tube-like space in the skin called a hair follicle.

◆ The papilla(e) forms the lower part of the follicles. These are supplied with nerves and blood vessels, which nourish the cellular activity.

◆ The **germinal matrix** surrounds each papilla and consists of actively forming hair cells.

◆ As the hair cells develop, the lowest, thicker part is shaped into the **hair bulb**.

◆ The cells gradually harden and die. The hair is formed of dead tissue. It retains its elasticity due to its chemical composition.

◆ The cells continue to push up from the papilla and push along the follicle until they appear at the skin surface as a tapered hair.

Sebaceous glands

The oil gland, or **sebaceous gland**, is located within the skin and secretes natural oil, sebum, into the follicle and onto the hair and skin surface. Sebum helps to prevent the skin and hair from drying and helps the hair and skin to stay pliable. Sebum is slightly acid – about pH 5.6 – and forms a protective antibacterial covering for the skin.

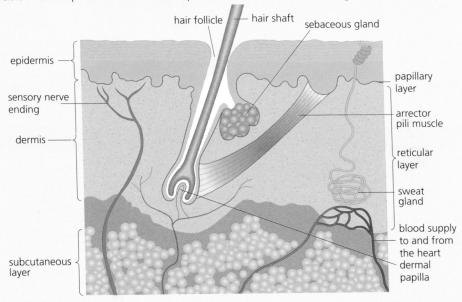

The hair in the skin

Sweat glands

The sweat gland secretes sweat, which passes out through the sweat ducts. Sweat appears at the surface of the skin through tiny pores. There are two types of sweat gland: the larger, associated closely with the hair follicles, are the **apocrine glands**; the smaller, found over most of the skin's surface, are the eccrine glands.

Arrector pili muscle

The **arrector pili muscle** is attached at one end to the hair follicle and at the other to the underlying tissue of the epidermis. When it contracts, it pulls the hair and follicle upright. This occurs when we feel cold as the 'upright' hairs trap a warm layer of air around the skin. This also produces dimples at the surface of the skin at the point where the muscle contracts; we call this sensation 'goose bumps'.

Hair growth

The hair on our head is called **terminal hair**: that means that it grows in specific terms or stages. Healthy hair will grow continually at a rate of 12.5mm per month, for a period of between one and six years, and then after the active growth stages it stops, rests and degenerates before finally falling out. However, before the hair leaves the follicle, the new hair is normally ready to replace it.

There are three main stages of hair growth:

◆ **Anagen**: the hair is actively growing.

◆ **Catagen**: the stage where changes occur (transitional stage).

◆ **Telogen**: the stage where the follicle 'rests' and no hair is growing.

Anagen stage

◆ Hair grows at 12.5mm per month.

◆ Longest growing phase (affects 85 per cent of hair at any one time).

◆ Average growing phase lasts one to six years.

◆ People with long hair have a longer anagen cycle.

◆ People with a shorter anagen cycle will never have long hair.

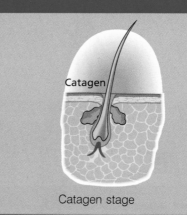

Anagen stage

Catagen stage

◆ At the end of the anagen phase, hair growth stops.

◆ The catagen phase lasts approximately two weeks.

◆ No new cells are produced in dermal papilla.

◆ Hair follicle shrinks to one sixth of its original length.

Catagen stage

Telogen stage

◆ This is the resting period for the hair follicle and dermal papilla.

◆ Telogen lasts roughly 10 to 12 weeks.

◆ Approximately 10–15 per cent of follicles are in the telogen stage at any one time.

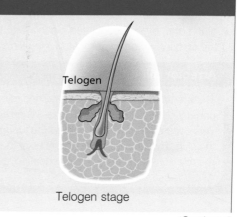

Telogen stage

(Continued)

(Continued)

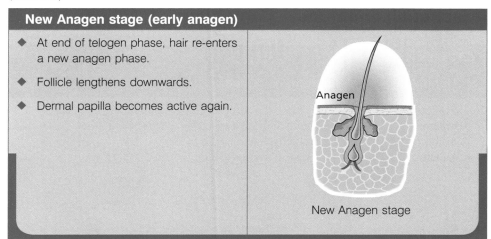

New Anagen stage (early anagen)

◆ At end of telogen phase, hair re-enters a new anagen phase.

◆ Follicle lengthens downwards.

◆ Dermal papilla becomes active again.

New Anagen stage

Hair and scalp diseases, conditions and defects

Consultation is the process of finding out what the client wants and seeing if there is any reason why that cannot be done. In many cases, the planned service will be able to go ahead as scheduled, but there are occasions where you will find contra-indications during the consultation and this will influence what you do next.

◆ Sometimes you will be able to carry out your planned service providing that you prepare the hair in a certain way. That is, conditioning treatments, styling, **straightening**, etc.

◆ Sometimes you will have to carry out tests before you proceed any further.

◆ Sometimes you will need to refer your client to someone else: a senior stylist, a pharmacist, their own GP or another salon.

◆ On other occasions, you may not be able to do their hair at all!

An initial examination must take place before any hairdressing process occurs, so that any adverse conditions are identified. If this is not done a variety of serious outcomes could occur. However, not all hair and scalp conditions are dangerous, some non-infectious conditions can be treated within the salon. This section looks at an array of hair and skin contra-indications: some of them will be **contagious**, others are non-contagious, but all must be recognized during consultation, so that cross-infection, cross-infestation, hair and skin damage can all be avoided.

Infectious conditions – Contagious

Infectious diseases – bacterial diseases					
Image	Condition	Symptoms	Cause	Action	Infectious
Courtesy of Mediscan Folliculitis	**Folliculitis Inflammation of the hair follicles**	Inflamed follicles, a common symptom of certain skin diseases.	A contact bacterial infection, or due to chemical or physical action.	Medical **referral** to GP.	**No**
Courtesy of Mediscan Impetigo	**Impetigo A bacterial infection of the upper skin layers**	At first a burning sensation, followed by spots becoming dry; honey-coloured, crusts form and spread.	A staphylococcal or streptococcal infection.	Medical referral to GP.	**Yes**
Prof. Andrew Wright, Dermatologist Bradford Sycosis	**Sycosis A bacterial infection of the hairy parts of the face**	Small, yellow spots around the follicle mouth, burning, irritation and general inflammation.	Bacteria attack the upper part of the hair follicle, spreading to the lower follicle.	Medical referral to GP.	**No**
Prof. Andrew Wright, Dermatologist Bradford Furunculosis	**Furunculosis Boils or abscesses**	Raised, inflamed, pus-filled spots, irritation, swelling and pain.	An infection of the hair follicles by staphylococcal bacteria.	Medical referral to GP.	**No**

Infectious diseases – Viral diseases

Condition	Symptoms	Cause	Action	Infectious
Herpes simplex (cold sore) A viral infection of the skin. Herpes simplex	Burning, irritation, swelling and inflammation precede the appearance of fluid-filled blisters, usually on the lips and surrounding areas.	Possibly exposure to extreme heat or cold, or a reaction to food or drugs: the skin may carry the **virus** for years without exhibiting any symptoms.	Medical referral to Pharmacist.	**Yes**
Warts A viral infection of the skin. Warts	Raised, roughened skin, often brown or discoloured. There may be irritation and soreness. Warts are common on the hands and face.	The lower epidermis is attacked by the virus, which causes the skin to harden and skin cells to multiply.	Medical referral to Pharmacist.	**Yes**

Infectious infestations – Animal (parasite) infestations

Condition	Symptoms	Cause	Action	Infectious
Head lice (pediculosis capitis) Infestation of the hair and scalp by head lice. Head lice	An itchy reaction to the biting head louse, 'peppering' on pillowcases and minute egg cases (nits) attached to the upper hair shaft close to the scalp.	The head louse bites the scalp, feeding on the victim's blood. Breeding produces eggs, which are laid and cemented onto the hair shaft for incubation until the immature louse emerges.	Referral to a pharmacist.	**Yes**
Scabies An allergic reaction to the itch mite. Scabies	A rash in the skin folds around the midriff and on the inside of the thighs, extremely itchy at night.	The itch mite burrows under the skin where it lays eggs.	Medical referral to GP.	**Yes**

Infectious – Fungal diseases

Tinea capitis **Ringworm** of the head. Tinea capitis	Circular bald patch of grey or whitish skin surrounded by red, active rings; hairs broken close to the skin, which looks dull and rough. The fungus lives off the keratin in the skin and hair. This disease is common in children.	Fungal infection of the skin or hair.	Medical referral.	**Yes**

Non-infectious conditions – Non Contagious

Non-infectious – Conditions of the hair and skin

Condition	Symptoms	Cause	Action	Infectious
Acne Disorder affecting the hair follicles and sebaceous glands. Acne	Raised spots and bumps within the skin, commonly upon the face in adolescents.	Increased sebum and other secretions block the follicle and a skin reaction occurs.	Medical referral to GP.	**No**
Eczema and **dermatitis** In its simplest form a reddening of the skin. Eczema	Ranging from slightly inflamed areas of the skin to severe splitting and weeping areas with irritation and soreness.	Many possible causes, eczema often associated with internal factors, i.e. allergies or stress. Dermatitis a reaction or allergy to external factors.	Medical referral to GP.	**No**
Dandruff (Pityriasis Capitis). Dandruff	Dry, small, irritating flakes.	Fungal (yeast-like) infection, or physical or chemical irritants.	Anti-dandruff treatments.	**No**

(Continued)

(Continued)

Non-infectious – Conditions of the hair and skin

Condition	Symptoms	Cause	Action	Infectious
Seborrhea 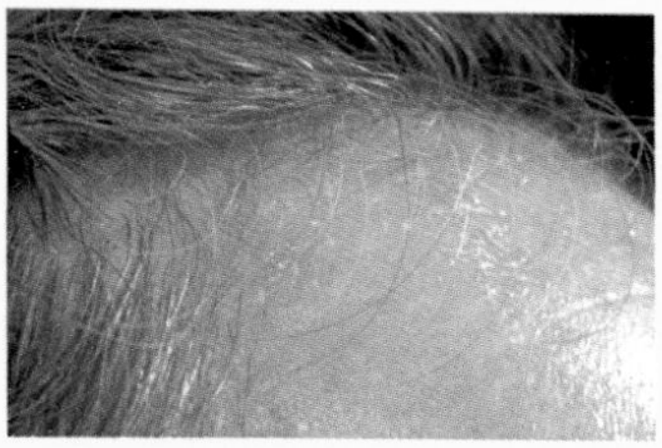 Seborrhea	Very greasy, lank hair and greasy skin, making styling difficult.	Over-production of sebum.	**Astringent** shampoos.	**No**
Psoriasis An inflamed, abnormal thickening of the skin. 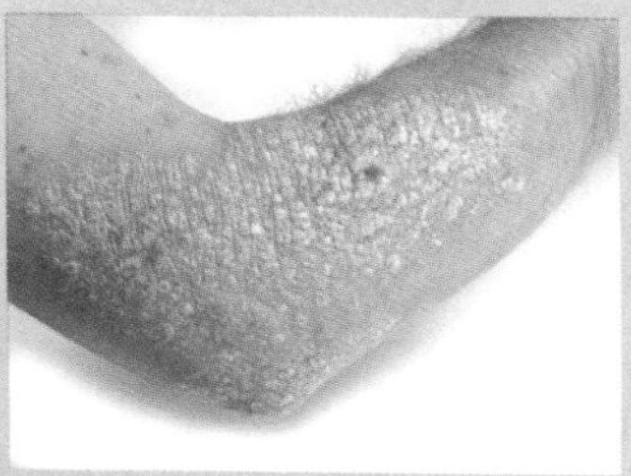 Psoriasis	Areas of thickened skin, often raised and patchy. Often on the scalp and also at the joints (arms and legs).	Unknown	Medical referral to GP.	No

Defects of the hair

Condition	Symptom	Cause	Action
Split ends (fragilitas crinium) Fragile, poorly conditioned hair. 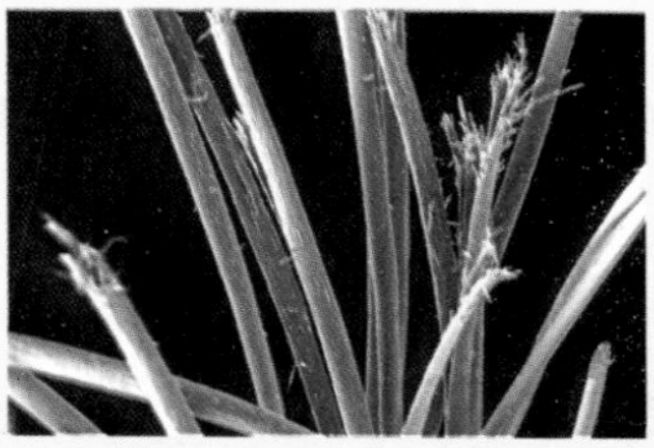 Split ends	Dry, splitting hair ends.	Harsh physical or chemical treatments.	Cutting off or special treatment conditioners.
Monilethrix Beaded hair. 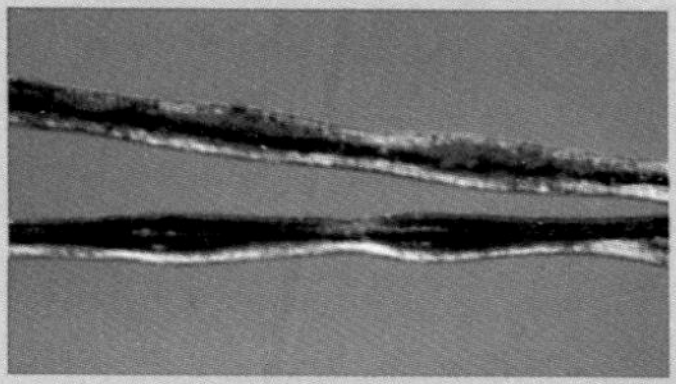 Monilethrix	Beadlike swellings along the hair shaft, hair often breaks at weaker points.	Irregular development of the hair formed during cellular production.	None

(Continued)

(Continued)

Defects of the hair

Condition	Symptom	Cause	Action
Trichorrhexis nodosa Nodules forming on the hair shaft. Trichorrhex is nodosa	Areas of swelling at locations along the hair shaft, splitting and rupturing the cuticle layer.	Harsh physical or chemical processing.	None, although cutting and conditioning may help.
Sebaceous cyst Swelling of the oil gland. Sebaceous cyst	Bumps, lumps and swellings on the scalp containing fluid, soft to the touch.	Sebaceous gland becomes blocked allowing a build-up of fluid to take place.	Medical referral.
Damaged cuticle Broken, split, torn hair. Damaged cuticle	Rough, raised, missing areas of cuticle; hair loses its moisture and becomes dry and porous.	Harsh physical or chemical processes.	None, although cutting and conditioning may help.

Hair loss – Alopecia

Other conditions – Alopecia (hair loss)

	Symptoms	Action
Alopecia areata Alopecia areata	The name given to balding patches over the scalp. Often starts around or above the ears, circular in pattern ranging from 1–2.5cm in diameter.	Trichological referral.

(Continued)

(Continued)

Other conditions – Alopecia (hair loss)

	Symptoms	Action
Traction alopecia Traction alopecia	Hair loss as a result of excessive pulling at the roots from brushing, curling and straightening. Very often seen with younger girls tying, plaiting or braiding long hair.	None
Alopecia totalis Alopecia totalis	Complete hair loss sometimes as a result of alopecia areata spreading and joining up across the scalp.	Trichological referral.
Cicatricial alopecia Cicatricial alopecia	**Baldness** due to scarring of the skin arising from chemical or physical injury. The hair follicle is damaged and permanent baldness results.	None
Male pattern baldness Male pattern baldness	Premature male pattern baldness occurs in teens or early 20s. Senile pattern baldness occurs in late 30s–50s. Hair recedes at the hairline or loss at the crown area. Condition is hereditary (passed on in families).	Remedies currently being developed.

Courtesy of Mediscan

Hair and skin tests

Earlier in this chapter we said that consultation is a process of finding out what the client wants and seeing if there is any reason why that cannot be carried out. Here we look at the variety of tests that you need to carry out in order to help diagnose the condition and likely reaction of your client's skin and hair. These tests will help you to decide what action to take before, during and after the application of hairdressing processes.

Tensile strength test

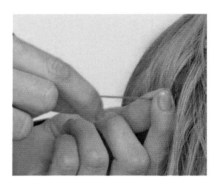

Elasticity Test

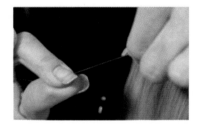

Porosity test

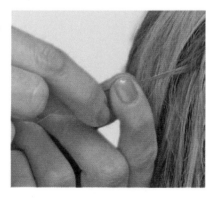

You will need to carry out and record all the results from these tests immediately after the test has been carried out. This is essential as your salon will need recorded details for:

◆ Future reference – for other services or treatments.

◆ Salon policy demonstrating professional practice – showing good customer care and details of periodic testing.

◆ Legal reasons – if there are any problems that lead to pursuance by insurers and any court action.

Type of test	Reasons for testing	How to test
Hair condition tests		
Tensile strength test	This test is used to find out how strong the hair is by testing it to 'snapping' point. This is particularly useful for: ◆ Coloured ◆ Lightened ◆ Highlighted ◆ Previously permed ◆ Delicate/weakened ◆ Fine ◆ Damaged ◆ Porous hair types and conditions.	1 Test a single strand of hair from the client's head in the area where you have concerns or doubts about its strength. 2 Take the hair between the thumb and forefinger of both hands and gently pull. 3 Continue to stretch the hair until the breaking point occurs. 4 Complete a client record of the date, time and results of the test. The resistance and flexibility of the hair should be noted as this has a direct bearing on the way that the hair will respond under many styling or chemical processes.
Elasticity test	This test is used to test both the inner hair strength and the condition of the cortex in relation to a range of hairdressing processes. This is particularly useful for: ◆ Coloured ◆ Lightened ◆ Highlighted ◆ Previously permed ◆ Delicate/weakened ◆ Fine ◆ Damaged ◆ Porous hair types and conditions.	Do this test on a dry, single strand of hair. 1 Take the hair between the thumb and forefinger of both hands and gently pull. 2 If the hair stretches to nearly a third more than its original length, then the hair is too stretchy and over elastic (often a problem with chemically processed hair, particularly lightened hair). 3 If the hair doesn't stretch much before it snaps it will show that the hair has no or very little elasticity and denotes hair in very poor condition. This has serious implications for many hairdressing services. 4 Complete a client record of the date, time and results of the test.
Porosity test	This test will indicate the condition (or damage) of the outer cuticle of the hair. A smooth cuticle surface will shine and indicate that the hair is in a normal condition and should have a reasonable resistance to absorption of chemicals and moisture. Conversely, a roughened cuticle surface will indicate that the cuticle scales are raised and will absorb moisture and chemicals too readily, causing product saturation and/or over processing.	Do this test on a dry, single strand of hair. 1 Test a single strand of hair on the client's head and hold it between the thumb and forefinger at the points end (not the root end). 2 Now run your finger/thumb back towards the roots to feel the roughness of the cuticle. 3 The rougher the feeling the more damage or raised the cuticle layers are. You may expect to get some slight roughness as you will be testing the hair against the natural lie.

(Continued)

(Continued)

Type of test	Reasons for testing	How to test
Porosity test continued		Cuticle scales have their 'free' edges pointing to-wards the point ends of the hair. To gauge this correctly you should repeat this on hair in good condition (with a tightly packed cuti-cle) to prove your result. You may wish to record this on your client record card for future reference.
Colouring tests		
Strand test	A strand test or hair strand colour test is used **during** processing to check the development of the colour process.	1 Put on your disposable vinyl gloves. 2 Following the manufacturer's instructions, mix and apply a small amount of the target shade to a section of hair. 3 After development, rub the strand of hair with the back of a tail comb to remove surplus colour. 4 Check to see whether the product has developed properly and achieved the target effect. 5 Complete a client record of the date, time and results of the test. Remember that in the case of a test cutting there will be no body heat and may affect the processing timings.
Test cutting	A test cutting is used as a **trial** test to find out what the colour effect will be on a strand or section of hair after colour has been processed and developed.	
Skin test /or Patch test	FOR **ALL** NEW CLIENTS WHO ARE CONSIDERING PERMANENT AND QUASI-PERMANENT COLOUR. The skin sensitivity test is used to assess the reaction of the skin to chemicals or chemical products. A growing number of people are allergic to contact with the colouring chemical; **PPD** (**P**ara**p**henylene**d**iamine: used in the formulation of permanent and quasi-permanent colour). Contact with this chemical can cause permanent scarring of skin tissue and/or hair loss. To find out whether a client's skin reacts to chemicals in permanent colours, the following test should be **carried out 24–48 hours prior to the chemical process.** *Note: Skin testing is not just for new clients, it has now been found that clients can develop sensitivity to chemicals through prolonged use of the same or similar products. Therefore periodic testing for adverse reactions is essential and should be carried out routinely two or three times a year (as recommended by the manufacturer).* You will be more likely to get a true test response by using natural base colours (**especially darker shades)** because these contain more PPD.	1 Put on your disposable vinyl gloves. 2 Apply a small amount of the (darkest shade, e.g. 1.0) colour within the range, (e.g. Majirel, Koleston Perfection, NXT, etc.) that you plan to use on to the tip of a cotton wool bud. 3 Prepare and clean a small area of skin behind the ear. 4 Apply a little of the colour to the skin. 5 **Complete a client record of the date and time of the skin test.** 6 Ask your client to report any discomfort or irritation that occurs over the next 48 hours. Arrange to see your client at the end of this time so that you can check for signs of reaction. 7 **Update your client record with the details.** ◆ If there is a *positive reaction*, i.e. a skin reaction such as inflammation, soreness, swelling, irritation or discomfort, YOU MUST NOT proceed with the intended service. Never ignore the result of a skin test. If a skin test showed a reaction and you carried on anyway, there might be a more serious reaction which could affect the whole body and lead to legal prosecution. ◆ If there is a *negative reaction*, i.e. no reaction to the chemicals, then the service can be carried out as planned.

(Continued)

Type of test	Reasons for testing	How to test
Tests for Colour and perms		
Incompatibility test	Some chemicals will not work together and will cause a **chemical reaction** if brought into contact with each other. The vast majority of hairdressing products are based upon '**organic**' chemistry, i.e. based upon carbon, hydrogen and oxygen. However a small amount of compound dyes, colour restorers still exist and these are based on 'inorganic' chemistry. These products contain metallic salts and will react violently on contact with organic-based chemicals. You should carry out an incompatibility test before colouring, lightening or perming if you are in any doubt about the products used previously on the client's hair.	1 Put on your disposable vinyl gloves. 2 Mix together in a bowl 40ml of 20 volume 6 per cent hydrogen peroxide and 5ml of alkaline perming solution (containing **ammonium thioglycolate**). 3 Place a small amount of the client's hair in the solution and wait for any changes. 4 If any heat is generated (you will feel this by holding the bowl) or the lotion fizzes and the hair breaks, disintegrates or changes colour you have a *positive reaction* to the test. 5 Complete a client record of the date, time and results of the test. ◆ If there is a positive reaction, YOU MUST NOT proceed with the intended service ◆ If there is a *negative reaction*, i.e. no reaction to the chemicals, then the service can be carried out as planned.
Perming tests		
Pre-perm test curl	A pre-perm test curl will enable you to see how your client's hair will react to permanent waving. A perm rod of the selected size is used for the following: ◆ Coloured ◆ Lightened ◆ Highlighted ◆ Previously permed ◆ Delicate/weakened ◆ Lank ◆ Fine ◆ Porous hair types and conditions.	Note: It is not always possible to conduct this test on the client's head so a section of hair may have to be cut. 1 Put on your disposable vinyl gloves. 2 Wind a section of hair around the chosen target curler/perm rod. 3 Apply a small amount of the selected perming solution and develop for the recommended time. 4 Carry out a development test curl and if processing has achieved sufficient movement, rinse and neutralize for the specified time by the manufacturer. 5 Complete a client record of the date, time and results of the test.
Development test curl	This test is used to check the processing of the perm and to see if the desired movement or curl has been achieved.	1 Put on your disposable vinyl gloves. 2 Remove the cap (if used) and holding a rod near the crown; undo the rubber fastener. 3 Unwind the curler by a couple of turns (without stretching the hair). 4 Push the hair back towards the scalp – allowing it to recoil back into an 'S' wave.

(Continued)

(Continued)

Type of test	Reasons for testing	How to test
		5 If the recoil of the hair is definitely occurring without too much assistance and the 'S' wave corresponds to the size of the curler, then processing may be complete.
		6 Check the development in a couple of other areas to see if the result is the same. If it is, then the hair is ready for neutralizing.
Relaxing tests		
Pre-relaxer test	This is done before a relaxing treatment to check the suitability of: ◆ Relaxing products ◆ Development times and to see if the result matches the client's desired effect.	1 Put on your disposable vinyl gloves. 2 Put a small amount of relaxer into a plastic bowl. 3 Take a small section of hair from the most resistant area. 4 Pull the section through a meche of foil with a pre-cut slit in it. 5 Fix the foil into place, masking the scalp with flat sectioning clips. 6 Apply the relaxing product to the strand of hair with a brush and leave for the specified time. If the treatment is a one-step process remove the product according to manufacturer's instructions. If it is a two-step process you will need to re-balance the hair by neutralizing. If you continue to carry out the service then the previously processed area cannot be processed again.

TOP TIP

Cuticles have their 'free' edges pointing towards the point ends of the hair.

BEST PRACTICE

Tests are a vital part of general hairdressing services. If they are missed or ignored you and the salon run the risk of a potential disaster.

Incompatible chemistry

Henna is still widely used throughout the world as a hair- and skin-dyeing compound. In the UK people using natural henna will often add other ingredients such as coffee, wine, lemon juice, etc. to intensify the final colour. However, other countries also add compounds to henna; e.g. India and Turkey sometimes add iron ore deposits which are crushed into the powder to increase the 'reddening' effect. If this mixture were to come into contact with hydrogen peroxide (either through colouring or perming), a chemical reaction would take place and in that exchange permanent damage and breakage would occur.

The pH Scale

Hair and beauty products often make references to **pH levels**. Perm lotions may be called acid waves and skin care products refer to being acid-balanced, but what does this really mean?

The degree of acidity or alkalinity of a hairdressing product can be measured on the pH scale. The scale ranges from pH1 to pH14, where pH1 denotes a very strong acid and pH14 at the opposite end of the scale denotes a very strong alkali. The mid-way point along this scale at pH7 is neutral, i.e. being neither acid nor alkaline.

The acid mantle

The illustration below shows the pH of the hair and skin. Here, sweat and sebum combine to produce a slightly acid film called the **acid mantle** which is 4.5–5.5. This is particularly beneficial to our skin as it helps prevent infection by creating a natural barrier to bacteria and fungi by providing an environment that does not help to develop their growth.

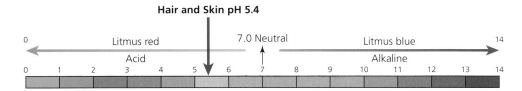

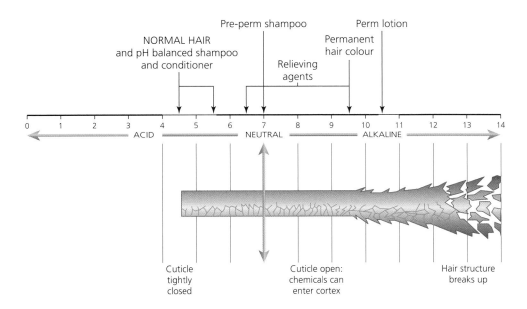

At the other end of the scale, alkali solutions open the cuticle scales, making the hair look rough and dull. Hairdressing chemical processes such as perming, lightening, colouring and straightening are all alkaline, because they have to lift the cuticle scale in order to penetrate the cortex and perform their chemical action.

You can see from the illustration that mild acid solutions have a tightening effect on the hair shaft; this closes the cuticle scales so they lay flatter which helps to improve the shine too. Therefore, any conditioning product that has an acid pH (4–6) (an **acid conditioner**) will tend to leave the hair in a shiny, smooth condition.

Alkalis play an important part in beauty treatments as they are used in hair removal creams and provide an alternative solution to shaving and waxing. Alkalis swell the hair shaft and break down its structure, which destroys the hair, removing it from the surface of the epidermis. The professional name used for this group of products is **depilatories.**

TOP TIP

Acid rinse conditioners.
Many conditioning treatments use mild acidic solutions such as acetic acid and fruit acids to make the hair shiny and smooth.

pH effects on hair

Effects of pH on hair

◆ Acidic products are kind to the hair since they help to close the cuticles.

◆ Mildly alkaline products will open the hair cuticles, allowing colour to penetrate the hair more easily.

◆ Highly alkaline products are very damaging to the hair since they will break up the hair structure.

You must ALWAYS consider the pH of the products you use and the potential damage they may cause to your client's hair.

Benefits of anti-oxidant conditioners

Anti-oxident conditioners

Permanent and quasi-permanent hair colours are alkaline in their composition and open the cuticles; therefore, an **anti-oxidant conditioner** is recommended for use after the colour has been shampooed from the hair.

An anti-oxidant conditioner will:

◆ Return the hair to its normal pH of 4.5 – 5.5 (slightly acidic).

◆ Add moisture to the hair.

◆ Stop further oxidation taking place (since this will damage the hair) '**creeping oxidization'**.

◆ Close the cuticles.

◆ Add/improve shine.

Client records

Accurate, up to date client records are essential for any salon; they help to ensure that the salon has a professional image and that the staff demonstrate good customer service.

By keeping accurate, up to date records, you will show that you are providing:

◆ A professional service based on advice, matched to the client's individual needs.

◆ Useful information that will help in the planning of future services or treatments.

◆ A full client service history.

◆ A formal document that may be used if there were any later dispute or legal action taken against the salon.

The records also give vital information should there be any later client complaints or worse, if there was any legal case taken against the salon.

Client record cards

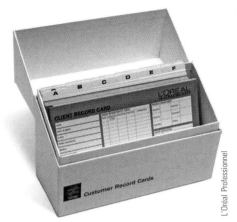

L'Oréal Professionnel

Records may be kept as: manual, card index files, computerized **databases** or point of sale applications (e.g. I Salon, Salon Genius, Salon Iris). All of these record systems must be kept secure and safe and your clients' rights are maintained and protected by law, under the Data Protection Act 1998.

Client records – A basic client record system should contain the following information:

◆ Relevant client details – name, address, contact numbers, ID.

◆ Date of services, treatments and tests provided.

◆ A description of the services or treatments provided.

◆ Details of any chemical services and products that have been used.

◆ Details about any tests that have been carried out.

◆ Contra-indications and courses of action.

◆ Recommendations or referrals.

A computerized recording system may also contain:

◆ Billings and sales history.

◆ Details of any purchases made.

◆ Details relating to hair type, tendency, length, natural colour, etc.

TOP TIP

Client records are personal and private information, they must be handled confidentially and you have a duty to uphold the rights of your clients if you keep their personal information on file. The information that we record about our clients is protected by the Data Protection Act (1998).

TOP TIP

If this information is handled and managed by the staff within the salon, then the salon is responsible by law (For more information see Data Protection Act (1998) in the Appendix at the end of this chapter) to keep this secure and to not misuse the information without expressed consent of the person(s) to which the information relates to.

BEST PRACTICE

Make sure that records are found prior to consultation and used to check on previous client history. Update the records in line with your actions taken after consultation.

A computerized system has several benefits over a manual system

◆ They are easier to keep secure.

◆ Provide marketing information about purchasing preferences.

◆ Keep track of sales, movements and products.

◆ Provide reports for stock management, promotions, purchasing habits, etc.

◆ Identify trends.

◆ Create financial budgets and forecasts.

SUMMARY

As a final reflection on what you have covered in this chapter, you should now have a clearer picture of all the essential aspects for providing consultation and advice to clients. In particular, you should now have a basic understanding of the key principles of:

1 How good communication is used to provide a professional consultation service.

2 The importance of why you should identify and recognize all the contra-indications to planned customer services.

3 Using a range of different communication methods during consultation, such as questioning techniques, visual aids, summarizing key points and negotiating suitable courses of action.

4 The structure of hair and skin and the functions that they perform.

5 Hair and scalp diseases and disorders.

6 Carrying out tests before services and treatments are provided.

And collectively, how these principles will enable you to provide a knowledgeable and professional consultation service for all of your clients.

ASSESSMENT OF KNOWLEDGE AND UNDERSTANDING

Project

For this project you will need to gather information from a variety of sources. List the services, treatments and products that are available in your salon. Then for each one listed explain:

1 What the features and benefits are to the client.

2 How you would go about explaining these to clients.

3 The costs of each of these.

Revision questions

A selection of different types of questions to check your consultation and advice knowledge.

Q1	The three stages of hair growth are anagen, _____ and telogen.	Fill in the blank
Q2	The cortex is the outermost layer of the hair.	True or false
Q3	Which of the following are infectious diseases (select all that apply)?	Multi selection

	Impetigo	☐ 1
	Scalp ringworm	☐ 2
	Alopecia	☐ 3
	Head lice	☐ 4
	Psoriasis	☐ 5
	Eczema	☐ 6

Q4   The natural colour of hair depends on the amount of melanin within it.   True or false

Q5   Which of the following is commonly known as split ends?   Multi choice

Trichorrhexis nodosa   O a

Monilethrix   O b

Tinea capitis   O c

Fragilitas crinium   O d

Q6   Dandruff is a condition of the scalp usually caused by fungal infection.   True or False

Q7   Which of the following tests are carried out *during* technical services?   Multi selection

Skin test   ☐ 1

Strand test   ☐ 2

Development test curl   ☐ 3

Incompatibility test   ☐ 4

Porosity test   ☐ 5

Test cutting   ☐ 6

Q8   The layer of the skin below the epidermis is called the _____.   Fill in the blank

Q9   Which face shape suits most hair styles and lengths?   Multi choice

Square   O a

Oblong   O b

Oval   O c

Triangular   O d

Q10   During consultation and hair analysis, a contra-indication will not allow   True or false
the planned service to be carried out.

Appendix

Data Protection Act 1998 – Plain-language summary of key principles

This section provides a quick overview of what the key principles of information-handling practice mean. The key principles themselves are discussed below in the context of their definition in law.

◆ Data may only be used for the specific purposes for which it was collected.

◆ Data must not be disclosed to other parties without the consent of the individual whom it is about, unless there is legislation or other overriding legitimate reason to share the information (e.g. the prevention or detection of crime). It is an offence for other parties to obtain this personal data without authorization.

◆ Individuals have a right of access to the information held about them, subject to certain exceptions (e.g. information held for the prevention or detection of crime).

◆ Personal information may be kept for no longer than is necessary and must be kept up to date.

◆ Personal information may not be sent outside the European Economic Area unless the individual whom it is about has consented or adequate protection is in place, e.g. by the use of a prescribed form of contract to govern the transmission of the data.

◆ Subject to some exceptions for organizations that only do very simple processing, and for domestic use, all entities that process personal information must register with the Information Commissioner's Office.

◆ The departments of a company that are holding personal information are required to have adequate security measures in place. Those include technical measures (such as firewalls) and organizational measures (such as staff training).

◆ Subjects have the right to have factually incorrect information corrected (note: this does not extend to matters of opinion).

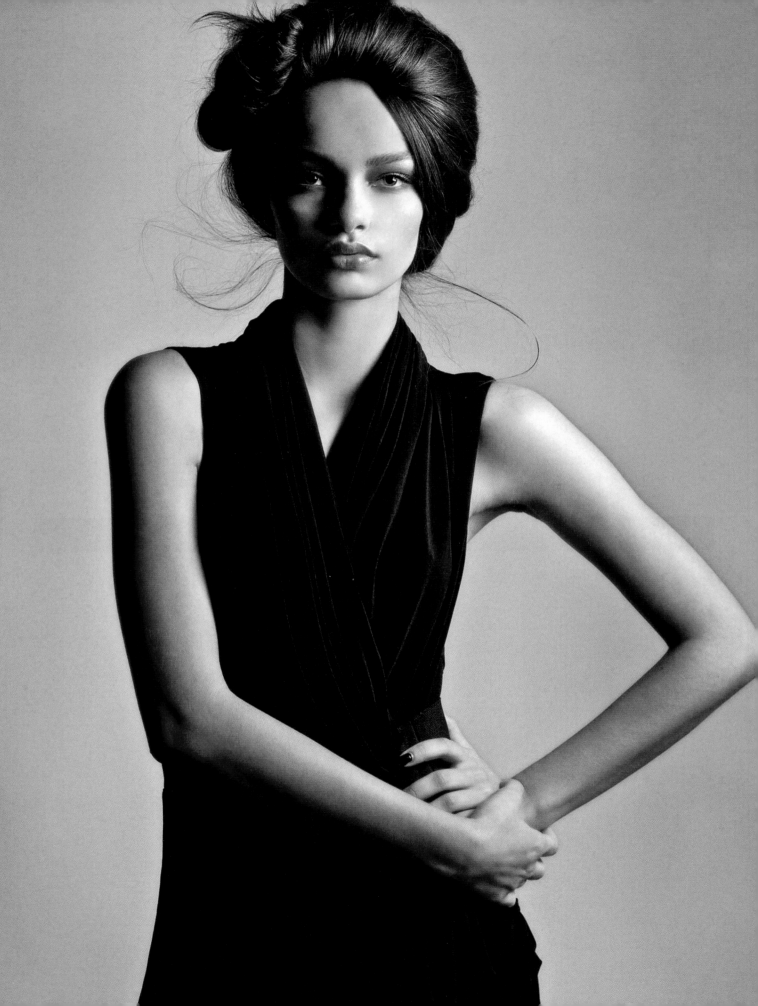

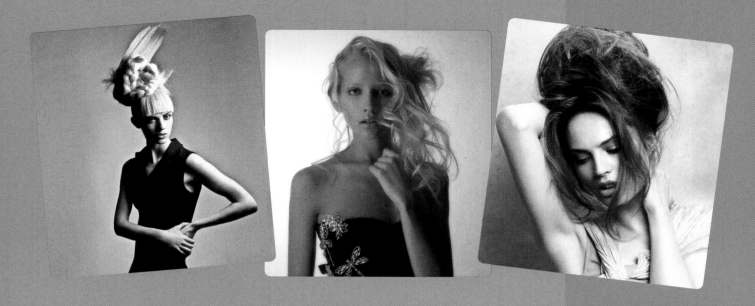

PART TWO

Technical Skills

This section provides you with the knowledge about the practical areas of hairdressing and barbering. Each chapter has a comprehensive format that starts out by telling you what it is about, and then extends to show you the techniques involved and the ways in which you can work to achieve the desired results for the level.

You will also find that many practices are linked in some way to each other, and may therefore benefit from looking at them collectively, and not in isolation. For example, it's one thing creating a beautiful haircut, but without the blow-dry, the client won't be able to see the finished effect.

7 Shampooing and conditioning hair

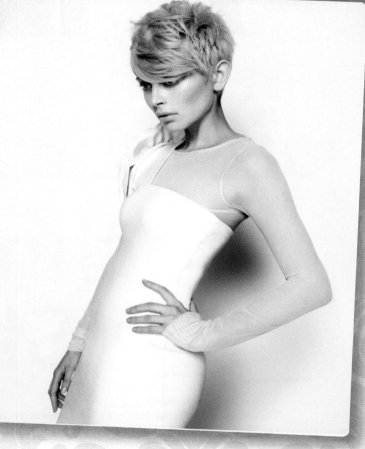

LEARNING OBJECTIVES

◆ Be able to maintain effective and safe methods of working when providing the services

◆ Be able to shampoo the hair and scalp

◆ Be able to condition and treat the hair and scalp

◆ Know how to work safely, effectively and hygienically when providing the services

◆ Understand the basic science for shampooing and conditioning

◆ Know the products and equipment that the salon uses

◆ Know how and when to use a variety of massage techniques for shampooing and conditioning

KEY TERMS

abrasion

aftercare advice

aloe vera (shampoo ingredient)

anti-dandruff treatment

anti-oxidant (conditioner)

camomile (shampoo ingredient)

caustic

cleanser

coarse hair

coconut (shampoo ingredient)

dermis

detergent

disentangling

greasy hair

hard water

hot towels

humectant

hydrophilic

hydrophobic

jojoba (shampoo ingredient)

lemon (shampoo ingredient)

medicated shampoo

microorganisms

mint (shampoo ingredient)

neck wool

oil (shampoo ingredient)

penetrating conditioner

Pityriasis capitis

portfolio

pre-perm treatment

restructurant

root lift mousse

soya (shampoo ingredient)

straighteners (chemical)

surfactant

tea tree oil (shampoo ingredient)

wetting agent

Unit topic

Shampoo, condition and treat hair.

INTRODUCTION

The shampooing and conditioning services are, more often than not, the first of the physical services that a client receives on their visit to a salon. Admittedly, the receptionist will have greeted them and they would have had a consultation with their stylist beforehand. But the impression that they get from services provided by you, at the basin, will have a long, lasting effect.

Quite simply:

◆ If shampooing and conditioning is done properly, the client feels valued and receives a stimulating, therapeutic experience.

◆ If done poorly, the client feels like they are on a production line, being processed by people who have no interest in either them, or their job!

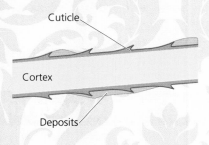

Dirt on hair cuticle

Purposes of shampooing and conditioning hair

Shampooing prepares the hair and skin by:

◆ Removing natural oil, dead skin cells and dirt

◆ Removing the product build-up caused by styling and finishing products

Shampooing and conditioning prepares the hair for:

◆ Further salon services

◆ Further salon treatments

Shampooing and conditioning

PRACTICAL SKILLS

Learn how to prepare the client and yourself

Learn how to recognize hair and scalp conditions, and know their causes

Learn about a range of shampooing and conditioning products and their suitability for your client's hair

Learn how to use a range of shampooing and conditioning products

Learn how to use equipment relevant to the shampooing and conditioning services

Learn how to adapt the massage techniques to suit the client's hair

UNDERPINNING KNOWLEDGE

Preparing and maintaining the work area

Recommending suitable products to the client

Using effleurage, petrissage and rotary massage techniques

Controlling the water pressure and temperature during the service

Disentangling the client's hair in preparation for the next service

Providing suitable aftercare advice

Learn about the pH of shampooing and conditioning products and their effect upon the hair

Learn how the action of shampooing works to cleanse the hair

Effective and safe methods of working

You may not think of shampooing or conditioning being a hazardous service, but like many other processes in hairdressing and barbering, nothing is ever that straightforward.

Think carefully and work safely throughout the process – this will avoid:	
Putting the client at risk from:	◆ Causing pain or injury to their neck by not adjusting the basin to suit their needs.
	◆ Causing back pain or discomfort by not adjusting the basin to suit their needs.
	◆ Burning their scalp by not controlling the water temperature correctly.
	◆ Soaking their clothes by not ensuring that the towel is correctly placed around their neck.
	◆ Staining their clothes by not cleaning the basins properly after chemical processes.
	◆ Cross-infection or cross-infestation from poor hygiene.
	◆ Slipping, from not clearing spilled water or other products.
Putting yourself at risk from:	◆ Causing pain or injury from bad posture; not standing correctly, while you work.
	◆ Developing dermatitis, by not wearing the correct PPE.
	◆ Cross-infection or cross-infestation from poor hygiene.

Cleaning and maintaining the shampoo and conditioning area

You should make sure that you always follow the manufacturer's instructions when handling any chemicals or equipment, as your health and safety and that of your clients, is vitally important. You must remember that shampoos and conditioners are chemicals and you need to wear adequate protection to remove any risk of developing dermatitis.

The wash-point is a very busy area and must be kept clean and tidy at all times. All waste items such as cotton **neck wool**, foils, meche, etc. should be removed from the basins and disposed of in a sealed bin. Used or dirty towels, gowns, plastic capes, etc. need to be removed and put ready for washing in the laundry. Always use the cleaning materials provided by the salon to clean the wash-point areas, this will ensure that only hygienic sprays etc. are used in areas where there is a risk to public health from cross-infection, as bacteria will quickly multiply.

The basins are in continual use and the clients may be coming and going back to these during different services. For example, a client who is having a cut and blow-dry will have their hair washed at the beginning of the services, whereas a client having a colour will arrive at the basin much later in the process. So, with all these different types of services going on, lots of different situations occur. A client who has had a full head colour may have been sat at the basin and the neck part of the basin may have colour stains where they were sat.

The basin and chair must be cleaned before the next client sits there, as it is not only unprofessional, but may even stain their clothes or hair. Always keep a check on the levels of wash-point products and materials too; towels, shampoos and conditioners will get used up and these will need replacing at different times, throughout the day.

BEST PRACTICE

If the shampoo doesn't remove all of the styling products that have been previously applied, they could block products used as part of the next service that you want to carry out. For example, hair wax that is applied on a daily basis will stick to the hair and is difficult to remove.

Prepare the tools, equipment and protective clothing The tools and equipment must be prepared before the client arrives. How do you think you would look to the client if you start running off to find things that you need and they are already sat at the basin? You need to work efficiently and safely at all times and you can only do this if you have made the right preparation beforehand.

Start by collecting all the tools and equipment you are going to need before the client service begins. The tools must be sterilized for each new client and the protective clothing must be fresh and clean for each client. You must check that the basin area where the shampoo services are taking place is clean and tidy and free from hair.

If you are going to do a conditioning treatment you will also need to clean and prepare a trolley and the electrical equipment involved: i.e. Climazone™ or steamer (remembering to refill the header tank with water and clean the inside of the hood). You can then move the equipment to the styling location where the treatment is to be applied.

You will need to prepare the following tools:

Tools & equipment

◆ Detangling combs
◆ Flat, wide tooth brushes
◆ Sectioning clips
◆ Bowls, applicators or brushes.

You will need to prepare the following for the client:

◆ Clean, fresh gowns
◆ Plastic cape
◆ Clean fresh towels

You will need to prepare your:

◆ Disposable non-latex gloves
◆ Plastic apron

You will need to prepare the following equipment:

◆ A trolley
◆ Climazone™
◆ Steamer

Steamer A steamer is a machine that produces **moist** heat instead of **dry** heat. It looks like a portable hood dryer with a water reservoir on the top and the water tank is removable and can be filled with tap water. The tank is replaced into the machine and a heating element boils the water when it is switched on. As the water boils within the machine, the steam travels to the transparent hood part of the steamer. A series of small holes within the lower, rear hood area of the steamer allow steam to emerge and provide a hot, moist heat which is delivered to the person seated beneath.

Moist heat (steam) opens the cuticle more effectively than dry heat, and therefore helps the treatment to penetrate deeper into the hair, which enables it to develop more quickly too.

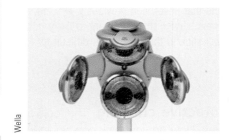

Wella

TOP TIP

Make sure that you match the correct products to the identified hair and scalp conditions. If you use the wrong products, you will probably be making the condition worse than it is. If in doubt, ask someone else.

BEST PRACTICE

If oily deposits remain on hair they may cause a barrier to other chemical processes. If you believe that the client's hair has build-up, you can use a clarifying shampoo as a deep **cleanser** first.

Precautions A steamer is an electrical piece of equipment, so always check the condition of the plug and lead before turning it on. When it is in use, keep an eye on the levels of water within the reservoir and always check with the client to make sure that the temperature is comfortable and not too hot.

The machine can be used for conditioning treatments and some lightening and colouring services, such as highlights and root application oil-based lightening products. When a steamer is used within a lightening service, the moist heat stops the lightening product from drying out too quickly, so keeps it working longer.

Preparation and protection for you and the client The client (and their clothes) must be protected from spills, stains and splashes throughout all the services that they receive in the salon. Their coat, scarves and any other outer garments or unnecessary baggage should be put away safely during salon services. They should be wearing a clean, freshly laundered gown at all times, and as added protection, a fresh clean towel is placed around their shoulders. This can be fixed in position with a sectioning clip so that it doesn't slip or fall away. You should also keep a lookout throughout shampooing and conditioning processes for the position of the towel in relation to the basin and the client's neck. If the towel slips down, then water can seep down the client's neck and wet their clothes.

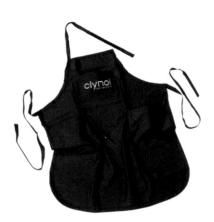 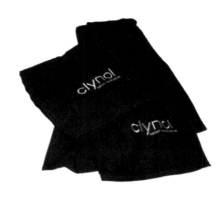

Some services require further protection so you may need to apply a plastic cape over the towel, particularly during chemical services or special conditioning treatments.

It is very important that after sitting the client at the basin, you make sure that they are comfortable and that their back and neck is fully supported by the position that they are in at the basin. When the client is sat correctly, the basin should form a supportive barrier at the nape of the neck that neither pinches, causing discomfort, nor allows water to leak over the rim.

Your salon uniform provides the ideal workwear and basic protection for you, it should be clean and ironed and you should be wearing low-heeled shoes. You should remove any rings and loose fitting or dangling jewellery and your hair needs to be clean and tidy or 'put-up' out of the way.

Your posture is equally important from your safety's point of view too. You should be standing up straight without having to twist, your shoulders should be level and positioned above the torso and hips without having to lean forwards. You need to maintain this posture, otherwise you will be exposing yourself to the risk of injury and longer term back condition or fatigue.

TOP TIP

A pre-treatment conditioner should be used before chemical processes to prepare the hair and even out the porosity of the hair before the process is carried out.

Protective Personal Equipment and relevant services

		Shampooing	Conditioning	Perming	Colouring	Lightening	Relaxing	Extensions
For you	Non-latex gloves	✓	✓	✓	✓	✓	✓	
	Plastic apron		✓	✓	✓	✓	✓	✓
	Uniform and low shoes	✓	✓	✓	✓	✓	✓	✓
For the client	Clean, fresh gown	✓	✓	✓	✓	✓	✓	✓
	Clean, fresh cape	✓	✓	✓				
	Clean, fresh towels	✓	✓	✓	✓	✓	✓	
		✓	✓	✓	✓	✓	✓	✓

For you

- Disposable non-latex gloves

- Shampooing, Conditioning treatments, Perming, Colouring, Lightening, Relaxing,

- Plastic apron

- Conditioning treatments Perming, Colouring, Lightening, Relaxing, Extensions,

- Uniform and (low-heeled) shoes

- Shampooing, Surface conditioning, Conditioning treatments, Perming, Colouring, Lightening, Relaxing, Extensions

For the client

- Clean, fresh (sleeved,) gown

- Shampooing, Conditioning treatments, Setting, Dressing, Cutting, Plaiting, Perming, Colouring, Lightening, Relaxing, Extensions,

- Clean, fresh towels

- Shampooing, Surface conditioning, Conditioning treatments, Perming, Colouring, Lightening, Relaxing,

- Plastic cape

- Conditioning treatments, Perming, Colouring, Lightening, Relaxing, Extensions

TOP TIP

A post-treatment; pH balancing conditioner is used after chemical processes to add shine and return the hair back to its natural pH-balanced state.

Hair and scalp conditions and causes

Clients need products that match the needs of their hair. That may sound obvious, but clients buy products to use at home for many reasons:

◆ They like the smell.

◆ They recognize the brand or manufacturer.

◆ They know who the model or celebrity is who promotes the product in advertising.

◆ The products happened to be on a multi-buy: *buy one get one free*.

◆ They like the packaging.

Do these factors guarantee any success for them?

These should not be the reasons for buying products from supermarkets and chemists, they need solutions to their problems:

◆ Hair condition.

◆ Scalp condition.

◆ Hair type.

◆ Hair texture.

◆ Previous hairdressing services.

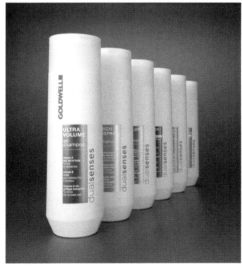

Goldwell

Professional recommendation

This is where you come in. You should be recommending the right product regime, based upon the clients' needs – how it will actually benefit their hair.

The table below looks at a variety of hair and scalp conditions, the possible reasons for those conditions and the main things that need to be addressed in order to correct the problems.

TOP TIP

Dandruff can sometimes in its simplest form be mistaken for a dry scalp. If your client is suffering from dandruff you will need to use an **anti-dandruff treatment**.

Hair condition	Possible reasons for the condition	Corrective action
Dry/porous	◆ Chemical treatments raising cuticle scale – i.e. colouring, perming, lightening, relaxers. ◆ Poor maintenance/handling, heat styling – i.e. **straighteners**, blow-drying, tongs. ◆ Environmental effects – excessive sunlight, wind damage (on longer hair), swimming (from chemicals in swimming pools).	◆ Hair needs lasting moisture from penetrating treatments, cuticle needs sealing/smoothing. ◆ Hair needs moisture and heat protection. ◆ Hair needs protection – from UV rays, from tangling/knotting. ◆ Hair needs demineralizing treatments.
Greasy	◆ Product build up – where subsequent washing is not removing previous styling products from the hair.	◆ Clarifying shampoos that are stronger than frequent use shampoos and will clean the hair.
Normal	◆ Virgin hair, i.e. no chemical services. ◆ Good hair management and correct use of products.	◆ None needed – provide client with recommendations and advice for maintenance.
Damaged	◆ Chemical damage – colouring, perming, lightening, relaxers. ◆ Physical damage – heat styling, i.e. straighteners, blow-drying, tongs, rough handling, i.e. brushing and combing, hair getting caught in clothing.	◆ Hair needs lasting moisture from penetrating treatments. ◆ Hair needs heat protection and strengthening treatments.
Scalp condition	**Possible reasons for the condition**	**Corrective action**
Greasy	◆ Overactive sebaceous glands.	◆ Scalp treatments to reduce natural oils. ◆ Shampoos for **greasy hair**/scalp.
Dry	◆ Overproduction of epidermal skin cells – i.e. dandruff/psoriasis. ◆ Reaction to chemical services changing skin pH – i.e. colouring, perming, lightening, relaxers.	◆ Scalp treatments to treat dandruff and/or infections. ◆ pH balancing and moisturizing scalp treatments.

BEST PRACTICE

When treating conditions of very oily scalps or dandruff, it is best to try one product at a time, giving it the full opportunity to do its job. It is all too easy to give up on a new introduction before it has had time to make a difference.

Shampoos

Shampoos have a variety of properties, like their *features*: i.e. the smell, the packaging, the frequency and ease of use. Then there are the *benefits* and more importantly, how they will actually help the client.

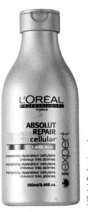

L'Oréal Professionnel

All shampoos have something in common and combine two main properties:

◆ A shampoo base – a chemical formulation that makes it work.

◆ Natural essences or oils – that provide specific benefits to the hair.

The **shampoo base** relates to a variety of chemicals that:

◆ Contain a foaming agent that will create a lather.

◆ Contain **detergent** that will clean the hair.

◆ Prevent 'sludge' occurring when grease and dirt is emulsified in water.

◆ Rinse away easily in water without creating a scum.

◆ Contain preservatives and stabilizers that provide a long and safe period of use when opened.

Typical ingredients of a shampoo base

Water – for suspending the following chemicals in solution.

Sodium Laureth Sulfate* (S.L.S.) – a detergent that cleans the hair by removing dirt and grease.

Cocamide DEA * – a foaming agent that creates a lather.

Cocamidopropyl Betaine * – a mild **surfactant** that reduces the irritation of stronger detergents (Sodium laureth Sulfate) and provides anti-static control.

Sodium Chloride – natural salt for softening water.

DMDM Hydantoin * – a preservative that controls/prevents growth of **microorganisms**.

Citric acid – a mild acid that helps to *soften* water.

Tetrasodium EDTA – stabilizing agent, reduces lime scale.

Note: The chemicals marked with an * are known allergens and may cause contact dermatitis.

BEST PRACTICE

At the end of the process you need to update all treatment records, including what shampoos and conditioners were used, for future purposes.

The **natural ingredients** in a shampoo are the components that provide the benefits to the client's hair: Henna, **camomile**, rosemary, **jojoba**, **aloe vera** and **mint** are just a few typical varieties available in the supermarkets today.

Choosing the right shampoo for the client's hair condition or for following a chemical service is important. If the wrong choice is made the hair may become difficult to manage afterwards and may become brittle, flyaway (static), oily or even dry.

Different types of shampoo

Shampoo ingredients	Benefits to the hair	Suitable for
Tea tree oil	A natural essential oil which is like an antiseptic and which will fight infections on the scalp.	Anti-bacterial/Dandruff
Medicated shampoo	Helps to maintain the normal state of the hair and scalp: contains antiseptics such as juniper or tea tree oil.	Dandruff
Jojoba	A natural base that is better on normal to dryer hair types.	Dry
Nut oils	Can contain a range of natural nut oils such as pine, palm, almond: these are used to smooth and soften dryer hair and scalps.	Dry
Coconut	Contains an emollient which helps dry hair to regain its smoothness and elasticity.	Dry/Coarser hair
Beer	Helps to provide body and shine to finer hair types.	Fine hair/Normal
Camomile	Better on oily scalps; has a natural lightening effect.	Greasy
Mint	A natural base suited to normal to slightly oily scalps, often used as a frequent use shampoo.	Greasy
Clarifying	Strong, deep-acting, often used prior to chemical services to remove build-up of styling products and dirt.	Greasy/build-up
Egg and lemon	Contains citric acid; ideal for sensitive scalp types.	Mild greasiness/Sensitive scalps
Aloe vera	A popular, mild, natural base ideal for healthy hair and scalps that can be used on a frequent basis.	Normal
Soya	Helps to lock in moisture for the hair and scalp.	Normal/Dry

Making the right choices about shampoos

HEALTH & SAFETY

Some injuries or neck complaints prevent the client from lying back at the basin. Ask your client if they have reasons for not lying backwards.

Making the right choices	
Texture, amount and condition of hair	◆ *Fine hair* (without product build-up) requires a single wash shampoo that will not make it too dry or fluffy. Choose a shampoo that will add body and volume.
	◆ **Coarse hair** usually requires two washes with a shampoo that will tend to soften it and make it more pliable.
	◆ *Thicker hair* usually requires two washes with shampoo that will penetrate and make good contact with all the hair and scalp.
Frequency of shampooing	◆ If hair is washed once or more daily, choose a shampoo specially designed for frequent use.

(Continued)

(Continued)

Making the right choices	
Water quality	◆ If the water in the salon is in a **hard water** area, more shampoo is needed to form a good lather. ◆ In soft water areas shampoos foam more easily, so less shampoo is required to do the job.
Shampoo purpose	◆ Is the shampoo intended just for cleaning the hair? ◆ Is it to treat the scalp, or condition the hair? ◆ Is it to follow on from a colouring of the hair?
Planned services	◆ What are you going to do with the hair later? Some shampoo ingredients (Pro V or dimethicone) produce a flexible coating on the hair shaft. This could be beneficial in adding protection and locking in moisture or, conversely, in the case of conditioning-type shampoos and most conditioners, it could prevent or prolong the processing of some treatments such as perms.

Planning your day

At the beginning of the day
Collect and put ready clean, laundered towels and gowns
Clean and prepare combs, brushes and electrical equipment
Clean and prepare the basins and seating
Top-up the products

Throughout the day
Clean and prepare the basins for the next client
Clean the combs, brushes bowls, etc.
Check stock levels; towels, gowns, shampoo and conditioners
Top-up the products as and when necessary

Replenishing and reordering stock

Although the basins are constantly in use, you will need to keep an eye on the items that will be needed by everyone throughout the day. As more clients are shampooed and conditioned, the more those things will run out. You will need to make sure that there are plenty of clean gowns and towels close at hand and that the products are replaced when they are running low.

In a college salon, the products are 'topped-up' in the dispensary. Shampoo dispensers can be cleaned and the pump tops can be rinsed in water. A funnel helps to refill each empty bottle from the 'bulk' supplies without spilling or wasting any. The pump tops are replaced and they can be taken back to the basin area.

If during stock replenishment you notice that the bulk items are running low, you should make sure that they get replaced in time, without any disruption to normal services.

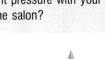

ACTIVITY

Hard, scratching and circulatory massage movements are uncomfortable for the client. Why not practise the right pressure with your colleagues at the salon?

BEST PRACTICE

Always record the products that you have used on the client's record card so that they can be charged for and used again in the future.

You need to make sure that all relevant records and stock systems are updated to avoid products being *out-of-stock*.

Completing client records All salons have some form of client service records and conditioning treatments are just one of many services that need to be monitored by management. You need to make sure that every client's record is updated accurately and efficiently after the treatment has been provided.

When should this be done? Client records are always updated at the end of the process and you will need to record all treatments or services provided, including the products that were used.

If you think of the normal repeat intervals for clients being at least six weeks, it will be impossible to remember what was used on their last visit, and next time, some other member of the team may be conducting the wash-point operations. What if the client asks for the same treatment as last time? The first person they will approach is you, because the client will say: *'Jenny did it last time'.*

Remember, without accurate up-to-date information the business will not be able to:

◆ Provide a consistent service to the client next time they visit.

◆ Recognize patterns of business for product sales or promotions.

◆ Manage the stock control and replenishment so efficiently.

BEST PRACTICE

Shampooing dos and don'ts:
◆ Always use clean, fresh towels and gowns.
◆ Make sure that your hands and nails are hygienic and clean.
◆ Wear non-latex disposable gloves.
◆ Avoid splashing water or shampoo lather onto the client's face or near their eyes as the chemicals will cause discomfort if not injury.
◆ Always keep your hand in contact with the water while rinsing so that you can detect any sudden change in its temperature.
◆ Always direct the water spray away from the hairlines and into the basin.
◆ Carefully comb the hair after shampooing to remove any tangles.
◆ After using the basin, always clear and clean the area before it is used again.
◆ Turn off the water in-between shampoos and conditioning to avoid wastage.
◆ Rinse and dry your hands afterwards to remove any shampoo or conditioning chemicals and reapply a barrier cream.

How does shampoo work?

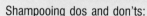

All shampoos contain a mild detergent which is the cleaning agent in a shampoo. The detergent is also a **wetting agent** and this helps to spread the water through even the thickest hair. However, a detergent on its own will not lather, so a foaming agent is included in the solution to produce a good lather and keep the detergent in close contact with the hair and skin.

Hydrophylic head
(Negative charge)

Hydrophobic tail

Detergent molecule

Detergent is a *'polar'* molecule with two opposing ends. One end is **hydrophilic** (i.e. water-loving) and the other is **hydrophobic** (water-hating). These produce a hydrophilic head and a hydrophobic tail. When detergent is introduced to hair during the action of shampooing the *water-hating* hydrophobic end penetrates the grease on the hair and the *water-loving* hydrophilic end is attracted to the water. The *surface tension* of the dirt and grease (i.e. the ability of the grease to stick to a surface) is broken and the grease rolls up into a globule and is lifted away from the surface of the hair. It is then suspended in the water as an emulsion. The *oil-in-water* emulsion containing the dirt is rinsed away with water, leaving the hair clean.

Detergent surrounding grease

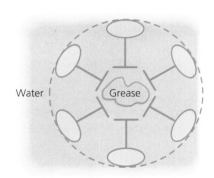

Water

Grease

Conditioners

Conditioning is a vital part of maintaining the health, look, feel and handling properties of the hair. We see the benefits of conditioning in the way that it improves the visual appearance of hair, i.e. by adding shine and revealing the beautiful colours. Also in physical ways: by having good elasticity and flexibility. These are the main factors that affect style durability and manageability. Quite simply, if we can maintain the condition of our clients' hair, then they will be able to look after it and manage it too.

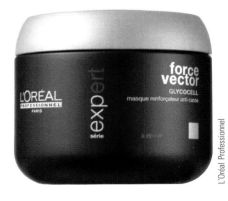

L'Oréal Professionnel

Other people will notice the quality of our clients' hair and ask them where they had it done. This recommendation is good for business and your reputation too!

Like shampoos, conditioners have two main properties:

◆ A conditioner base – a chemical formulation that makes it work.

◆ Natural essences or oils – that provide specific benefits to the hair.

Typical ingredients of a conditioner base
Water – for suspending the following chemicals in solution.
Cetyl Alcohol – an emollient and thickener for conditioning bases.
Stearyl Alcohol – an emollient that will coat and smooth the cuticle.
PEG-40 – a spreading agent that will disperse the chemicals evenly along the hair.
DMDM Hydantoin* – a preservative that controls/prevents growth of microorganisms.
Stearalkonium Chloride – anti-static agent, prevents flyaway hair.
Cetrimonium Chloride – antiseptic conditioning agent.
Note: The items marked * are known allergens and may cause contact dermatitis.

The **conditioner base** relates to a variety of chemicals that:

◆ Contain moisturizing emollients that will fill and smooth raised cuticles.

◆ Contain dispersants that will allow conditioning agents to spread evenly along the hair.

◆ Contain antiseptic properties inhibiting the growth of microorganisms.

Again, like shampoos, the **natural ingredients** are the components in a conditioner that provide the benefits to the client's hair: e.g. Henna, camomile, rosemary, jojoba, aloe vera and mint are just a few typical varieties available in the supermarkets today.

Go to shampoo ingredients on p. 198 to find out more about the benefits of natural ingredients.

How do conditioners work?

Conditioners use a combination of chemical and electrical (ionic charged) properties to achieve their effects. They can balance and counteract the effects that the chemical services and physical processes have upon the hair. There are two ways in which they bond with the hair:

◆ *Absorption* – This relies upon the natural state of the hair. Dry and porous hair has many tiny spaces within the hair's internal structure. These areas suck in the conditioning agents by capillary action, just as water is drawn into a sponge.

◆ *Attraction* – This occurs after the hair has been shampooed. The action of the detergent on the hair during shampooing ensures that all product, dirt and dust are removed. When these particles are removed it leaves the surface of the hair in a 'charged' state. This prepares the hair for the conditioner which is now attracted to the sites upon the hair that have been electrically charged. (This ionic attraction principle can be explained another way. Do you remember how you stick balloons to the wall or ceiling at a birthday party? After blowing the balloons up, you rub them vigorously on the sleeve of your jumper. This removes electrical particles and now makes the balloon stick to anything it comes into contact with, just like a magnet!)

BEST PRACTICE

If your client is in the habit of washing their hair every day advise them to use a mild frequent use shampoo. Anything else may be too strong or may create a build-up with regular use.

Different types of conditioner

There are three different types of hair conditioners:

◆ Surface conditioners.

◆ **Penetrating conditioners**.

◆ Scalp treatments.

Type of conditioner	How they act upon/within the hair	Typical ingredients
Surface conditioners *L'Oréal Professionnel*	These conditioners remain on the cuticle surface. Their main purpose is to coat the hair and improve the look and feel by adding shine and moisture. Some of these conditioning rinses are used after perms and chemical straighteners to return the hair back to its natural pH balance.	◆ Vegetable and mineral oils. ◆ Silicone. ◆ Fats and waxes. ◆ **Anti-oxidants** – rebalance the hair to pH 5.6 and close the cuticle. Often citric, or acetic-acid based.
Penetrating conditioners *Goldwell*	They enter the hair shaft through the cuticle layer and are deposited into the cortex by capillary action. This suction of the product is like a natural magnetism, drawing the product in to the cellular spaces within the hair. These penetrating conditioners, often called **restructurants**, are designed to repair the physical structure of the fibres within the cortex and damaged areas within the cuticle layers. Apart from smoothing the hair and adding shine, they tend to make the whole hair structure much stronger.	◆ Proteins – amino acids. ◆ **Humectants**, which lock in moisture to the hair. ◆ Emollients, which soften, smooth and moisturize and add shine to the hair. ◆ Chemical strengtheners which can make the cortex stronger.
Scalp treatments *L'Oréal Professionnel*	These are scalp-active treatments that are chemical preparations specifically developed to target disorders such as: ◆ Greasiness. ◆ Dandruff. ◆ Hair loss.	◆ Astringents and medicated, Tea tree oil. ◆ Zinc Pyrithone, Selenium, Coal tar. ◆ Monoxidil.

Pre-treatments and post-treatments Where the cuticle has been damaged, the hair cortex becomes more porous, like a sponge soaking up any chemicals applied to the hair. Older hair is more likely to be damaged than newer growth. The

HEALTH & SAFETY

Always report blocked pipes or basins immediately. Bacteria quickly contaminate standing waste water and it has an unpleasant smell too!

HEALTH & SAFETY

Steamers: Steam will only be produced when water is boiled at 100° centigrade. Therefore the moist heat can be very hot if the steamer is left unattended. Always check with the client to make sure that the equipment is not too hot.

HEALTH & SAFETY

If you do use the hot towel method for developing a treatment, always check that the temperature of the damp towel is not too hot, or that excess moisture is not dripping from it. The towel must be damp, but not wet.

porosity must be reduced and evened out along the hair shaft, before hair can be successfully permed or coloured. Pre-straighteners or **pre-perm treatments** will balance the porosity evenly through the hair. This enables the chemical service to be carried out in the confidence that no parts of the hair will be unduly damaged through the action of additional chemical application.

The pre-colouring treatments have a similar effect. These products will 'fill' the damaged sites along the hair shaft, repairing the cuticle layer and maintaining an even absorption, i.e. the 'take-up', of colouring products into the cortex.

After chemical services the hair may need rebalancing with a post-colour or perming treatment. The normal state of hair is slightly acidic (pH 5.6) and many of the processes use **caustic** – ammonium-based compounds – or corrosive – acid-based compounds. In these situations it is always advisable to use an *acid-balancing conditioner*. Acid-balancing conditioners will act either as an anti-oxidant (to remove unwanted 'free oxygen', which may be left in the hair after using hydrogen peroxide in operations such as neutralizing, colouring and lightening) or to reduce the alkaline state of hair with mild acidic compounds following perming and straightening.

What are the benefits of using conditioners? Professional products are formulated to protect and improve a range of different hair types and disorders.

The main benefits from using conditioners

◆ Smooths the cuticle edges.

◆ Improves handling and combing when the hair is both wet and dry.

◆ Temporarily repairs and fills damaged sites along the hair shaft or missing areas of the cuticle or cortex.

◆ Provides shine, lustre and sheen.

◆ Creates flexibility and movement by locking in moisture.

◆ Balances the pH value of the hair back to a slightly acid 5.5.

Scalp treatments

Dry scalps Dry scalps can often be mistaken for dandruff. A dry scalp has some of the symptoms of dandruff, such as flaking on the surface of the epidermis, but if wrongly diagnosed, the corrective treatment may make the problem worse. A dry scalp can occur for a number of reasons.

It may be from:

◆ A natural moisture imbalance within the client's skin.

◆ A reaction to unsuitable shampoos or styling products.

◆ A reaction or sensitivity to chemical services – colouring, perming, etc.

A dry skin condition is often a long-term problem; you should recommend a scalp-active treatment that will nourish and moisturize the scalp and that can be followed up, by the client, at home. The type of treatment will depend upon the condition of the hair too. If the client has a dry scalp it doesn't necessarily follow that the hair will be dry too. This will have a bearing on how the treatment is to be applied. If the hair is normal and healthy, you would not want to overload it with heavy moisturizers and emollients, so a 'lighter' treatment may be more suitable.

You will need to explain to the client that application has a lot to do with achieving a successful result. The product must target the problem and the hair will need to be divided and applied to the scalp, rather than just spread over their hair.

Dry scalps can occur from intolerance to hairdressing products. A client can get a reaction when they use something different on their hair. Ask them whether they have tried something new. A typical cause would be newly introduced styling and finishing products such as **root lift mousse** or heavy definition waxes. However, even a simple change of shampoo can cause dryness.

A dry scalp can also occur after chemical treatments. Many of the solutions we use in hairdressing have a quenching effect upon the skin. Alkaline solutions create this continual drying 'thirst' upon the scalp, so this is particularly relevant to perming and chemical straighteners. However, a reaction can be caused by any exposure to chemicals and you can prevent this by taking particular care when you apply any chemical service to the client.

Dandruff

Dandruff can sometimes in its simplest form be mistaken for a dry scalp. Unfortunately, if you wrongly diagnose this condition, you will either make the problem worse or have no effect at all.

Normally, the skin cells produced in the lower **dermis** take up to 30–45 days to work up through to the surface of the epidermis. Once there, the cells shed daily in the form of a fine visible dust. In the case of dandruff, though, this process becomes erratic.

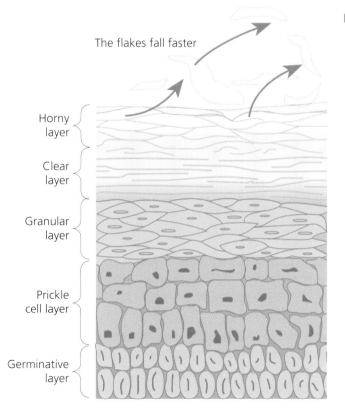

Diagram of shedding skin

The flakes fall faster

Horny layer

Clear layer

Granular layer

Prickle cell layer

Germinative layer

In the diagram you can see that, as the cells in the lower layers of the epidermis work up towards the surface layers of the epidermis, they eventually 'lift' and come away as 'shedding'. This is commonly noticeable as 'scurf', white skin cells, when you brush or comb the client's hair. More often, it appears on their clothes.

Dandruff or **Pityriasis capitis** is caused by the overproduction of skin cells. It initially appears as small white flakes that loosen and continually shed from the scalp, rather as is the case with dry skin. A secondary condition occurs if the problem isn't rectified: the scalp becomes infected by bacteria and larger yellower, waxy flakes now appear that usually stick to the scalp. When dandruff has progressed to this stage, you often smell it too! This condition is often more prevalent in people with oilier scalps.

In tackling this problem in its earliest stages, you should ask the client if they have or have had a dry skin condition. If they say no, then the scurf is probably due to this skin production imbalance. This can be rectified over a period of time by regular home use of the correct shampoos and conditioners.

If the dandruff has progressed to the second stage, it must be treated initially in the salon, and then with a follow-up at home over a longer period in time. The first objective would be to combat the bacterial infection, then to clear the scalp of the scaly build-up. This degree of infection cannot be rectified by one scalp-active application. It will usually involve a course of treatments often in liquid forms applied onto pre-sectioned hair, directly onto the infected areas.

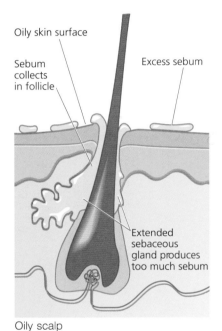

Oily skin surface

Sebum collects in follicle

Excess sebum

Extended sebaceous gland produces too much sebum

Oily scalp

Oily scalps

Oily scalps   An oily scalp, or 'seborrhoea', is caused by overproduction of natural oil (sebum) from the skin. The sebaceous gland in a normal state produces moderate amounts of oil, which is generally sufficient to lubricate the hair shaft and create natural moisture for the skin. This moisture, in turn, keeps the skin supple and helps to 'lock in' flexibility and elasticity. When the glands work overtime, then the imbalance of moisture becomes a nuisance. This is seen as excessively greasy hair and scalps that require frequent washing to give lank hair volume and body.

The normal approach to combating oily scalps is to shampoo it every day. When a client is asked how often they wash their hair and they give the answer 'at least once a day', there is a strong likelihood that there's a reason behind it. Sometimes people wash their hair every day because they fall into the routine of doing it when they take a shower. This is particularly obvious if they have easy-to-manage hair styles, their lifestyle dictates it or they just have short hair.

pH and the effects of alkaline and acidic compounds on the hair and skin

The normal pH of the hair and the skin's surface is 5.5. This is referred to as the skin's 'acid mantle'. The acidity is due in part to the sebum, the natural oil produced by the skin. Sebum production is an important skin function. Skin protects the underlying tissue, acting as a barrier – it prevents liquid loss from inside and keeps excess liquid outside the body. It also protects the body from infection. An acid skin surface inhibits, i.e. slows down, the growth of bacteria and makes them less likely to enter the skin. If the acidity of the skin is reduced and rises above pH 5.6 infection is more likely to occur.

Hairdressing procedures can affect this natural equilibrium, so pH-balancing products are used after perming and straightening, to return the skin to the natural acid mantle.

TOP TIP

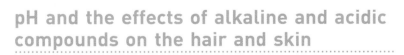

Effleurage is a smooth, soothing stroking action, performed with firm but gentle movements of the hands. You should use it before and after the more vigorous movements. It improves skin functions, soothes and stimulates nerves and relaxes tensed muscles.

Effects of alkaline acidic products

Alkaline products	Acid products
◆ Swell the cuticle. ◆ Enables products to penetrate deeper into the cortex.	◆ Close raised cuticle scales – make hair smoother. ◆ Restore hair to a natural pH after chemical treatments. ◆ Help to lock-in moisture.

Substance	pH value
Acid	0.1–6.9
Alkali	7.1–14.0
Neutral solutions	7.0
Normal hair and scalp	5.0–5.6
pH balanced shampoos and conditioners	5.6

Following manufacturers' instructions Always read the manufacturer's instructions on the bottle, or its packaging or any supplied information contained with it on a leaflet, etc. This will ensure a successful service and allows the product to achieve its optimum performance. Remember that the storage conditions, i.e. temperature, location, light, may have an effect on the life of the product.

If you fail to follow these instructions, it could lead to legal action against the salon.

Shampooing and conditioning step by step techniques

Shampooing

Shampooing is supposed to be a therapeutic service. In other words it is a calming, beneficial and relaxing service. So bearing this in mind, we can look at the process and the effects of the massage techniques and water temperature upon the client.

Effleurage This is the first and last massage technique – used in both shampooing and conditioning. It uses the palms of the hand to apply an even pressure across the head in a stroking, smoothing action when shampoo or conditioner is applied to the hair.

The technique is started at the centre of the hairline above the forehead, with the palms of the hand. The hands move slowly backwards towards the crown area and then down

TOP TIP

Petrissage is a deeper, circular, kneading movement. It assists the removal of waste build-up and promotes the flow of nutrients to the skin. It is normally used in conditioning and hand scalp massage.

TOP TIP

Always spread the product evenly between the palms of the hands before applying it to the client's hair.

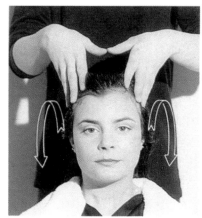
Effleurage

to the nape of the neck. They are then brought upwards around the sides towards the sides of the head – above the ears and then again backwards towards to the nape. The same process is repeated several times to makes sure that the product is evenly applied over the head and that pressure and contact is maintained throughout.

Rotary Rotary massage is used during the shampooing process to provide a therapeutic massage and to clean the hair. It is done with the hands in a loose 'claw' shape – where the pads of the fingers make contact with the head. The massage starts at the front hairline with hands balancing the pressure evenly on both sides. The fingers remain in contact with the head throughout the process, and as the massage continues the fingers work in a circulatory movement over the scalp. Similarly to effleurage, the fingers work backwards to the crown and down into the nape, then up around the sides of the head, to the temporal area and back up to the front. The process is repeated several times before the lather is rinsed from the hair.

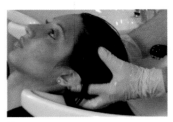

Rotatary

In situations where:

◆ The hair has product build up;

◆ Is dirty or greasy;

◆ Is very thick;

◆ Or in areas of *hard* water,

it may be advisable to provide a second shampoo.

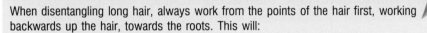

BEST PRACTICE

When disentangling long hair, always work from the points of the hair first, working backwards up the hair, towards the roots. This will:

◆ Make combing far easier and quicker.
◆ Eliminate harsh, painful pulling.
◆ Reduce tearing and further damage to the hair.
◆ Minimize any discomfort to the client.

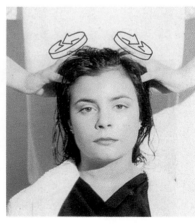

Petrissage

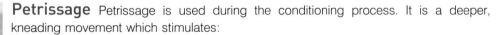

Petrissage Petrissage is used during the conditioning process. It is a deeper, kneading movement which stimulates:

◆ The sebaceous glands – to secrete the natural oil sebum.

◆ The blood supply – promoting the delivery of nutrients to the dermal papilla.

It also relieves the stress and tension of a tight scalp by relaxing the muscles that cover the cranium. Petrissage requires a firmer application of pressure than rotary and this can be achieved by keeping the elbows out, in - line with each other, at either side of the head. The massage starts as a very slow, circular movement that 'picks up' and gently squeezes in a kneading action, the flesh across the scalp. Similar to the other two techniques, the fingers work backwards from the frontal area, back across to the crown, down into the nape and forwards again around the sides of the head. The process is slower and firmer and provides a relaxing end to the conditioning treatment.

Contra-indications to massage

Do not provide scalp massage if:

◆ There are any cuts or **abrasions** on the scalp.

◆ The client feels unwell or has a headache.

◆ The client has oily scalp/hair – as this will encourage more oil to be produced.

◆ The client has infections or infestations.

BEST PRACTICE

After completing the shampooing and conditioning treatments you should provide the client with some recommendations on how they can manage their hair themselves.

Water and its effects on the hair and scalp You must control the temperature and pressure of the water throughout the shampooing and conditioning processes.

Remember the effects of water	
Test the water temperature	◆ Do this at several points throughout the service to ensure that the water is neither too hot nor too cold for the client. ◆ Do this by directing the water spray onto your wrist to test the temperature. ◆ Ask the client if the water temperature suits them – different people like different temperatures.
Adjust the water pressure	◆ Make sure that the pressure is correct and doesn't splash the client throughout rinsing and damping.
Cool water	◆ Closes the cuticle scale and makes the hair shinier. ◆ Causes discomfort to some clients. ◆ Can be invigorating as a final rinse for those that like it. ◆ Can be soothing on some conditions like dandruff.
Cold water	◆ Causes discomfort to some clients.
Warm water	◆ Opens the cuticle – allows products to penetrate further.
Hot water	◆ Will burn the client's scalp. ◆ Will stimulate the sebaceous glands, making the hair greasier.

Massage techniques of shampooing and conditioning

Massage technique	Used during	Description	Remember
Effleurage	Shampooing Conditioning	A smooth, soothing, stroking action used during the application of product.	◆ Take care with damaged hair, could make problem worse.
Rotary	Shampooing	A relatively firm, stimulating, circular movement using the pads of fingers. This agitates the detergent, produces lather and removes dirt/grease.	◆ May cause long hair to tangle ◆ Use firmer rotary on thick hair and lighter rotary on finer types. ◆ Use lighter rotary on greasy scalps, can make it worse. ◆ Use former rotary on dry to stimulate oil glands.
Petrissage	Conditioning	A slow, kneading action using the fingertips on the scalp. Can be done as a gentle or firm massage but is applied with an even pressure to produce a rotating and rhythmic sequence.	◆ Use lighter rotary on greasy scalps, could make it worse. ◆ Use firmer rotary on dry to stimulate oil glands.

CourseMate video: Shampoo and Condition

TOP TIP

Always use a wide tooth comb for detangling hair.

STEP-BY-STEP: SHAMPOOING TECHNIQUE

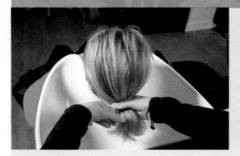

1 Prepare the client with a clean, fresh gown and towel.

Sit the client at the basin and detangle their hair.

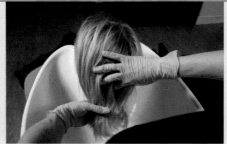

2 Loosen the lengths and make sure that all the hair is in the basin and none is caught around the nape area.

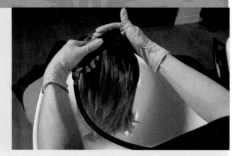

3 Check and adjust the water pressure and temperature. Ask the client if it is OK.

Create a shield with one hand and dampen the hair working from the front to the back.

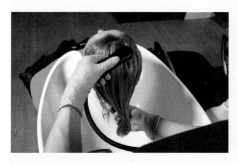

4 Ensure that all the hair is wet.

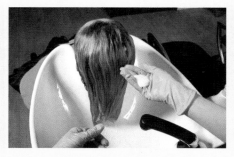

5 Select the correct shampoo for the client's hair, then apply a small amount from the dispenser to the palm of your hand.

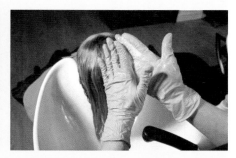

6 Spread evenly over your hands.

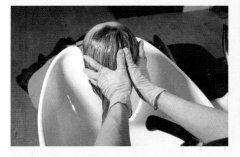

7 Apply the shampoo evenly to the hair with effleurage.

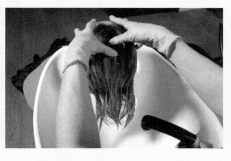

8 Start the rotary massage technique at the front with your hands in a 'claw like' position.

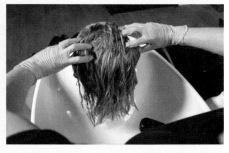

9 Gently move your fingers in circulatory movement around the head.

Ask the client how firm a pressure they would like.

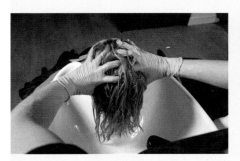

10 Work from the front, over the top, over the crown, down to the back of the head and then around to the sides.

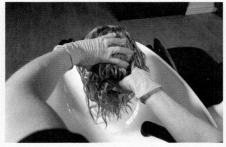

11 Work from the front, over the top, over the crown, down to the back of the head and then around to the sides.

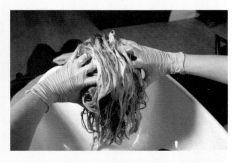

12 Work the massage until a lather increases, this will show that the hair is being cleansed.

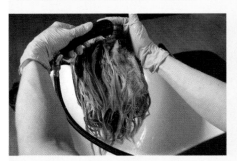

13 After shampooing, recheck the water temperature and pressure and rinse the lather away.

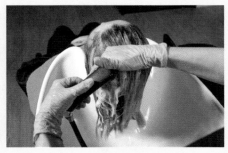

14 Repeat the whole process if a second shampoo is required.

Normally on short hair one shampoo will do and take around five minutes.

Longer hair will need a second shampoo and take proportionally longer.

Conditioning

Each conditioning treatment is specific to the task in hand. It is therefore extremely important to follow the manufacturer's instructions so that the product can do its job. Some (like a dandruff treatment) require the hair to be divided and lotions to be applied directly to the scalp. Others require heat assisted from **hot towels** or a steamer for deeper penetration into more damaged types of hair.

STEP-BY-STEP: CONDITIONING TECHNIQUE

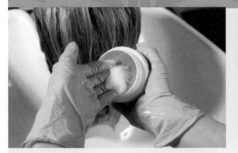

1 After shampooing, remove the excess moisture from the hair and take a small amount of the treatment.

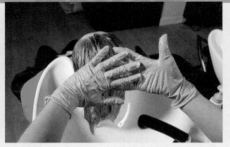

2 Spread the hair treatment evenly between your hands.

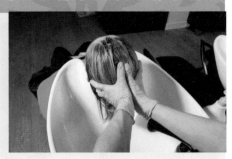

3 Apply the treatment to the hair evenly using effleurage.

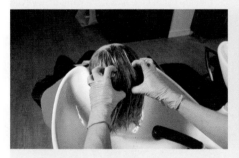

4 Now using deeper stroking movements – draw the treatment through the underlying sections of hair to ensure a comprehensive coverage.

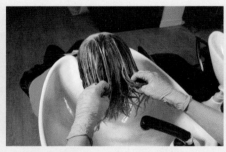

5 Use effleurage to massage the treatment into the hair.

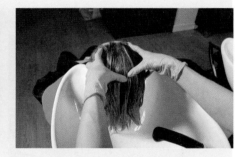

6 Remember that the treatment is a therapeutic service – with the product evenly applied, now work with petrissage movements from the frontal area.

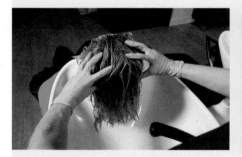

7 Over the top towards the crown.

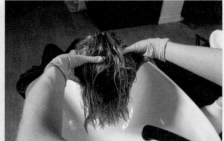

8 Then, back around the ears – through to the nape of the neck.
Repeat this sequence 6, 7 and 8 several times.

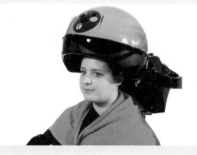

8a Note* If the treatment needs to be developed with the aid of a steamer, move the client to a styling section to allow for full processing.

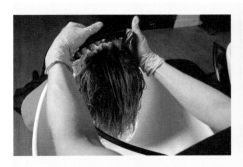

9 When the processing is complete – rinse away the excess at the basin.

Remember to shield the client's hairline to avoid splashing their face.

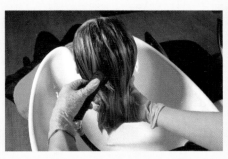

10 Rinse until the hair feels clean.

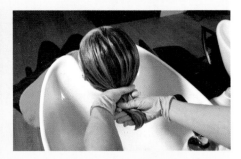

11 After thorough rinsing – carefully squeeze out the excess.

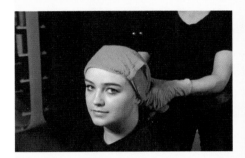

12 Carefully envelop the hair in a clean towel and move the client to the styling section for further services.

Applying treatments

Step-by-Step: Hair and Scalp Treatments The following sequence provides guidelines for applying scalp tonics or hair treatments.

1 Prepare electrical equipment and (for steamer) fill reservoir with tap water. Plug in appliance and pre-heat machine to warm up ready for the treatment. Prepare the trolley with the selected treatment, sectioning clips and comb.

2 After shampooing at the basin, squeeze out excess moisture from the hair. Disentangle with a wide-toothed comb and wrap a clean towel around the client's hair. Secure with a sectioning clip.

3 Move the client to the prepared workstation.

4 Place another towel around the client's shoulder and secure with a clip. Over this place a plastic cape around the client's shoulders and secure. Take down the towel around the hair and separate the lengths.

5 Separate the hair into a 'hot-cross-bun' – then on longer hair – apply the treatment from roots to ends with a brush, working through the four quadrants in small horizontal sections.

6   If the treatment is a scalp application, you will need to separate each section and apply the treatment directly to the required area.

7   When all of the hair (or scalp) has been evenly treated, remove any excess.

8   If required by the manufacturer, start petrissage movements over the scalp from the frontal area, over the top and down through to the nape. Repeat this circular process several times. (If a scalp treatment go to step 10.)

9   Using a wide-toothed conditioning comb, start disentangling the hair once again, working at the points of the hair first and then gradually working a little further up the hair, until the hair can be combed easily from roots to ends.

10 Now move the steamer into position and check the temperature and water reservoir, before positioning the hood over the client's hair. Note that on longer hair you may need to fasten the hair loosely, so that all the hair can benefit from the moist, penetrating heat.

11 Develop the treatment for the recommended time.

12 Finally, remove the steamer hood and switch off the machine. Move the client back to the basin and remove the traces of unabsorbed treatment following the manufacturer's instructions.

13 Move the client to a clean workstation and proceed to disentangle and prepare the hair for the next service.

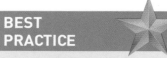

BEST PRACTICE

Always update the client's record immediately after the service.

Detangling the hair

After the shampoo and conditioning process the client is moved back to the workstation. Their towel can be removed and the excess moisture is gently squeezed into the towel so that the hair remains moist but not dripping wet. Then, another clean dry towel can be placed around the shoulders and the client's hair can be loosely separated with your fingers.

Finally, taking a wide-toothed detangling comb, you can detangle the hair in preparation for the next service. If the client's hair is short, it should comb through quite easily. However, if the client has longer hair, you should start combing through nearer the ends of the hair and then carefully work back up the hair until it can all be combed through without tangling.

Conversely, if you were to start combing nearer the scalp, the wet hair will knot and you could be causing damage to the cuticle layer as well as causing the client a lot of pain.

Aftercare advice

After completing the shampooing and conditioning treatments, you should provide the client with some recommendations on how they can manage their hair themselves.

You need to tell them about:

◆   The ways and reasons for combing and brushing their hair.

◆   Different sorts of products that would be beneficial to them.

◆   How often they should use these products at home.

The ways in which the client should comb and brush their hair

You need to tell the client how they can make their hair easier to manage and maintain a good condition for a longer period of time. Most hairstyles require some sort of styling or finishing product and we have already explained that shampooing aims to remove this type of product build-up.

Many clients aren't aware that they should be brushing or combing their hair on a daily basis, and that's regardless of whether they are washing it or not. The action of styling and most finishing products on the hair will lock the cuticle together in some way and it is this principle which enables the hair to stay in style/place. But unless this is detangled in the morning after lying on it, it will start to damage those areas that are locked together by tearing layers of cuticle away from the hair. So it is essential that the hair is detangled. Initially this is done by separating the main tangles with the fingers and then when roughly loosened, the hair can be brushed or combed.

If the client has long hair recommend that they start brushing near the ends of the hair first. If the hair is brushed from the root area first, all the locking points down the hair will be squeezed to the same point, causing a large knotted area that will be difficult to remove without damaging the hair. As the ends become free, the client can slowly work backwards, up the hair shaft to the mid-length and ends and then finally the roots.

Hair should always be combed or brushed downwards. If you have ever attempted to back-comb dry hair, you may have noticed some resistance. This is because the cuticles' free edges all point towards the ends of the hair. So when you push against them they will tangle together. But that makes combing hair out much simpler. When we comb through conditioners we always detangle the ends first, working back up the lengths. This helps the cuticle edges to slip over one another, making the whole process far less painful.

The different sorts of products that would be beneficial to the client

Your recommendations for products are based upon what you decided to use during the shampooing and conditioning process. Salons want their clients to make the most of the services that they offer and that includes the retail ranges that it may offer too. Most forward thinking salons use the same products at the wash-point as those available within their retail items – this backs up the salon's services by giving the client the opportunity to have similar experiences at home as they do in the salon.

You should always make a point of telling the client what products you are using on their hair and more importantly, why you are using them. This professional practice will stimulate interest and can lead to important additional sales too.

Good advice is invaluable, you should be telling the client what would happen if they use the wrong products.

For example, if they use the wrong products on their hair it may:

◆ Become static (flyaway) and be very difficult to manage.

◆ Create a film or barrier on the hair that would impair the effectiveness of chemical services.

◆ Make it dry, brittle or unmanageable.

◆ Make it greasy, lank and dull.

How often the client should use these products at home

Finally, after providing the client with information about what products they should be using, you should also be giving them some idea of how frequently their product regimen should be used. Many people are locked into washing their hair on a daily basis and in most cases, this is unnecessary. Very few people need to wash their hair every day but it becomes part of a habit, particularly if in having a shower every day they find it's just as quick to wash their hair too. If their own particular needs point towards not washing every day, then you should tell them. For example if the client has dry, porous and damaged hair, they certainly will not benefit from excessive washing, although the conditioning aspect will be particularly beneficial. Similarly, a client who has an excessively oily scalp may have to shampoo every day, but then may not benefit from using a regular surface conditioner. As you can see, each client must be considered on an individual basis as they have individual needs. Your advice will go a long way to helping them counter their own particular problems.

SUMMARY

As a final reflection on what you have covered in this chapter, you should now have a clearer picture of all the essential aspects for providing a shampooing and conditioning. In particular, you should now have a basic understanding of the key principles of:

1 The pH values and how this affects hair and skin.

2 The common ingredients used within shampoos and conditioners and how they work, what they do and how they can benefit the client.

3 How the shampooing and conditioning service affects the client and the other salon services.

4 Providing advice to the clients about their hair maintenance.

And collectively, how these principles will enable you to provide a service that benefits the client, the salon and yourself.

ASSESSMENT OF KNOWLEDGE AND UNDERSTANDING

Project

This project relates to the techniques of shampooing and conditioning and the differences between types of conditioner.

Describe in your own words when you would use the following techniques:

1 Rotary

2 Effleurage

3 Petrissage

How would you adapt the techniques for clients with very long hair?

What is the purpose of the following types of conditioner?

1 Surface-acting

2 Penetrating

Write your answers in your **portfolio**.

Revision questions

A selection of different types of questions to check your knowledge.

Q1	Coarser, _____ hair takes longer to dampen than finer, oilier hair during shampooing.	Fill in the blank
Q2	Petrissage is commonly used during shampooing.	True or false
Q3	What factors should you consider during shampooing and conditioning? (Select all that apply.)	Multi selection

Water hardness	☐ 1
Water pressure	☐ 2
Water softness	☐ 3
Water temperature	☐ 4
Water wastage	☐ 5
Water wetness	☐ 6

Q4	Effleurage is a massage movement of circulatory movements.	True or false
Q5	The pH value of pH-balanced shampoos and conditioners is:	Multi choice

3.5–4.5	○ a
4.5–6.0	○ b
5.5–6.5	○ c
7.0–7.5	○ d

Q6	Dandruff is a condition of the scalp usually treated by shampoo.	True or false
Q7	Which of the following would take place after chemical processing? (Select all that apply.)	Multi selection

Pre-perm shampoo	☐ 1
Anti-oxidant conditioning	☐ 2
Medicated treatment	☐ 3
Conditioning rinse	☐ 4
Anti-dandruff shampoo	☐ 5
Pre-perm treatment	☐ 6

Q8	When conditioning long hair it is important to apply to the mid-lengths and _____.	Fill in the blank
Q9	A shampoo for dry hair would typically contain?	Multi choice

Critical acids	○ a
Oils	○ b
Medicating agents	○ c
Anti-dandruff agents	○ d

Q10	During conditioning it is always necessary to leave the treatment on.	True or false

8 Style and finish hair

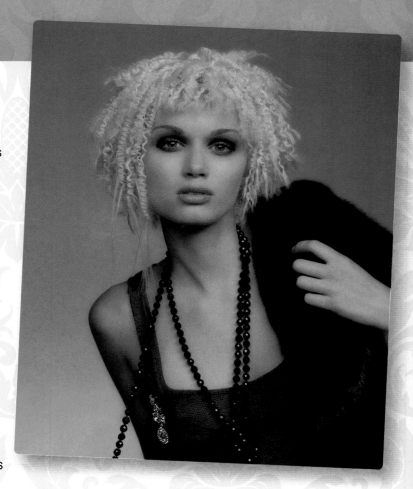

LEARNING OBJECTIVES

◆ Be able to maintain effective and safe methods of working

◆ Be able to blow-dry hair into shape

◆ Be able to finger-dry hair into shape

◆ Be able to finish hair with heated styling equipment

◆ Know how to work safely, effectively and hygienically

◆ Understand the effects of styling and finishing techniques on the hair

◆ Know how to use styling products and equipment

◆ Know how to provide aftercare advice to clients

KEY TERMS

added hair
barrel curls
brick wind
cane rows
chignon
cohesive setting
dexterity
finger waves
fish hook

fish tail plait (herringbone plait)
flat brush
flat twists
french plait
French pleat
heat protection sprays
heated rollers
heated tongs
layering (layered cut)

linear patterns
scalp plaits
Senegalese twist
serums
style line
tail or pin comb
temporary bonds
velcro rollers

Unit topic

Style and finish hair.

INTRODUCTION

This chapter looks at the creative area of styling and finishing hair. It incorporates a variety of techniques including blow-drying, setting, dressing, finger-drying and plaiting hair. In the past, these techniques have been separated out and students have '*latched onto*' their favourites and tried to avoid their dislikes. So blow-drying has been the most popular, setting has been the least popular and plaiting has proved the most difficult.

In reality, these disciplines merge, and in the salon, skills learnt to do one thing actually cross over into another. For example, blow-drying with a radial brush is similar to setting with rollers and the skills needed in dressing out one, are the same in the other. So logically, and at last, the different skills combine and now you will learn all of them.

Style and finish hair

PRACTICAL SKILLS

Learn how to prepare the client and yourself correctly

Learn how to analyze the client's hair and recognize any influencing factors

Learn about the suitability for using different styling products matched to your client's needs

Learn how to work safely and hygienically

Learn about the suitability of different styling, dressing and finishing techniques matched to your client's needs

Learn about hair and skin tests and how they affect intended services

Learn how to prepare your client's hair for different styling effects

Learn how to apply suitable accessories and ornamentation to your client's hair

Learn how to communicate effectively and professionally

UNDERPINNING KNOWLEDGE

Assessing the client's needs and suggesting appropriate styling or dressings

Using a range of different styling tools and equipment

Carrying out a range of different styling, dressing and finishing techniques

Using the appropriate products to achieve the desired effects

Providing suitable aftercare advice

Client preparation – care and attention

Setting and blow-drying are final styling services for our clients and these are the culmination of everything that has gone before. We want their last experience to be as good as any of the others, so we need to be extra careful with our professionalism and our courtesy. We need to be thinking about the client sat in front of us, and not the next one waiting in reception. We don't want to *cut any corners* and we want them to leave on a high, as well as dry!

One of the things that we can do is to make sure, if the towel is removed, that the client's hair will not drip. It's bad enough when saturated short hair drips down on to the gown and soaks the client's clothes, but this becomes even worse and far more uncomfortable if the client has long hair. If you can, the best way to tackle any service is with the client's hair in a slightly damp, i.e. semi-dry state and this goes for setting, blow-drying or cutting for that matter. Working with damp hair is far more comfortable for the client and cuts down a lot of time for busy stylists.

Why work with damp partially dried hair?

In blow-drying or setting, the hairstyle is fixed into shape as the **alpha keratin** changes to **beta keratin**. This takes place at the point where hair changes state from moist to dry. So when blow-drying, finger-drying and setting it is better to work with hair that is damp as it cuts down the drying time and maximizes your efficiency and the amount of time spent on each client. Hair that is saturated still has to be dried, and using the hood dryer on maximum heat (or in blow-drying at top speed) and scorching the hair dry is definitely not the solution.

This is because:

For alpha and beta keratin, go to *The principles of heat styling* on pp. 225–226.

◆ It is uncomfortable for the client.

◆ It will probably cause damage to the client's hair.

◆ It may even burn their scalp too.

Your client's seating position

Client positioning has a lot to do with your safety too. If a client is slouched in the chair, they are a danger not only to themselves but to you too. Client comfort should extend to the point where it makes the salon visit a welcome and pleasurable experience, but not to the point where their belongings clutter the floor (around the styling chair) with bags, magazines and shopping. Anything that can safely be stored away should be.

Salon chairs are designed with comfort and safety in mind; your client should be seated with their back flat against the back of the chair and the chair at a height at which it is comfortable for you to work. You need to be able to get to all parts of the head, so the chair's height should be adjusted to suit the particular height of the client. Don't be afraid of asking the client to sit up: it is in their best interest too.

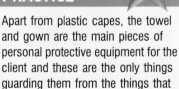

BEST PRACTICE

Always dry the client's hair well to remove the excess water before combing, blow-drying or finger-drying.

Your client's protection

Make sure that the gown is still on and properly fastened around the neck. It should cover and protect the client's clothes and come up high enough to cover collars and necklines. Don't make the fastening too tight, but it should be close enough at least to stop things going down the back of the neck.

If you can style and dry hair with a towel around the client's shoulders, do so. But in some situations, this is not possible as the length of the hair can get in the way of the styling or drying technique.

BEST PRACTICE

Apart from plastic capes, the towel and gown are the main pieces of personal protective equipment for the client and these are the only things guarding them from the things that you do.

Your working position and posture

Hairdressing involves a lot of standing and, because of this, you need to be comfortable in your work. You should always adopt a comfortable but safe work position, although sometimes comfortable and safe are not necessarily the same thing.

A naturally comfortable position for work should allow you to stand close enough to the styling chair without touching it. This should allow you to position your shoulders and body directly above your hips and feet and to distribute your weight evenly over them.

You shouldn't have to twist at any point, as you can easily work around the chair or get your client to turn their head slightly towards you. You should always wear flat shoes, so that your body weight is supported comfortably on the widest parts of the feet. This will allow you to work for longer periods without risk of injury.

Always make a point of lifting your arms to check the work height for your client. If you have to raise your arms anywhere near horizontal during your work, you will find that your arms will start to ache very quickly. Make your adjustments to the styling chair, either up or down to suit your needs. Don't forget to tell the client what you are doing, if only out of courtesy, as it might be a little shocking for them to find themselves being *'jacked'* up to the ceiling!

Your personal hygiene

You may have already covered this in a previous chapter, but here is a quick reminder of the main aspects.

BEST PRACTICE

Work with semi-dry hair during styling, as this enables the natural tendencies of the hair to be seen.

BEST PRACTICE

Look out for ways and things that can make your client's visit more comfortable and pleasurable. This is the first step in providing a better customer service.

Health, safety and hygiene
◆ Always wash your hands before attending to any clients.
◆ Only wear the minimum of jewellery as it can catch or tangle in the client's hair.
◆ Wear flat (and not open-toed) shoes when on the salon floor.
◆ Remember bad breath is offensive – use breath fresheners.
◆ Remember BO is offensive – shower daily.
◆ Make sure your workwear/uniform is clean, fresh and neatly pressed.
◆ Look professional, make sure you have clean tidy hair and neatly trimmed nails.
◆ Work safely and reduce the risk of cross-infection to others.

BEST PRACTICE

Tell the client that you are adjusting the chair height, they might be a little shocked in the belief that it's going to give way!

HEALTH & SAFETY

Portable appliance testing (PAT). All items of electrical equipment have to be tested and certified fit for use by a competent person. The items are tested, labelled and recorded and a compiled list is made available for inspection.

Working efficiently, safely and effectively

Working efficiently and maximizing your time is essential, so making the most of the resources available should occur naturally. But how can you do that? One way of making the most of the salon's resources is being careful in the way that you handle the equipment and the products that you use. Always treat the salon's materials in the same way that you would look after your own equipment. Always try to minimize waste, be careful of how much product you use: it's pointless using an amount of mousse the size of a football if a small orange will do! It only needs a bit of care and control when you dispense the products from their containers. Only use what you need, any excess styling products is wasteful, it's like throwing money away.

Work in a tidy and organized way, you should have *all* the tools and equipment that you need at hand, along with the products that you want to use. You need to be thinking about all of the things that you need before you need them. This is a good exercise in self-organization and shows others that you are a professional and thinking about your work.

Safety with electrical equipment

Dos	Don'ts
✓ Do check the plugs and leads to make sure they are not loose or damaged before use.	✗ Don't use electrical equipment with wet hands.
✓ Do put the equipment back after every time it is used.	✗ Don't use any piece of equipment for any purpose other than that for which it was intended.
✓ Do unravel and straighten the leads properly before you plug them in.	✗ Don't ravel up leads tightly around the equipment: it could work the connection loose.
✓ Do switch off electrical items when they are not in use.	✗ Don't put hot, heated styling equipment down onto an unprotected work surface.
✓ Do check heated styling equipment such as straighteners and tongs before applying them to the client's hair.	✗ Don't tangle equipment flexes around or over your client – keep them out of their way.

Styling consultation

Choosing the appropriate styling options for your client is essential for achieving a satisfactory result. In other words, if you use the wrong styling method, you have little chance of pleasing the client. You need to be realistic about what the client's hair will do and if it matches their expectations. It would be pointless trying to blow-dry body and volume into very fine, sparse hair, when you should be using heated rollers to achieve the result. Similarly, if a client with long hair, wanted a **French plait**, you wouldn't dream of 'wet setting' it first, particularly when a quick wash and blow-dry will prep the hair in a fraction of the time.

You do need to think about other contra-indications too. The following information relates to consultation and the considerations you should make for hair styling.

For more information about suitability, hair and scalp diseases, conditions and defects go to CHAPTER 6 on Consultation p. 169.

Styling consultation: Your method of working

Things or aspects to look for	Things you could ask the client	Why do I need to ask this?
Look at the hair shape	'How would you like your hair styled?'	You can see if the style is achievable from the length and layering patterns as you brush through the hair and what sorts of products you will need to help style it.
Look for conditions of the scalp that will stop you from carrying on	'Have you had any problems with your hair or scalp recently?'	If the client has had problems it gives you the prompt to investigate further.
Look at the type and tendency of the hair	'Is your hair naturally wavy (or curly)?'	If there is movement in the hair you need to find out if it is natural to get an idea of which brushes you need to use and whether you will need to use other heated styling equipment too.
Look at the amount and texture of the hair	'Does your hair take long to dry and style?'	Thicker hair and some hair textures take longer to dry. You need to find out if there are any condition issues first.

(Continued)

(Continued)

Styling consultation: Your method of working		
Things or aspects to look for	**Things you could ask the client**	**Why do I need to ask this?**
Look at the head and facial shape	'Do you find that some styles suit you better than others?'	Find out whether the client naturally chooses and wears styles that are aesthetically correct for them.
Look at the natural partings	'Is this the way that your hair usually falls?'	If the natural parting is not where the client wants it, you need to point out the pitfalls of working against the natural fall of the hair.
Look at the quality of the hair and the way that it lies	'Do you normally use a finishing or defining product on your hair?'	Will the final look be improved by definition, **serums** or other finishing products?
Likes and dislikes, visual aids/pictures	'Would you like something along these lines or do you prefer a simpler style?'	You must get the client to confirm the desired effect before you start.

Other factors affecting styling options

The client's physical features and their lifestyle have an impact on the choice of styling. Their face and head shape may not be suitable for what they have in mind. Similarly, if their job or leisure activities limit the options available to them, then you do need to point these aspects out.

The basic rules for styles and face shape suitability are:

For more information on lifestyle factors and hair growth, Go to **CHAPTER 6** on Consultation p. 168.

◆ Face shapes

◆ Lifestyle

◆ Hair growth patterns.

Face shapes	
Oval face shape	An oval-shaped face suits any hairstyle, so these facial shapes present the fewest problems and style selection limitations.
Round face shape	Rounder facial features are diminished by height, this compensates for the width of the face. Hairstyles that finish at a point just below the ears tend to draw a focus to that point and therefore longer lengths at the side are a better option.

(Continued)

(Continued)

Face shapes

Long facial shape	Shorter profile lengths improve longer facial shapes with added width as opposed to added height. Sides can be worn forwards with softer, feathered edges to reduce any angular effects.
Square face shape	Squarer face shapes need rounder styled edges with texture on to the face to soften the corners or heavier jawlines. Longer lengths also are favourable and these tend to create a frame focus elsewhere.
Triangular or 'heart' shaped face	The width of the face at the temples is *balanced* with height. These facial shapes tend to have a pointed chin. So avoid short perimeters with solid angles, as this will accentuate this feature, whereas longer lengths at the sides with fullness and movement will diminish it.

HEALTH & SAFETY

Look out! Hairdryers will suck in the client's hair from the back if you get too close.

Alpha and Beta Keratin – the principles of heat styling (the temporary set)

Both setting and blow-drying provide methods for fixing hair into shape on a temporary basis. By using these methods, you can make hair straighter, curlier, fuller, flatter or wavier.

Both methods involve the placing and positioning of damp/wet hair (either around a roller, or onto a brush) in to selected positions, and fixing the movement in to it, by using heat. This simple way of starting with damp hair and drying it into a stretched or tensioned shape, forms the principle of temporary setting. (Also referred to as **cohesive setting**)

The following sequence explains what is happening inside the hair structure during the changes from alpha to beta keratin

Alpha and beta keratin

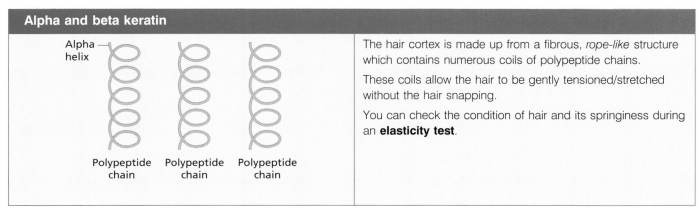

The hair cortex is made up from a fibrous, *rope-like* structure which contains numerous coils of polypeptide chains.

These coils allow the hair to be gently tensioned/stretched without the hair snapping.

You can check the condition of hair and its springiness during an **elasticity test**.

(Continued)

(Continued)

Alpha and beta keratin

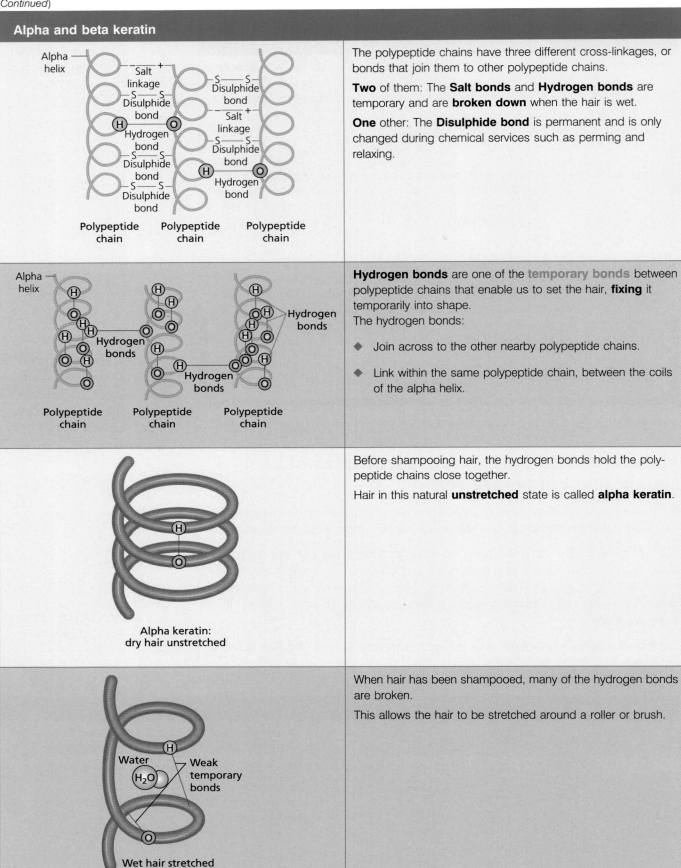

The polypeptide chains have three different cross-linkages, or bonds that join them to other polypeptide chains.

Two of them: The **Salt bonds** and **Hydrogen bonds** are temporary and are **broken down** when the hair is wet.

One other: The **Disulphide bond** is permanent and is only changed during chemical services such as perming and relaxing.

Hydrogen bonds are one of the temporary bonds between polypeptide chains that enable us to set the hair, **fixing** it temporarily into shape.
The hydrogen bonds:

◆ Join across to the other nearby polypeptide chains.

◆ Link within the same polypeptide chain, between the coils of the alpha helix.

Before shampooing hair, the hydrogen bonds hold the polypeptide chains close together.

Hair in this natural **unstretched** state is called **alpha keratin**.

When hair has been shampooed, many of the hydrogen bonds are broken.

This allows the hair to be stretched around a roller or brush.

(Continued)

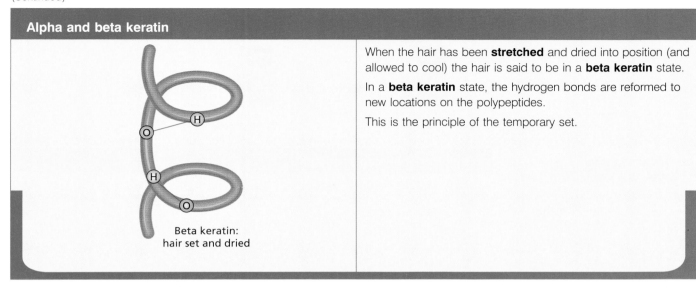

Alpha and beta keratin

Beta keratin:
hair set and dried

When the hair has been **stretched** and dried into position (and allowed to cool) the hair is said to be in a **beta keratin** state.

In a **beta keratin** state, the hydrogen bonds are reformed to new locations on the polypeptides.

This is the principle of the temporary set.

When hair is wet the hydrogen bonds are broken, they reform when the hair is dried. This principle enables hair in good condition to hold a set or blow-dry very well, or at least until the hair gets wet again **or** absorbs moisture from the atmosphere.

So, in order for hair to be styled correctly, it has to be moistened and dried with tension into its new shape. After drying the brush or roller needs to cool down, as this fixes the curl into position. If not, then hot hair can 'relax' back to its previous state.

The effects of humidity on the hair

Blow-drying and setting produce only a temporary change in hair structure, the fixed or set effect is soon lost if/when moisture is absorbed or introduced to the hair. You have probably already discovered this yourself: if, after having your hair done, you take a bath in a steamy bathroom, what happens to the hair style?

BEST PRACTICE

Moisture is all around us in the atmosphere and, in more extremes of humidity, it is seen as mist and fog. Moisture allows beta keratin to change back to its alpha state and will allow a style to drop. There is a wide variety of setting and styling products that resist/repel moisture on hair and you can recommend them to your clients to prevent this from happening.

Go to **CHAPTER 13** Perming pp. 406–408 for more information on the Disulphide bond.

TOP TIP

Hair is hygroscopic – it absorbs moisture from the atmosphere.

BEST PRACTICE

A cool shot helps during blow-drying to fix the curl into position.

Styling products

There is an ever-growing range of styling and finishing products available to the profession. In recent years, this has been the major growth area and careful research and technological advances have ensured that each product is specifically designed to do a particular job. This can be particularly confusing for our clients and this is where your help and advice is useful, as without it, they could be putting anything on their hair!

Styling products contain setting agents that hold and support the hair in its shape. Apart from hold, they often have other additives that can:

◆ Lock-in, or repel, moisture.

◆ Provide protective UV sunscreens.

◆ Add shine and lustre.

◆ Add definition and shape.

TOP TIP

Some hair conditions are more suited to setting techniques. If the client's hair is too porous or lightened, dry setting or heated rollers would be a good alternative.

Features of styling products

When used before styling a styling product will:

◆ Give hold.

◆ Add volume.

◆ Provide body, shine, lustre.

◆ Reduce frizz and static.

◆ Smooth and straighten.

◆ Provide a protective barrier, prevent moisture penetrating hair, protect from sunlight.

◆ Aid the longevity/durability of a style.

◆ **Setting solutions** – such as mousses, or thermal setting sprays, protect the hair from excessive heat. They increase the time that the hair is held in shape and the volume and/or movement created, all while being exposed to the blast from the dryer's nozzle. They can be in a variety of different strengths for differing hair types and holds.

◆ **Finishing products** – are products that enhance the hair by adding shine or gloss, and improve handling and control by removing static, fluffiness or frizziness from the hair. Certain finishing products like waxes will define the movement in hair, giving texture or spikiness. Some products laminate the outer cuticle layer, protecting it from the environment, sun, sea and elements. Look out for **Argan Oil** (Moroccan Oil™).

◆ **Heat protection** – many products provide protection from heat styling. Regular use of straightening irons could damage the hair so there are a number of products that can be applied to eliminate any long-term effects. Other products provide protection from harsh UV rays in sunlight in a variety of 'leave-in' treatments that can be used at any time. They are put on before exposure to harsh sunlight and can be removed after by washing. This is particularly useful for clients who have coloured hair, as the lightening effects of sunlight will quickly remove colour.

◆ **Other protective products** – like demineralizing treatments have the ability to resist or remove the effects of minerals on the hair such as chlorine from swimming pools. This is particularly useful, as blonde hair that is exposed to chlorine, tends to look green!

Styling products

Product	What is it for?	How is it applied?	When do you use it?
Styling mousse Goldwell	A general styling aid for adding volume and providing hold.	Apply a blob the size of a small orange evenly to the lengths.	Use on dampened hair before sectioning and drying.
Root lift mousse L'Oréal Professionnel	A special mousse that has a directional nozzle allowing you to apply foam at or near to the roots.	Lift and separate sections of dampened hair so that the root area is exposed. Hold the can so that the nozzle aims the foam near the root.	On hair that needs body but doesn't require setting hold at the mid-lengths and points.
Styling gel/glaze L'Oréal Professionnel	A wet look firm hold finish on shorter hair-styles.	Apply a small 'pea-size' amount from the finger-tips all over evenly. (You can always add more if necessary.)	Not easy to blow-dry with but can be used in finger-drying and scrunch-dry techniques.
Moulding clay L'Oréal Professionnel	A dual purpose product for styling or finishing that bonds the hair with firm hold.	(On damp hair) Apply a small 'pea-size' amount from the fingertips all over evenly. (On dry hair) Apply with fingertips to the points of the hair for texture and definition. (You can always add more if necessary.)	Used to give a firm textural bond on most lengths of hair.

(Continued)

(*Continued*)

Styling products

Product	What is it for?	How is it applied?	When do you use it?
Defining crème *L'Oréal Professionnel*	A finishing product that provides control on un-ruly hair.	(On dry hair) Apply small 'droplet' amounts a little at a time with fingertips. (You can always add more if necessary.)	Used throughout the lengths of the hair for smooth control and conditioning.
Defining wax *L'Oréal Professionnel*	A slightly greasy finish-ing product that pro-vides textural effects to short to longer hair.	(On dry hair) Apply small 'pea-size' amounts a lit-tle at a time with finger-tips. (You can always add more if necessary.)	Used throughout the ends of the hair for style definition and/or textural effects.
Serum *Goldwell*	A slightly oily finishing product that provides improved handling and shine.	(On dry hair) Apply small droplet amounts a little at a time with fingertips. (You can always add more if necessary.)	Used throughout the lengths of the hair for smooth control and better conditioning.
Hairspray *L'Oréal Professionnel*	A finishing product that is available in a variety of holds/strengths from either a pump or aero-sol spray.	Apply mist to hair from about 30–40cm away from the hair for a 'fixed' hold on dry hair.	Used as a final fixative, as an overall sealer or applied as a scrunch-ing, textural finish.

(Continued)

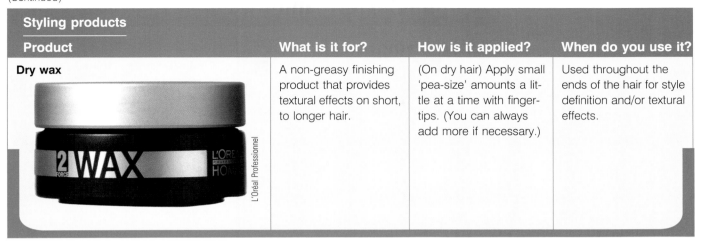

Styling products

Product	What is it for?	How is it applied?	When do you use it?
Dry wax	A non-greasy finishing product that provides textural effects on short, to longer hair.	(On dry hair) Apply small 'pea-size' amounts a little at a time with fingertips. (You can always add more if necessary.)	Used throughout the ends of the hair for style definition and/or textural effects.

L'Oréal Professionnel

Tools and equipment

You will be using a wide variety of tools and equipment in blow-drying and setting.

For more information on blow-drying and setting tools and equipment, go to CHAPTER 1 Your tools and equipment box, p. 6.

Setting equipment

Tools and equipment

◆ Setting rollers
◆ **Velcro rollers**
◆ **Heated rollers**
◆ **Heated tongs**
◆ **Tail or pin comb**

◆ Straight combs
◆ **Flat brushes**
◆ Pin clips
◆ Grips and setting pins

Blow-drying equipment

Tools and equipment

◆ Denman Classic Styling brush
◆ Vented brush
◆ Paddle (flat) brush
◆ Radial brush

◆ Diffuser (although not a brush it is a piece of equipment used to style the hair)

The styling techniques

Blow-drying

Blow-drying is the most popular way of styling hair: it involves the tensioning, drying and positioning of hair into place with just a brush and the blow-dryer. The technique requires a reasonable amount of skill and manual **dexterity**, so it is quite difficult to pick up at first.

A blow-dryer is fitted with a nozzle that focuses the blast of air/heat on the work area. This stops the dryer from randomly blowing other hair, or things about and is the professional way in which to use it. As you progress through a style, the nozzle can be rotated, so that the client's scalp can be shielded from being burned, and other sections of hair (awaiting styling) are not disturbed by the stream of air.

The best idea would be to start at the bottom or nape area and to fasten any hair not being styled out of the way neatly. Then as each section is completed, you work upwards to the next section so that **newly dried** and styled hair is placed upon **previously dried** sections. This is the *time tested* approach and ensures that the hair style is progressed in a methodical way.

Before the client's hair is blow-dried, any excess moisture should be removed, so that:

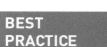

BEST PRACTICE

You need to work upon hair that is damp rather than wet, so pre-blow-dry any areas that need it first.

◆ Only **damp** and not saturated sections are worked upon.

◆ The benefits of styling products are not lost/diluted by excess water.

◆ The client's hair is not unduly or excessively overheated.

◆ The client remains comfortable and dry throughout the process rather than getting wet and cold.

To select the product to use, go to the **styling product table** on p. 229.

Apply the styling product After towel-drying the client's hair, use a wide-tooth comb to find the parting and detangle the hair lengths. And remember, if the hair is long you will need to work from the point ends first, then through the lengths, back towards the roots.

Select your product and apply to the hair. Distribute the product evenly throughout the hair, trying not to overload any particular areas and work through the lengths so that the product is evenly distributed through the hair.

Drying the hair – roots to points You should only work on relatively small areas at any one time; these sections should never be any larger than the *'footprint'* area of any type of brush that you will be using. If the sections are too large, you will not be able to dry each mesh of hair properly and this will affect how long the style will last.

Brush footprint area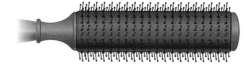

Be careful not to overheat any sections of the hair while you are drying, the effects would be long term and very damaging to the condition of the hair.

Start the blow-dry at the lower back by sectioning out of the way any surplus hair and securing it with a clip. Then, taking your dryer in one hand, offer the dryer across to the section so that you can see whether the angle of the nozzle will create a parallel jet stream of air to the angle of the hair. Then after any adjustments, take your brush in the other hand and introduce the bristles to the hair somewhere near to the root area. Pick and turn the brush so that the hair is caught across the bristles, turn on the dryer and now aiming across the brush, follow the brush downwards with the dryer holding it about 4–6cm away.

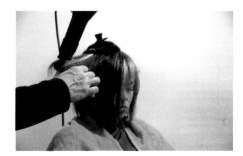

Focusing the jet stream The hair can only dry if the blast from the dryer is working over the surface of it. So bearing this in mind, carefully aim the flat, jet stream of heated air across the surface of the brush, shielding the heat from the back (scalp) side of the brush. As you move the brush down, move the dryer down so that it mirrors the position of the brush at always the same distance away. Blow-drying from root to point ensures that the cuticle lays flat therefore reducing flyaway frizz and smoothing the overall result.

Water moisture will naturally fall down the hair shaft with gravity, so starting near the root area will always quicken the drying process. After a couple of passes through the hair, the section will be dry.

If you are using a radial type brush, you will find that you need to take a section (like that of rollering) and wind the hair around the brush. Again, focus the jet stream over the curved surfaces of the brush, but this time from both sides. This will enable the hair to dry around the brush forming part of the wave. Then after drying and while still warm, use a cool shot from the dryer (or use blast only without heat settings) to 'freeze' and fix the wave into place. (This is similar in setting; when rollers are allowed to cool down before removal and final brushing and dressing out.) If you do not allow the meshes of hair to cool, it will result in a less firm result and will not last as long.

Finally, with the section dry you can take down another mesh, ready for drying into position.

Working with tensioned hair You have to maintain an even tension to the meshes of hair throughout the blow-drying service. This ensures that the hair will dry with a smooth, sleeker effect without frizzes or crimped areas. If you do create a kinked, uneven result, you can lightly mist (spray down) the hair with a water spray and start again. Look out for the hair in the sectioning clips waiting to be dried too: If the hair has a natural tendency to wave or curl it might *crimp* it before you can style it. Again, lightly mist it down with water and start over.

BEST PRACTICE

Hot styling tools can make hair static and flyaway, **heat protection sprays** control this and protect the hair from being excessively overheated.

Blow-drying dos and don'ts

Dos	Don'ts
✓ Do dry off the hair well so that it's moist but not wet before starting the blow-dry.	✕ Don't leave damp towels around the client's shoulders.
✓ Do take small enough sections that you can control and dry evenly throughout.	✕ Don't leave the dryer running while you resection the hair.
✓ Do try to direct the flow of air away from the client.	✕ Don't use the top heat setting unless it's really necessary.
✓ Do adjust the chair height so you can reach the top of the client's head without overstretching.	✕ Don't pass the brushes to the client for them to hold in between sectioning.
✓ Do ask the client to adjust their head position if you need to.	✕ Don't try to use the same hand for brush work on both sides of the head.
✓ Do clip out of the way any sections that are not yet being worked on.	✕ Don't over-dry the hair as this will cause permanent damage.

TOP TIP

Scrunch-drying is a way of drying hair more naturally with a diffuser. It uses the natural body or movement within the hair to create tousled and casual effects.

CourseMate video: Long Hair Blow Dry and Straighten

STEP-BY-STEP: BLOW-DRYING WITH A FLAT BRUSH

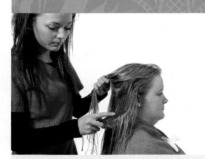

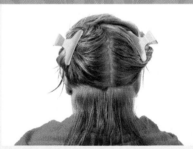

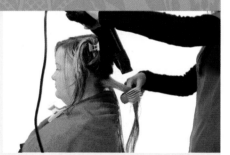

1 Move your client to the workstation and carefully disentangle their hair.

2 So starting at the bottom – take a horizontal section about 3cm above the nape hairline. Secure the remainder out of the way neatly.

3 With nozzle attached and parallel with the section held in the brush, start drying from roots through to the ends.

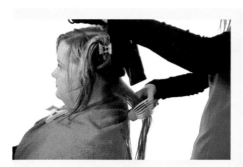

4 Remember to maintain an even tension upon the hair as you work through each section, taking care not to overheat or burn the hair.

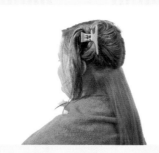

5 The dried section should look smooth and be evenly dried before you take down further sections to work on.

Repeat the process as you work up through the hair.

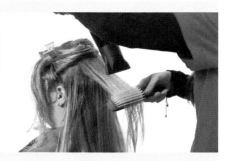

6 You should dry all of the back in the same way before starting the sides.

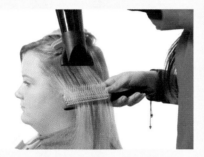

7 Moving around to the sides – start again at the lower sections, drying each one fully before moving on.

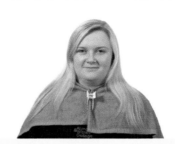

8 With all the hair dry – you are now ready to finish off with the straighteners.

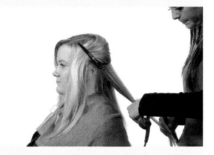

9 Start again at the back of the head at the lowest sections.

Make sure that the straighteners are not too hot (adjust the temperature according to the hair. For example, finer hair needs less heat – 170°–180° Coarser, curlier hair needs more heat 200°–210°).

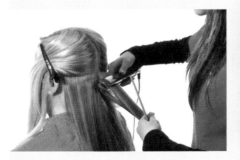

10 With the correct temperature, continue to work up through the sections – laying warm, recently straightened sections down onto previously straightened sections.

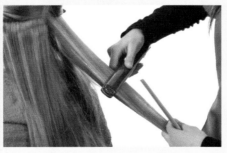

11 Be careful to use the straighteners correctly by passing the heated plates over the hair and downwards in ONE SMOOTH, CONTROLLED PASS over the hair at the same speed.

TOP TIP

DO NOT ALLOW the straighteners to overheat any particular areas. YOU WILL DAMAGE THE HAIR PERMANENTLY!

STEP-BY-STEP: BLOW-DRYING WITH A RADIAL BRUSH

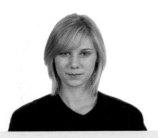

1 Gown and prepare your client, then shampoo and condition their hair.

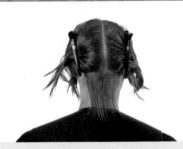

2 Rough-dry the excess moisture and detangle the hair.

Start at the nape area and section off the lower perimeter length.

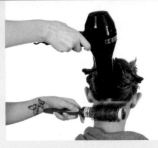

3 Wrap the client's hair around the brush and dry the hair from above and below to ensure that each section of hair is thoroughly dry before moving on.

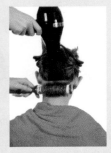

4 Be careful with the direction of the air from the dryer nozzle as it is easy to burn the client.

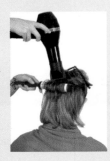

5 Carry on taking sections down and dry each one in a similar way.

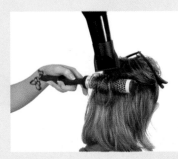

6 As the hair gets longer you will need to dry the root area first before attempting to dry the ends.

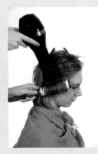

7 Start with the lower side sections first, building the shape and volume in the same way with the brush.

Work up through to the parting area and dry the fringe across, but with less volume.

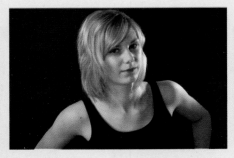

8 Final effect.

STEP-BY-STEP: STYLE WITH A DIFFUSER

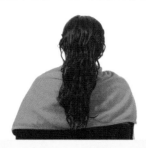

1 Towel-dry and remove excess moisture before you start.

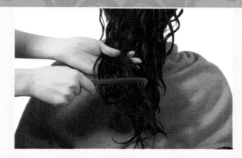

2 Detangle any knots with a wide tooth comb.

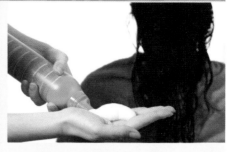

3 Apply some mousse to help hold the style.

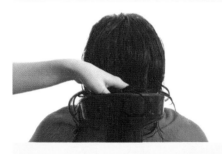

4 After rough-drying the hair – Fit a diffuser on to the end of the blow-dryer and hold the lengths of the hair onto the diffuser prongs.

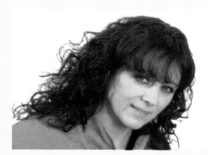

5 As the hair dries further, bulk the lengths together to finish drying the lengths.
(This prevents the hair from separating too much and becoming fuzzy or fluffy.)

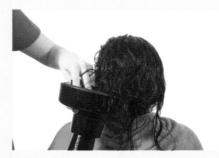

6 Final effect.

Finishing off

After blow-drying the client's hair, you will need to do something to finish the look, even if it is only to brush the final effect through. More often than not, there is a lot more to do. This could be to:

◆ Apply finishing products to the hair.

◆ Use other heated equipment to finish the effect.

Applying finishing products to the hair Choosing the correct finish really depends on the look you are trying to achieve. It would be easy to get it all wrong at this stage and choose something that works against you. Sometimes it's the right product but wrongly applied, but often it's the wrong product and wrongly applied!

Most styling products like mousse or setting lotion do not create an immediate build-up upon the hair. They might be a little tackier than you had expected, or they might give a firmer hold than you had wanted. But in either case, when the hair is dry, a little too much won't have a critical impact on the finished effect. However, if you apply too

HEALTH & SAFETY

Always follow the manufacturer's instructions for using setting and dressing products within the salon.

much serum or wax on the hair you will find yourself having to wash and start all over again!

This can be easily avoided if you add product to your final effect in small steps. In other words, you build up the desired effect slowly by adding a little more until the result is achieved.

How do heat protecting products work?

Previously we said that you need to protect the hair from moisture in the atmosphere: well that's not the only thing. Blow-dryers can get very hot, but heated styling equipment is another thing altogether. Straightening irons and tongs have been very popular with male and female clients and neither seem to really understand the damage that they can do.

Heat-protecting sprays will put a heat-resistant layer upon the hair by doing two things.

For more information on finishing products, see the section on **Styling products** on p. 229.

◆ They improve the surface of the hair by smoothing it and enabling the heated equipment to slip over the surface without grabbing in any areas (like a non-stick coating on cooking pots and pans).

◆ They resist high temperatures from styling surfaces long enough for the hair bonds to be rearranged in the new shape.

For more information on the effects of heat on the hair, go to the section on **Alpha and beta keratin** on p. 225.

Keeping the heated styling equipment clean

With prolonged use, the surfaces on tongs and straighteners can get product build-up themselves. This should always be looked for as any residue of styling products such as wax, hair sprays and gels, serums, etc. will stick to the slippy, smooth surfaces and create roughened areas that will grab and lock-on to the hair when they are hot. This is damaging as it *will* burn the hair!

TOP TIP

Moisture is the enemy of any finished set. It weakens the hold and therefore how long the overall effect will last.

Heated equipment: straightening irons and tongs

Electric curling tongs, heated brushes and straightening irons are a popular way of applying finish to a hairstyle. They are particularly useful in situations where:

◆ Setting or blow-drying will not achieve the desired look.

◆ The hair is not in a suitable condition to be dried into shape.

Sometimes you will not achieve the result that you or the client is expecting. When extra volume, movement or curl is needed, heated tongs and/or brushes will provide a quick solution. They can be bought in a variety of different sizes (i.e. diameters and widths), which give different levels of movement and finish.

To learn more about using ceramic straighteners, go to **Step-by-step – Blow-drying with a flat brush** on pp. 234–235 above.

Professional heated tongs and straighteners have a thermostatic temperature control. This is particularly useful as you can 'dial up' the heat setting required to match the client's hair type. This reduces the risk of damage to the hair from excess heat.

STEP-BY-STEP: CURLING USING SPIRAL TONGS

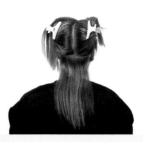 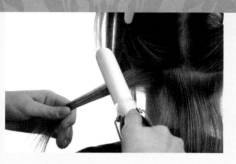 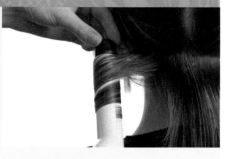

1 The majority of hairdressing services are started at the back.

Section off and secure the hair at the nape.

2 Dial up the correct temperature for the hair type, then place the barrel of the tongs near the root end and start to turn.

3 As you turn slightly open and close the tongs so that hair is drawn in to the barrel of the tongs.

Note: This produces a far more effective spiral curl than trying to wind points to roots.

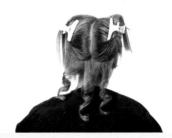 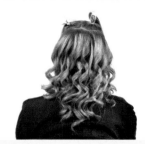 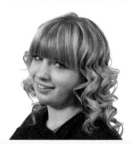

4 With the lower section done, carry on working up through the hair until all of the back is complete.

By starting at the bottom you lay new warm curls down onto cooler, previously curled hair.

5 The back should start to look like this – continue the same patterning into the sides.

6 Final effect.

CourseMate video: Spiral Tongs

Straightening irons and particularly ceramic straightening irons have been a very popular way of calming unruly hair. They work by electrically heating two parallel plates so that the hair can be run between them in one movement from roots to ends, smoothing out the unwanted wave or frizz in the process.

Ceramic straighteners have been particularly successful as they heat up in just a few moments and have a higher operating temperature than metal irons (180°–200°C). This alarmingly high temperature is potentially damaging to hair but, because they have the ability to transfer heat quickly and smoothly to the hair without grabbing, they are very effective in creating smoother effects. But because of their temperature you must check them before you introduce them to the hair so that you don't permanently damage the client's hair.

When straightening is needed to complement the look on longer hair, it is sometimes better to straighten each section as the blow-dry proceeds. If you start underneath, each section is completely finished before you move on up the head. The hair will stay

TOP TIP

Very hot styling tools without a non-slip coating or ceramic surface, can often tend to stick when they are introduced to hair that has styling products on it.

TOP TIP

Hot styling tools can make hair static and flyaway. Heat protection sprays control this and protect the hair from being excessively overheated.

flatter from the start and each section will be totally dry, stopping the hair from reverting to its previous state.

Crimping irons The use of crimping irons tends to go through phases of popularity at least once every decade or so. They too have parallel fixed plates but these are wavy and produce flat 'S' waves on longer hair. They are a great styling accessory for competition and stage work, as crimped effects are visually striking and very unusual. In hairdressing shows, models with crimped hair will often accompany the look with strong fashion colours.

Unlike tongs and straightening irons, crimpers are not turned, twisted or drawn through the hair.

1 Each mesh of hair is started nearer the head and works down to the points of the hair.

2 The meshes should be no wider than the crimping irons and are crimped across the width of the plates.

3 After a few moments of heating each section of the mesh, the crimpers are moved to the last wave crest created and pressed again.

4 This is repeated down the lengths of the hair until all of the hair is crimped.

5 The final look should not be combed out or brushed, but allowed to fall in waved sections.

Crimping is not advisable on shorter, layered hair unless a frizzy, fluffy look is wanted. The most successful results are on longer, one-length hair.

Using electrical equipment

◆ Never get too close to the client's head with hot styling equipment.

◆ Never leave the styling equipment on one area of hair for more than a few moments.

◆ Always replace the styling tools into their holder at the workstation when not in use.

◆ Always check the filters on the back of hand dryers to make sure that they are not blocked (this will cause the dryer to overheat and possibly ignite).

◆ Look out for trailing flexes across the floor or around the back of styling chairs.

◆ Let tools cool down before putting them back into storage.

◆ Always check for damage or kinks in flexes or damaged plugs.

◆ Never use damaged equipment under any circumstances.

Setting Hair

Rollers – Rollering hair

There are various sizes and shapes of roller. When using rollers you need to decide on the size and shape, how you will curl the hair on to them and the position in which you will attach them to the base.

- ◆ Small rollers produce tight curls, giving hair more movement.

- ◆ Large rollers produce loose curls, making hair wavy as opposed to curly.

- ◆ On-base rollering produces root lift/volume and end curl.

- ◆ Off-base rollering produces end curl without root lift.

- ◆ The direction in which the hair is wound will affect the final style.

STEP-BY-STEP: ROLLERING

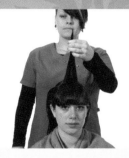

1 Wet setting can achieve similar effects to that of heated rollers.

In this wet set, **brick wind**, large curlers are used to produce a contemporary, long lasting effect.

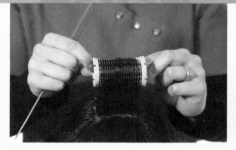

2 The first roller is placed centrally behind a full fringe area.

Care has been taken to ensure that the section taken is no wider or deeper than the roller's footprint.

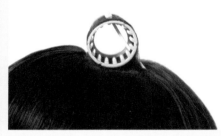

3 Side view – showing root lift and correct plastic pinning.

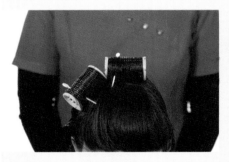

4 Another roller is wound adjacent to the first.

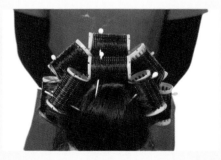

5 More rollers are placed to create a brick-work effect.

This will eliminate roller marks and stop the hair parting in the wrong position.

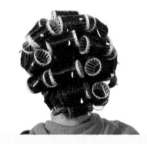

6 The hair set before putting under the dryer.

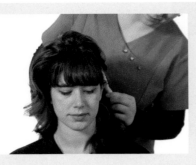

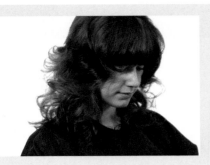

7 For a natural effect, more care is taken during combing out, so that the curls aren't unduly stretched.

A light brushing with a wide toothed brush.

8 The final effect.

1 Comb through to remove any tangles and apply the setting lotion evenly to the hair. Start by taking a clean, smooth section of hair – that is no longer or wider than the 'footprint' (size of the basal section) of the roller being used – straight out, but slightly forwards from the head.

2 Place the hair points centrally on to the roller. Use both hands to retain the hair section angle and keep the hair points in position.

3 As you turn the roller 'lock', the hair points against the body of the roller. Then continue winding down with an even tension until you reach the base of the section.

4 As you work, make sure that any shorter or wispy flyaway ends are included in the wound roller.

5 Place the wound roller centrally on to the sectioned base (i.e. 'on base') to achieve full height/volume from the set. Secure the roller by pinning through to stop it unravelling. Make sure that the pins are comfortable and link through to other rollers and not on to the client's scalp.

STEP-BY-STEP: HEATED ROLLERS

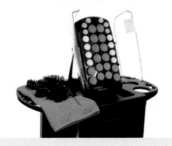

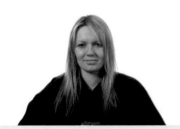

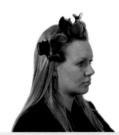

1 Heated rollers provide a softer option for contemporary set effects that cannot be achieved by blow-drying or wet setting.

Prepare your trolley with brushes, combs and the roller sizes that you want to use.

2 Prepare your client with a clean, fresh gown.

3 Start by placing the rollers into the hair from the front.

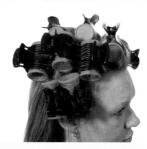

4 As you progress through the set, check with the client that the rollers aren't too hot.

If they are uncomfortable you can use pieces of neck wool as an insulator between the bottom of the roller and the scalp.

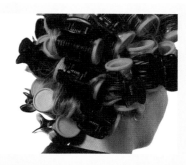

5 Leave the rollers in until all the rollers have cooled down.

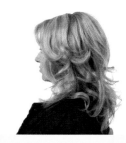

6 Then carefully remove the rollers starting at the bottom and not the top.

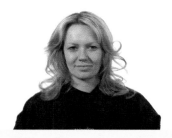

7 Work through with your fingers without brushing to create the looser natural, dressed effect.

Common rollering problems

- ◆ Rollers not secured properly on base, either dragged or flattened, will not produce lift and volume in the final style.

- ◆ Too large a hair section will produce reduced movement in the final effect.

- ◆ Too small a hair section will produce increased movement or curl in the final effect.

- ◆ Longer hair requires larger rollers unless tighter effects are wanted.

- ◆ Poorly positioned hair falling off the sides of the roller will have reduced/impaired movement in the final effect.

- ◆ Incorrectly wound hair around the roller will create **fish hook** ends.

- ◆ Twisted hair around the roller will distort the final movement of the style.

BEST PRACTICE

If you are not sure which size roller to use, go for the smaller. If necessary, you can brush out and stretch too tightly curled hair later. Loosely curled hair will drop more readily, so you may not achieve the style you were aiming for.

Pin-Curls – Curling

Curls add 'bounce' or lift to the hair, and control the direction in which the hair lies. Pin curling is the technique of winding hair into a series of curls or flat waves which are pinned in place with pin clips while drying. The two most common types of curl produced in this way are the barrel curl and the clock spring curl.

Each curl has a root, a stem, a body and a point. The curl base – the foundation shape produced between parted sections of hair – may be oblong, square or triangular. The shape depends on the size of the curl, the stem direction and the curl type. Different curl types produce different movements.

You can choose the shape, size and direction of the individual curls and this will affect the finished effect and how long it lasts. The type of curl you choose depends on the style you're aiming for:

◆ A high, lifted movement needs a raised curl stem.

◆ A low, smooth shape needs a flat curl.

You may need to use a combination of curl types and curling methods to achieve the desired style – for example, you might lift the hair on top of the head using large rollers, but keep the sides flatter using pin curls.

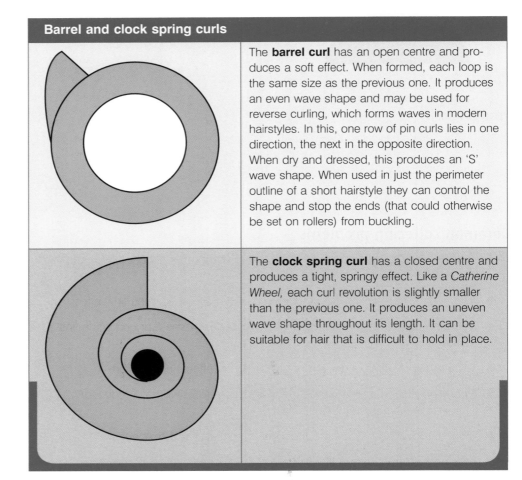

Barrel and clock spring curls

The **barrel curl** has an open centre and produces a soft effect. When formed, each loop is the same size as the previous one. It produces an even wave shape and may be used for reverse curling, which forms waves in modern hairstyles. In this, one row of pin curls lies in one direction, the next in the opposite direction. When dry and dressed, this produces an 'S' wave shape. When used in just the perimeter outline of a short hairstyle they can control the shape and stop the ends (that could otherwise be set on rollers) from buckling.

The **clock spring curl** has a closed centre and produces a tight, springy effect. Like a *Catherine Wheel*, each curl revolution is slightly smaller than the previous one. It produces an uneven wave shape throughout its length. It can be suitable for hair that is difficult to hold in place.

STEP-BY-STEP: PIN CURLING

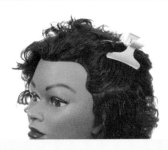

1 Pin curling is often thought to be difficult, although like anything else, it's about preparation and placement.

Pin curls should be started at the bottom and then work upwards, working on areas already completed.

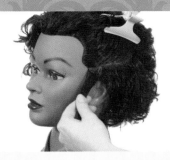

2 After sectioning off a horizontal row, subdivide the section into a square based stem.

Comb again to smooth it.

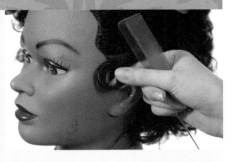

3 Now take the curl around and hold the points between your finger and thumb.

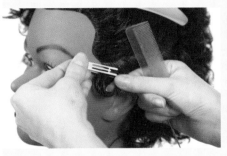

4 Taking a pin clip, now place the clip on the opposite side to where you would take another pin curl.

Repeat 2, 3 and 4 for as many as you want.

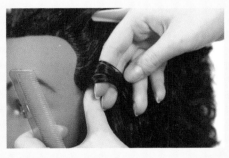

5 Another form of pin curl is the 'stand-up' pin curl. This forms small **barrel curls** which add movement and lift.

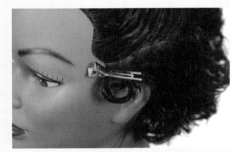

6 Take another square section and this time, turn it around your finger.

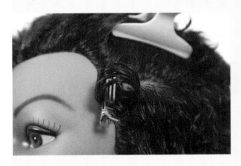

7 This is secured at the bottom of the base with a clip.

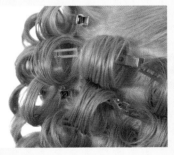

8 Several 'stand-up' pin curls.

CourseMate video: Pin Curling

Common pin curl faults

◆ Tangled hair is difficult to control. Comb well before starting.

◆ If the base is too large curling will be difficult.

◆ If you hold the curl stem in one direction but place it in another the curl will be misshapen and lift.

◆ If you don't turn your hand far enough it will be difficult to form concentric loops.

Curl body directions
A flat curl may turn either clockwise or anti-clockwise. The clockwise curl has a body that moves around to the right and the anti-clockwise a body that moves around to the left. Reverse curls are rows of alternating clockwise and anti-clockwise pin curls – these will produce a finish that has continuous 's' waves, similar to the effect of **finger waves** throughout the style. Stand-up pin curls, like rollers, have a body that lifts away from the scalp.

Putting your client under the dryer

1   After setting move your client to a hood dryer.

2   Make sure that the client is comfortable.

3   Set the dryer to a temperature that suits the client. (Although this can be over-ridden by the client as they can turn it down themselves.)

4   Set the timer for drying. You should allow around 15 minutes for short fine hair, and up to 45 minutes for longer, thick hair. The average is around 25–30 minutes.

5   Check the client after five minutes, to see if they are alright or need anything.

6   After drying has finished, remove the hood dryer and let the hair cool down for a short while.

7   Then check to see if the hair is dry by carefully removing one roller from the crown area, one from the nape and one from the front; if they are all dry carry on carefully removing all the pins and rollers, leaving the set curl carefully in its position without dragging or distorting the formed curl.

Dressing out

Dressing is the final styling process of setting. Whereas the setting process provides volume, curls or waves, the dressing-out now blends and smooths these pre-set movements into an overall flowing shape.

Dressing uses brushing and combing techniques and dressing aids such as dressing crèmes, and hairspray to keep the hair in place. If you have set the hair carefully and accurately, then only the minimum of dressing is required.

Step-by-step – brushing
Brushing blends the waves or curls by removing the partings or set marks created at the curl bases during rollering. It also removes the stiffness caused by setting lotions that aid the hold of the set.

1   Take a wide-toothed brush, so that it brushes through the hair comfortably.

2   Start at the lower nape area of the set, and brush through the roller marks.

3 Work up the head, towards the crown.

4 Brush through the waves or curls you have set, gradually moulding the hair into shape.

5 As you brush, pat or smooth the hair with your hand to guide the hair into shape. Remember, though, that overdressing and over-handling can ruin the set.

6 If the hair has static, stop brushing and apply a little dressing crème to calm down the 'flyaway' ends.

Back-brushing

Back-brushing is a technique used to give more height and volume to hair. By brushing backwards from the points to the roots, you roughen the cuticle of the hair. The hair will now tangle slightly and bind together to hold a fuller shape. The amount of hair back-brushed determines the fullness of the finished style.

Most textures of hair can be back-brushed and it adds bulk and makes the hair easier to manage. The technique is especially useful with fine hair.

Step-by-step – Back-brushing

1 Hold a section of hair out from the head: for maximum lift, hold the section straight out from the head and apply the back-brushing close to the roots.

2 Place the brush on the top of the held section at an angle slightly dipping in to the held section of hair.

3 Now, with a slight turn outwards with the wrist, turn and push down a small amount of hair towards the scalp.

4 Repeat this in a few nearby sections of hair.

5 Smooth out the longer lengths in the direction required, covering the tangled back-brushed hair beneath.

Alternatively, use Back-combing This technique is similar to back-brushing above: however, in this situation a comb is used rather than a brush to turn back the shorter hairs within a section. This provides firmer support and volume than back-brushing as back-combing is applied deeper toward the scalp; it provides a stronger, longer lasting result.

BEST PRACTICE

Back-combing is applied to the underside of the hair section. Don't let the comb penetrate too deeply otherwise the final dressing and smoothing out will remove the support you have put in.

Use the workstation mirror As you work, keep using the mirror to check the shape that you are creating. If you find that the outer **style line** is misshapen or lacking volume, don't be afraid to go back to re-section and back-brush/comb again. When you have finished the look, hold a back mirror at an angle to maximize what the client can see of their hairstyle.

Dressing Longer Hair

Many people find working with longer hair or doing non-routine services, like bridal work, quite daunting, but they needn't be. The main reason why someone finds any part of hairdressing difficult is because they are not doing those effects regularly enough.

The most important things to remember with long hair-ups are:

◆ Assessing whether a particular look or effect is going to suit the client.

◆ Agreeing the effect before you start.

◆ Having a plan of what you are trying to achieve.

◆ Building enough structure to support the look.

Assess a style's suitability for your client

In most cases, non-routine *hairdos* are for special situations, so our clients come to the salon for the things that they can't do themselves.

The problem from a suitability point of view is how will the client know if they are going to like their hair up if they seldom have it styled that way? For people who don't normally wear their hair in plaits, pleats or twists, there are always underlying reasons and these could be:

◆ Their hair is too thick.

◆ They don't like the shape of their ears.

◆ They feel that 'head-hugging' shapes make them more conspicuous.

◆ It makes their nose bigger.

◆ They prefer their hair to have volume so they don't like it scraped back.

◆ Their hair isn't really long enough.

Physical features→ Hair style↓	Head shapes				Protruding ears	Prominent nose	Short neck
	Oval	**Round**	**Triangular**	**Square**			
Vertical roll/pleat	✓	with height to compensate	with height to compensate	with height and width to compensate	Volume at the sides to cover	Volume at the sides	Needs to be sleek
Barrel curls	✓	✓	✓	✓	Volume at the sides to cover (not triangular)	Volume at the sides	Needs to be sleek
Low knot or chignon	✓	✓ with height	✗	with height	Volume at sides except triangular	✗	✗
High knot	✓	✓	✓	✓	Volume at sides except triangular	✗	Needs to be sleek
Plaits	✓	✓ with height	✓	✗	Volume at sides except triangular	✓	Needs to be sleek
Twists and cornrows	✓	✓ with height	✓	✓ use designs that involve curves and not straight lines/linear effects	Volume at sides except triangular	✓	Needs to be sleek

Agree the effect before you start

When you have selected a suitable look, you need to find examples of how this would look on the client. Visualization and, more importantly, self-visualization from the client's point of view is very difficult. You need to try to rearrange the hair loosely, so they can get an idea of the weight distribution, height and width. If you can convey to them roughly what it will look like when their face is exposed, and they like what they see, you are halfway there. It will save lots of time later and save you having to unpick everything that you have done.

Have a plan – get organized

If the client likes the effect in principle then you can set out a plan of how you will achieve it. You need to work out where you need to start, the midpoint in the styling and what the final touches will be. The starting point will be a position that you will be unlikely to get at and change later on, so it's a bit like making a cake.

- You start with a recipe – the style you want to create.
- You gather the ingredients – all the pins, grips, bands and accessories.
- Get out tools – get all the equipment you need together.
- Start preparing the mix – start the process.
- Place in the oven – mould and spray.
- Take out and ice the cake – finish off with the decoration/accessories.

Building a base structure for vertical rolls/pleats

Some styles need support; they cannot last and stay in without it. It needs to be secure as well as creative in its effect. It can only be secure if you use back-combing, grips, bands, etc. Do not be afraid to back-comb the hair. It may look as if the whole thing is getting too big, but don't forget you can take out as much as you like when you smooth the dressing. Back-combing provides you with a solid base that you can grip without the fear of the grips dropping out. As you become more experienced in handling long hair, you will find that you won't need to use much spray in the styling stage, but only later in the finishing off.

The other main tools for giving structure and support are grips. Kirby grips have one leg with a serrated profile; this helps them to stay in the hair much better.

Wherever possible ensure that you interlock (criss-cross) your grips, whether the patterning is in a straight line (e.g. in supporting and fixing a pleat) or whether it is placed in a complete interlocking circlet (e.g. in hair dressed in knots, chignons or any other centrally positioned dressings).

Vertical roll (French pleat)

The vertical roll or **French pleat** is a formal classic dressing that suits many special occasions. The hair can be enhanced further by the additions of ornaments, accessories or even fresh flowers. If you review the planning stages for putting hair up, you will see under 'building the support' that back-combing is an essential aspect for creating a solid foundation. This should be your starting point for the step-by-step procedure.

STEP-BY-STEP: VERTICAL ROLL (FRENCH PLEAT)

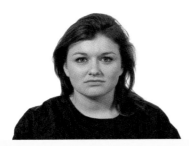

1 Before
Prepare the hair by brushing through smooth – you may have to consider straightening first if the hair is too curly.

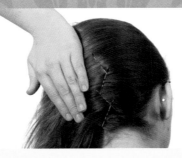

2 Place a vertical row of interlocking grips from the lower hairline to a position just below the crown.

Double row the interlocking grips if needs be.

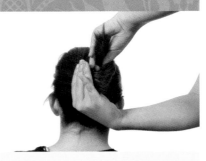

3 Smooth the hair across from the other side and hold with your hand pointing downwards and hair held in the palm of your hand.

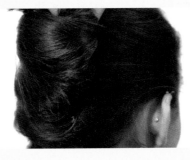

4 Turn inwards to form the pleat.

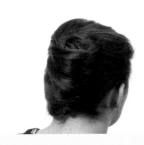

5 Now secure the side of the pleat with fine pins.

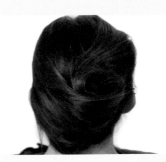

6 Finished effect.

CourseMate video: French Pleat informal

STEP-BY-STEP: PARTY HAIR UP STYLE

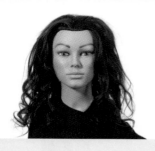

1 Before
The hair has been prepared by setting with heated rollers to give body and loose waves.

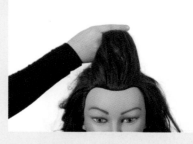

2 A section is taken at the front and back-combed to provide added volume.

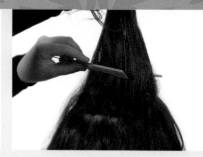

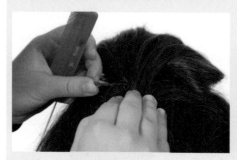

3 This section is secured into place with grips.

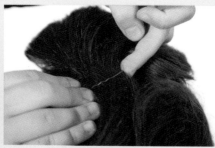

4 Use your mirror to ensure that the profile shape has the lift and balanced desired before finally fixing into place.

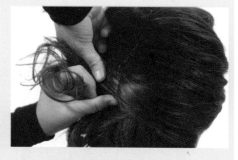

5 With the front done, the back can be worked on.

In this asymmetric effect the right hand side is brushed smooth and secured with interlocking grips (similar to a French pleat).

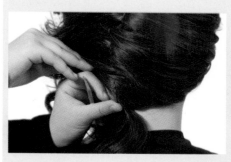

6 Fasten the lowest point of the hairstyle to stop the structure slipping while it is worn.

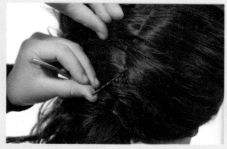

7 Secure the grips and hide the fixings by letting the longer hair fall back over the pleated area.

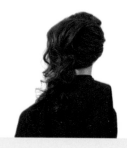

8 Final effect.

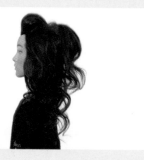

9 Final effect.

Plaiting hair

Plaiting is a method of intertwining three or more strands of hair to create a variety of woven hairstyles. When this work is done for specific occasions, it is often accompanied by ornamentation: fresh flowers, glass or plastic beads, coloured silks and **added hair** are also popular.

The numerous options for plaited effects are controlled by the following factors:

◆ Number of plaits or twists used.

◆ Positioning of the plait or twist across the scalp or around the head.

◆ The way in which the plaits are made (under or over).

◆ Any ornamentation/decoration or added hair applied.

BEST PRACTICE

In shops, people are more likely to buy things that they have handled, so make a point of passing the products that you use to the client so that it stimulates interest and conversation.

HEALTH & SAFETY

The tension used in plaiting can exert exceptional pressure on the hair follicle and scalp-type plaits/cornrows create more vulnerability than free-hanging plaits. In extreme cases hair loss may be caused by this continued pulling action – areas of hair become thin and even baldness may be result!

This condition is called traction alopecia and is particularly obvious at the temples of younger girls with long hair who regularly wear their hair up for school, sport or dancing.

'Plaits' usually refers to a free-hanging stem(s) of hair that is left to show hair length. This length can be natural or can be extended by adding hair during the plaiting process: an example is the 'French' or **fish tail plait**.

Step-by-step – Loose Plaiting – Three-Stem (Loose) Plait The basic three-stem plait demonstrates the fundamental principles of plaiting hair.

1 Divide the hair to be plaited into three equal sections.

2 Hold the hair with both hands, using your fingers to separate the sections.

3 Starting from either the left or the right, place the outside section over the centre one. Repeat this from the other side.

4 Continue placing the outside sections of hair over the centre ones until you reach the ends of the stems.

5 Secure the free ends with ribbon thread or braiding band.

STEP-BY-STEP: FISHTAIL PLAIT – FOUR-STEM (LOOSE) PLAIT

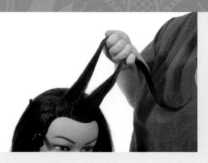

1 A fishtail plait differs from all the other plaiting techniques as it involves four stems and not three.

Start by separating the hair into two stems.

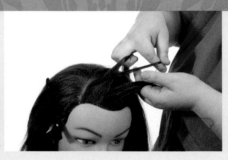

2 While holding each stem in each hand, sub-divide each one, taking the outer, narrower stem and passing it across the other and into the centre.

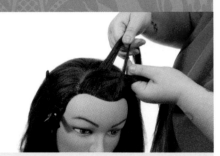

3 Do the same with the other side – sub-divide and pass the outer over and into the centre.

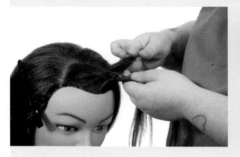

4 Repeat this movement and work down the hair length.

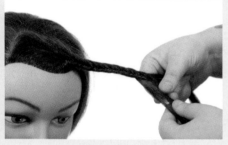

5 The fishtail now forms.

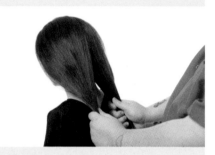

6 Now look at the same sequence when done at the back of the hair.

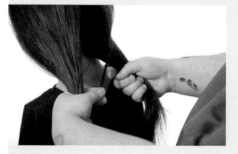

7 While holding each stem in each hand, sub-divide each one, taking the outer, narrower stem and passing it across the other and into the centre.

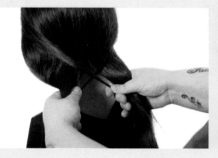

8 Do the same with the other side – sub-divide and pass the outer over and into the centre.

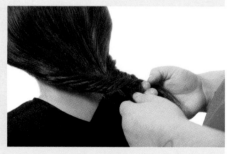

9 Repeat this movement and work down the hair length.

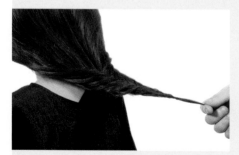

10 The fishtail now forms.

CourseMate video: Fish Tail Plait

STEP-BY-STEP: THREE-STEM 'FRENCH' PLAITING

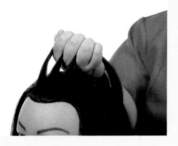

1 With the hair tilted backwards, divide the foremost hair into three equal sections.

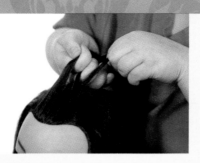

2 Hold them with one stem in one hand and two in the other, then pass one of the outer stems across and into the centre.

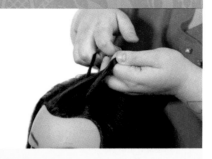

3 Do the same on the other side.

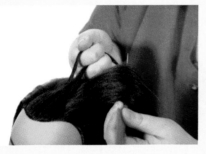

4 With the first part done, you now take an extra section on one side and join it in with the outer stem.

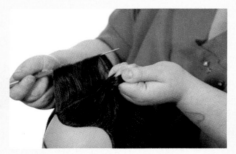

5 Do the same on the other side.

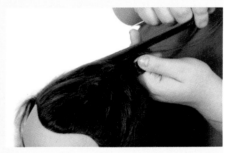

6 Continue the sequences 4 and 5 taking in a new section of hair from the hairline each time.

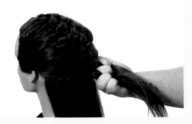

7 Your French plait will now form.

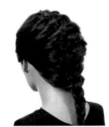

8 The finished effect.

Decorative plaits and twists

The corn row is another type of three-stem plait that is secured close to the scalp to create head-hugging patterned designs.

Cane rows, otherwise known as 'corn rows', is a technique that originated in Africa. Its ethnic origins have been a unique way of displaying hair art and design and have often incorporated complex patterns that historically indicated status or tribal connection. In fact, as this art form has been passed down by subsequent generations for thousands

CourseMate video: French Plait

of years, it is quite probable that the very first hairdressers worked on these elaborate techniques, as it is unlikely that people could do these themselves.

Cane rows create design patterns across the scalp by working along predefined channels of hair. These channels are secured to the scalp by interlocking each of the three sub-divided stems as the plaiting technique progresses.

Short, or even layered hair can be made to look longer still if hair is added, via extensions, during the process. The added hair is plaited into the style along each of the sections that create the plaited effect.

When cane rows have been applied to the hair, the effect can last for up to six weeks or more before they should be removed. Advice should be given on handling and maintaining the hair although regular shampooing can still be carefully achieved.

Preparation for corn rows and twists

Unlike loose plaits designed to last for just a day or so; the closer, tighter technique of plaiting lasts up to several weeks. Because of this, you need to make sure that you cover all the aspects of durability, maintenance and expected results with the client from the outset. This type of work takes a lot longer than basic loose plaits, so make sure that you also give the client a good idea of the costs involved.

A thorough consultation for this type of work is essential. All of these intricately designed effects take a lot of time and you need to have a clear idea of what you are trying to achieve before you start. Plaiting and twisting involves some additional tension on the hair and this can put the client's hair roots under considerable excess stress. Our clients want their hair designs to be neat, controlled and easy to manage and to last for as long as possible. Because of this it is very easy to cause traction alopecia.

As mentioned earlier, traction alopecia is caused by the excessive and continuous strain put on the roots by hairstyled effects such as plaits and twists. You need to make sure that you ask the client throughout the service if the work that you are doing is comfortable and not pulling at different areas across the scalp.

You need to be able to recognize during consultation any previous signs of traction alopecia. The first indications of traction alopecia can be seen around the front hairline, often around the temples. This shows as an area of thinned or missing hair and if the condition is recent, it will be sore and tender.

Before any plaiting, twisting or woven effects can be applied to the hair, you need to assess the suitability of this form of styling for the client.

Other factors affecting the service of plaited or twisted hairstyle. The following list provides you with a quick checklist of things that you should consider in addition to the normal consultation covered previously in this chapter.

- ◆ Style terminology.
- ◆ Style suitability.
- ◆ Hair condition.
- ◆ Hair length.
- ◆ Removal of previous plaits or braids.

Style terminology This is an important aspect for client consultation. It is all too easy for the client to understand a technical term as meaning one thing, while you know it to mean something completely different. This communication aspect may seem rather basic, but it is still the single main reason why clients end up being dissatisfied with a service. It is always better to get down to basics; try to refrain from using clever technical terms. It might be appropriate with your colleagues as you speak the same language, but often the terms used by clients (wrongly) are words picked up from magazines, TV and other people, such as friends or work colleagues. Different people have different ways of saying things – a corn row to one person could mean a **Senegalese twist** to another.

These complex ways of styling hair involve a lot of work and take a lot of time. In most cases, they would take considerable time to unravel and redress. So make sure that you both have a clear idea of what you are trying to achieve. Use visual aids – examples of pictures communicate effects that often cannot be put easily into words.

Style suitability This is an important aspect of consultation. Any work that you are planning to do should be really thought through beforehand. If you were to do a full head of **scalp plaits**, would they suit the client's head and face shape? It may look elaborate when it's finished, it may impress other people, but you do need to ask yourself whether the style enhances the client and is an improvement on what they looked like before. All of this type of work takes a lot of time and when it's done well, the final effects are long-lasting too.

Hair condition Test the hair for poor elasticity, look for damage or over-porous hair. Hair that is weakened for any reason is a contra-indication for plaiting or twisting. If the client is definitely intent on having some form of plait or twisted hair design work, think about recommending a course of restructurants or hair strengtheners beforehand.

Hair texture This is also a major consideration: if the hair is curly, it will need smoothing or straightening first, so that the hair is easier to handle and to improve the final look of the designed work. Remember, hair curl patterns can vary across the scalp: some areas such as the lower nape may be tighter than other areas, so make sure that you check the hair and scalp all over.

Hair length This is an obvious consideration. Make sure that the hair is long enough to produce the effect that you want to achieve. If not, would the hair benefit from added hair extensions?

Removal of previous plaiting If the client needs their previous design work removed, you should dissuade them from having a new set of plaits or twists put in straight after.

Extra care should always be taken when removing the old plaits, as the scalp may be quite tender, sensitive or even sore. Over time, products can build up around the scalp and this can bond the hair together making detangling quite difficult. In any event, you will need patience and care to disentangle or unravel the hair, so that it is not weakened, broken, or damaged any further.

Shampoo and condition the hair The hair must be shampooed and conditioned thoroughly before any plaiting or twisting service is done. You need to make sure that any traces of product – moisturizers, gels, serums and oils – are removed from the hair first.

Drying into shape

Drying into shape Both plaiting and twisting techniques tend to make the hair appear shorter, as with plaits, much of this length is used laterally (across and around the head) as decoration. So you would need to blow-dry the hair first, to make the most of its overall length. This is necessary anyway, as the hair needs to be dried and made smoother before any other work can take place. After blow-drying, the hair and scalp can be prepared with hair oils or dressings. Any moisturizing will be beneficial to the hair, making it more elastic, improving its brittleness, and making it more pliable.

The design that you create is based on a sort of graphical layout. Regardless of whether you are doing scalp plaits, singles or twists, the direction in which they flow is related to their starting position on the scalp and accurate sectioning creates this.

Cane/corn rows

Cane/corn rows Cane rows are a type of scalp plait that creates linear designs across the head. They will last anything from one week to a couple of months – although with washing and general wear and tear, they tend to look a little untidy after a couple of weeks. Cane rows create design patterns across the scalp by working along pre-defined channels of hair. These channels are secured to the scalp by interlocking each of the sub-divided stems as the plaiting technique progresses.

Short or even layered hair can be made to look longer still by adding hair extensions to the client's hair during the process. The added hair is plaited into the style along each of the sections that create the braided effect.

Advice should be given on handling and maintaining the hair although regular shampooing can still be carefully achieved. This type of work is ideal for natural hair as it can be worn with or without added hair extensions, even making short hair look long. They are easily removed although the smaller the plait stems and sections the more difficult and fiddly it becomes.

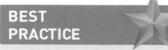

BEST PRACTICE

Always use flat clips for any braiding or twists, it keeps the hair smoother.

STEP-BY-STEP: METHOD OF CANE ROWING

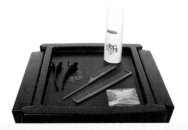

1 Prepare a your trolley with:

  1 Flat sectioning clips.

  2 A tail comb.

  3 A straight cutting comb.

  4 Braiding bands.

  5 Suitable styling products.

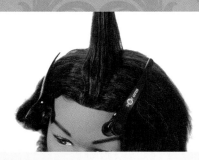

2 Decide on the linear design that you want to create first, as this will have an impact on where you start.

Section off a channel of hair – the length of the scalp plait required.

Section all the other hair out of the way with flat clips.

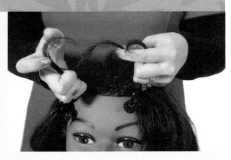

3 Take a small section from the front and divide into three stems.

Cross-over the left and right stems, under the central one.

Move the outer left stem over the central stem, now bring the right outer stem in and over the central stem.

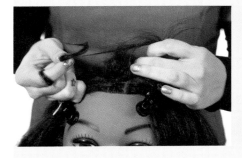

4 To progress along the scalp – pick up a small section and incorporate it into the left stem.

Move the outer left stem over the central stem, now bring the right outer stem in and over the central stem.

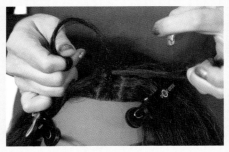

5 Repeat 4 until you have worked along the scalp to the desired point.

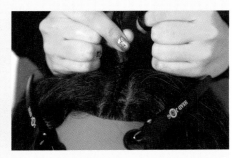

6 Remember to keep the plait taut with an even tension to avoid 'bagging'.

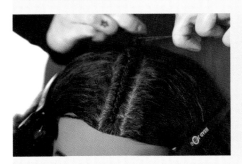

7 When you have reached the end of the plait, secure the remainder with a braiding band.

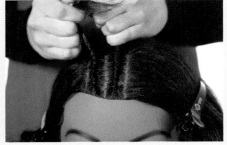

8 Complete the other corn rows in the same way.

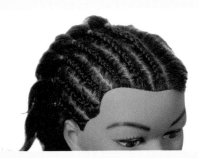

9 Final effect.

Method for adding hair into the cane row The method for adding or extending the hair is similar to the above except that narrow strands of hair extensions are taken and added to take the place of the two outer sections, i.e. it is looped across the client's natural hair to create the first and third stem of the braid. Then as each time the outer braid introduces part of the client's hair, the added hair is secured down to the scalp.

Added hair or extension hair can be made from a variety of materials that can be natural or synthetic. They come in a variety of different textures, types and colours and can be added to the client's natural hair for a variety of different styling reasons. Subtle, harmonizing tones and textures can be added to make the client's own hair appear longer than it is. Conversely, bright fashion colour extensions can be added to create dramatic, contrasting effects.

Single plaits Single plaits are a popular method of styling for men or women. They can be done on natural or chemically processed hair although the effects are more dramatic on longer hair. This doesn't mean that people with shorter hair can't have plaits – they are obvious candidates for extensions and added hair. Single plaits are quite durable and typically they will last for up to three months, but, like cane rows, their appearance deteriorates after a few weeks. The ends of the plaits should be secured with 'clear' (transparent) braiding bands.

Step-by-step – Method For Single Plaits

1   Wash, condition and pre-dry the hair straight.

2   Starting at the nape section the hair horizontally and secure the remainder.

3   Sub-divide the horizontal section into small 1cm by 1cm square sections and separate into three equal stems.

4   Hold the first section between the middle and third finger of the left hand and the next, middle section between the index finger and thumb. Now take the last or third section between the middle and third finger of the right hand.

5   Continue to cross the outer stem on the left over the centre stem, and then pass the outer stem on the right over what is now the centre stem.

6   Repeat this down to the ends of the hair and secure with a professional band.

7   Move to the next square section of hair and repeat steps 4–6.

8   Continue this by working up the back of the head, then to the lower sides and again up to the top of the head.

If added hair extensions are required, do the above steps 1 and 2, then at 3:

3   Sub-divide the horizontal section into smaller square sections, then attach extension hair to each of the stems of the client's hair and plait as normal as a three-stem plait above.

Twisting techniques

Twists are an alternative to plaited styles: they will last for up to a month before they become untidy. Unlike plaits, they don't involve any interlocking of hair, so they usually require an application of pomade or light styling gel to bond the hair while the twists are being formed.

BEST PRACTICE

Use products sparingly as it would be easy to apply too much product, which would make the hair feel greasy or dirty and mean that it would have to be washed again.

Twisting is achieved by using the fingers or a comb to twist the hair into strands. This can be done in **linear patterns** along the scalp such as **flat twists**, or off the scalp as with single twists or two-stem twists.

Flat twists Flat twists have a similar appearance at a distance to corn rows, but when you look more closely, you can see that the hair is not inter locked in the same way. The durability of the effects depends upon the type of hair, but as a rule of thumb, twists don't last as long as corn rows. But on a positive note, they don't take anything like the same amount of time to put in as tight, three-stem scalp plaits.

Step-by-step – Method For Creating A Flat Twist

Step 1 Shampoo, condition and dry the hair roughly into shape.

Step 2 After brushing the hair to remove any tangles, start the style at the front by dividing the hair with a tail comb.

Step 3 Twist the section of hair firmly but not too tightly back towards the crown area.

Step 4 Grip the twisted section into place before starting the next channel.

Step 5 Continue with the same technique on each of the channels.

Step 6 Twist the sections at the back from the nape up to the crown in the same way.

Step 7 Leave a section at the front to soften the hairline profile. Lightly back-comb the remaining hair to finish.

Step-by-step – Method For Creating Single Twists

1   Wash, condition and towel-dry the hair.

2   Divide the hair into four quadrants and secure with sectioning clips.

3   Section off horizontally at the nape and secure the remainder out of the way.

4   Sub-divide the horizontal sections into smaller areas of just a few millimetres across. (The smaller the sections the tidier the twist will look.)

5   Apply the gel or pomade throughout the length of the twist stem.

6   Place a tail comb into the stem close to the root and start to turn in either a continuous clockwise (or anti-clockwise) movement. Work down the section of hair to the end.

7   Continue on to the next twist in the horizontal section and repeat steps 5 and 6.

8   Continue working up the head.

9   When all of the twists have been completed, arrange them neatly in the direction of the desired style and place under a dryer for 20–30 minutes.

10 When completely dry, apply product, either a spray fixative or serum to complete the look.

METHOD FOR CREATING TWO-STEM TWISTS (ROPE TWISTS)

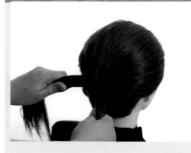

1 Fix the hair centrally at the back in a pony tail with a covered band.

Then divide the pony tail into two equal parts.

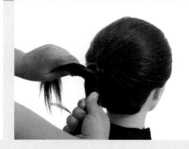

2 Both stems should be twisted in a clockwise direction.

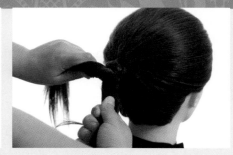

3 And then wound around each other.

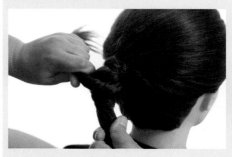

4 Continue twisting and then winding around each other.

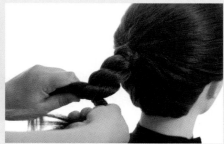

5 Continue twisting down the length of the pony tail.

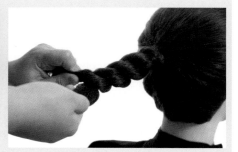

6 Repeat until you have twisted enough hair to finish the look.

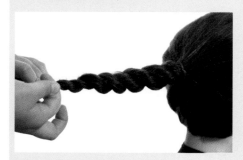

7 Use a braiding band to bond the ends together.

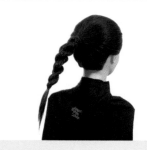

8 Final effect.

CourseMate video: Rope Plait

Senegalese twists Senegalese twists are a scalp twist effect – they consist of stems of hair that are always twisted in the same direction with hair crossing over and creating a rope effect.

Step-by-step – Method For Creating Senegalese Twists

1 Wash, condition and pre-dry the hair smooth.

2 Section out a channel of hair with a tail comb to create the direction and the design required.

3 Using the fingers, start close to the root, take a small section of hair and twist it in a clockwise movement.

4 As you work along the channel, pick up and work in more sections of hair to create the scalp twist effect.

5 When the channel of twisted hair is finished, secure until all of the others are finished.

6 The free ends of the twists can be interlocked together, and then after they have been dried under a dryer the effect can be thermally styled to complete the total effect.

Provide aftercare advice

Good service must always be supported through sound advice and recommendation. The work that you do in the salon needs to be cared for at home by the client too. What would be the point of creating something if the client doesn't know how to achieve and/or maintain the same effects at home?

Aftercare checklist

◆ Talk through the style as you work: that way the client sees how you handle different aspects of the look.

◆ Show and recommend the products/equipment that you use so that the client gets the right things to enable them to get the same effects.

◆ Explain how routine styling with tongs or straighteners can have detrimental effects.

◆ Demonstrate the techniques that you use so they can achieve that salon hair look too.

◆ When you have put the client's hair up, or provided a plaited or twisted effect, give them advice on how to take the style down/remove the plaits or twists.

Talk through the style as you work

It's very difficult to do two things at the same time and you have probably found this yourself at work. Have you noticed how a senior stylist chats with the client while they are working? On the other hand, have you noticed the difference when a less experienced stylist is trying to do a similar technical piece of work? It seems to go very quiet!

The client probably notices this too: that's because a less confident stylist will always divert their attention to the job in hand.

It's far easier to talk about the things that you are doing with the hair than to talk about the client's children at school, who may be taking their exams. Make a point of talking through your technique as you go:

1 it eliminates long periods of silence while you are working and, more importantly;

2 it is useful to the client as they get good advice on how to recreate a similar effect at home.

Show and recommend the products/ equipment that you use

As you talk about the ways in which you have styled the hair, make a point of talking through the products that you have used as well.

So when you use a particular product, why not hand it to them so they can have a closer look. This way they get to see, smell and feel the product too and subconsciously this has a very powerful effect on them. By doing this, you are involving the client in what you are doing by giving them a greater experience of the service. They will be able to see a direct link between what you are doing and the effects that you are achieving on their hair, with the added benefit of knowing that buying those particular products will help them to recreate a similar effect.

Explain how routine styling tools can have detrimental effects

Only hair in good condition is easy to maintain. You know how difficult it is to make dry, damaged hair look good. It tends to be lifeless, dull and sits there just like a wig! Your clients can recognize the difference between good and poor condition and given the choice, they will always choose hair that has lustre, shine, flexibility and strength.

With these known facts, you would be doing an injustice to your clients if you didn't warn them of the pitfalls of repeatedly using hot styling equipment, so make a point in asking them if they use them at home too. If they say that they use straighteners or tongs on a daily basis then tell them about the benefits of using heat protection sprays. Remember, the condition of their hair is directly proportional to the amount of heat applied to it. So if they are locked into using these styling tools their hair is going to need all the help it can get.

Demonstrate the techniques that you use

Clients want to be able to recreate the effects that you achieve in the salon and this is your chance to show them how to do it. Clients haven't had the benefit of your training: they don't know the little tricks and techniques that make it seem so simple. Show them how to do things: correct brushing, back-combing, twists or rolls. We have all seen the effects when these are not done properly, so make a point of giving them a few tips on how they can achieve a similar result.

Advise on how to take the style down

Damage occurs when the hair is mistreated and this is a simple fact that we all know. When hair is put up, it tends to use a lot of scaffolding in support. All that metalwork in pins, grips, ornaments and accessories or even rubber hair bands can have a damaging effect on the hair if they are not handled and removed in the proper way.

Tell your clients where they need to start: most people try to feel around the back and take out the first grip or pin that they come to. That's not the way to do it. You know that if the innermost hair sections are pulled out first then it creates a big knot and then everything just tangles together. If you were taking it down, you would start at the last area that was secured into place. Tell clients where they should start and the negative, damaging effects on their hair if they just pull the style apart.

Finally, tell your client about the things that they may need help with too. If you are doing a bridal hair-up, then it might involve a headdress too. Many brides will wear one through the ceremony and the reception after, but want to remove this at some point later in the evening. You know that if it isn't done carefully it could pull the whole hairstyle out of shape! Explain how the combs or accessories are positioned into the hair and the ways that they can be removed carefully without destroying the hairstyle.

SUMMARY

As a final reflection on what you have covered in this chapter, you should now have a clearer picture of all the essential aspects for styling and finishing hair. In particular, you should now have a basic understanding of the key principles of:

1 Why preparation is essential to the service.

2 The science aspects relating to styling and finishing hair.

3 The styling products available and the tools and equipment used within the service.

4 The techniques involved in blow-drying, setting and dressing hair and how heated styling equipment can be used to finish off the hairstyling effects.

5 How to use and maintain the tools and equipment associated with the different styling services.

6 Smoothing, curling, folding and fixing longer or shorter hair in a variety of different ways.

7 Providing advice to the clients about styling and maintaining their hair.

And collectively, how these principles will enable you to provide a comprehensive range of styling services to your clients.

ASSESSMENT OF KNOWLEDGE AND UNDERSTANDING

Project

For this project you will need to gather information from a variety of sources.

Collect together photographs, digital images and magazine clippings about styling, blow-drying, setting and dressing techniques.

Include styles for long hair as well as short: for weddings, special occasions and casual wear.

In your portfolio describe:

1 How the styles were achieved.

2 Why each is suitable for its purpose.

3 The equipment (with examples) that was used to create the effects.

4 The products (with examples) used to help hold or define the effects.

Revision questions

A selection of different types of questions to check your styling and finishing hair knowledge.

Q1 A round brush is also known as a _____ brush.   Fill in the blank

Q2 Humidity in the atmosphere will make a blow-dried finish drop.   True or false

Q3 Which of the following items are examples of heated styling equipment?   Multi selection

Tongs	☐	1
Vented brush	☐	2
Crimpers	☐	3
Thinners	☐	4
Grips	☐	5
Straighteners	☐	6

Q4 The keratin bonds of stretched hair are said to be in the beta keratin state.   True or false

Q5 Which chemical bonds within the hair are affected during heat styling?   Multi choice

Hydrogen bonds	O	a
Disulphide bonds	O	b
Sulphur bonds	O	c
Premium bonds	O	d

Q6 Ceramic straighteners can be used to curl hair.   True or false

Q7 Heated tongs will produce which of the following results and effects?   Multi selection

Increased body at the roots	☐	1
No body at the roots	☐	2
Curl at the ends	☐	3
Straighter effects	☐	4
Wavy effects	☐	5
Same as straightening irons	☐	6

Q8   A paddle brush is a type of _____ brush.   Fill in the blank

Q9   Which item of equipment would smooth and flatten frizzy, unruly hair best?   Multi choice

Curling tongs   ○ a

Ceramic straighteners   ○ b

Crimping irons   ○ c

Blow-dryer   ○ d

Q10   In blow-drying the hair should always be dried from root to points.   True or false

9 Men's styling

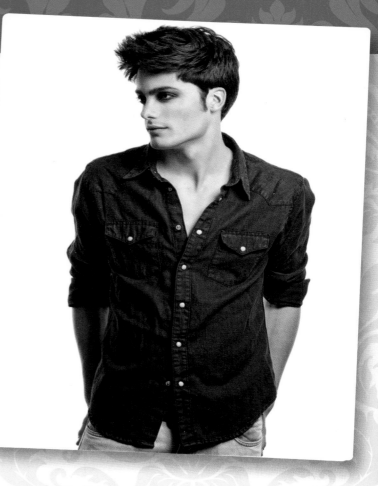

LEARNING OBJECTIVES

◆ Be able to maintain effective and safe methods of working

◆ Be able to dry and finish men's hair

◆ Know how to work safely, effectively and hygienically

◆ Understand the basic science that relates to drying and finishing hair

◆ Know how and when to use different drying and finishing techniques, products and equipment

◆ Know how to provide aftercare advice for clients

KEY TERMS

client consultation

defining crème

defining wax

dry wax

hairspray

moulding clay

posture

scrunch drying

Styling men's hair.

INTRODUCTION

The professional finish applied to men's hair after cutting is often something that is rushed, or poorly executed. This happens when most of the appointment time is given over to the cutting service, and the finishing off is simply a quick blast with a hair dryer to enable the client to walk out with dry hair.

This was, and should never be, the intention of men's styling. In fact, this quick, in and out approach to men's hairdressing has 'wrong-footed' the industry, in leading our male clients to think that this is the norm, and what they should be expecting. Wrong!

The time you take in providing a professional finish, the products that you use, along with the advice that you give your client, is going to have a huge impact on:

◆ The quality of service they receive.

◆ Their perception of you.

◆ The profits for the business.

And collectively, these factors will start to re-educate an underserved proportion of our clientele.

Shampooing and conditioning

PRACTICAL SKILLS

Learn how to prepare the client's hair before styling

Learn how to select the right products, tools and equipment

Learn how to recognize hair and skin conditions, defects and disorders

Learn about recognizing contra-indications and other things that can affect intended services

Learn about following safe and hygienic working practices

Learn how to communicate in a professional manner

Providing advice to clients about their hair

UNDERPINNING KNOWLEDGE

Styling men's hair using basic techniques

Using a range of appropriate styling products

Using a range of appropriate styling tools and equipment

Preparing to style men's hair

All of the things that you need to know about preparation are already covered elsewhere in this book. So to avoid unnecessary duplication, the following aspects can be found on the following pages.

◆ Gowning and preparing your client	**CHAPTER 10** Cutting Hair (Preparing to cut hair)
◆ **Posture** and safe working positions	
◆ Safe and organized work areas	
◆ Safe and effective use of tools	
◆ Shampooing and conditioning hair	**CHAPTER 7** Shampooing and conditioning
◆ Personal hygiene	**CHAPTER 2** Working in the hairdressing industry (personal effectiveness and professionalism)
◆ Client consultation	**CHAPTER 6** Client Consultation

TOP TIP

Most preparations for male clients are the same for female clients too. A client is a client.

Main differences for drying and finishing men's hair

The main differences in drying and finishing men's hair relate to the products that are specifically formulated with the male client in mind. There may be far fewer products available for him, but there are still sufficient options to cover all the styling needs and effects. So in other words, a modern man creates his fashionable looks from a toolkit of far fewer styling products. He creates his individualistic look by using a range of products that do specific jobs.

Product	Application	Purpose	Suitability
Dry wax *L'Oréal Professionnel*	Applied in small amounts by the fingertips into pre-dried hair.	A moderately firm hold providing a non-wet look or greasy finish. Ideal for men who really don't like the look of product on the hair, but need the benefits of the control it provides.	Suited to short- and medium-length hair: the effects need to be created carefully and slowly by adding more as needed. It is very easy to add too much and overload the hair, particularly on finer hair types.
Defining wax *Wella*	Work a small amount of product in your finger-tips and sculpt into dry hair. Shape and rework as desired.	A strong defining clay that allows styles to be reshaped and recreated.	Ideal for textured looks and short hair, styles can be used to define key areas.
Hair varnish/gloss *L'Oréal Professionnel*	Applied in small amounts by the fingertips into pre-dried hair. Care needs to be taken in applying the product evenly, throughout the hair.	A high-gloss look with a greasy texture. The styles created are moisture repelling. Ideal for men who do like product effects on their hair.	Suits short hair with long lasting low maintenance looks, suitable for sports etc. Again the effect needs to be created slowly: it is easy to overload the hair and these types of product do produce a build-up upon the hair.
Hair gel *Wella*	Distribute 1 or 2 pumps into your palms and work into the hair.	A styler that lifts, tex-turizes and tousles hair into many different styles with a pearl shine, finish and hold.	Can be used on dry hair. For extra lift in short hair, work into wet hair and blow dry.

(Continued)

(Continued)

Product	Application	Purpose	Suitability
Styling glaze *L'Oréal Professionnel*	Applied first to the hands and rubbed into wet or pre-dried hair all over. The hair is styled after and allowed to dry and fix into shape.	A wet look effect with firm to strong hold. Suitable for controlled or groomed looks with a mild, wet look effect.	Again like gel, you can't overload the hair as the look is based on 100 per cent coverage. The styles created are suited to short hair and are more resistant to moisture than gel but create less sculpted or high-hair effects than gel.
Moulding clay/Hair putty *Wella*	Work a small amount of product in your fingertips into dry hair to design your desired shape.	A matt styling paste to create casually textured styles.	Suitable on dry hair to add definition.
Defining crème *Wella*	Work a small amount of product in your fingertips into dry hair.	A moulding cream to construct a rugged texture with a strong matt definition.	Ideal for short hair for an edgy, matt finish.
Hairspray *Wella*	Applied to pre-dried hair by directional spraying from 30cm away.	Provides mild, moderate and firm hold, can be used as a final fixative or as a styling product when scrunched in.	Easy to apply, providing a long lasting effect on any hair length.

Choosing the right tools and equipment

Having the correct product, and using it in the right context, is essential and sometimes, this gets blurred. Often, fashion will dictate that we use the *latest and greatest* or *new improved formula*. These may seem like really compelling reasons for using a product, but if it's inappropriate for your client, you need to be providing the best possible advice that's *tailored* to their needs.

As a student stylist, you are learning what to use and when to use it and this is important. You may have already come into contact with the negative aspects of product build-up, and even struggled to get the client's hair to do what you want it to do, but the biggest sufferers of 'bad hair days' are men. This is probably more to do with poor maintenance and lack of knowledge, rather than a keen interest to walk around with dirty hair.

Unfortunately, some products are more prone to creating a build-up than others, and this makes it difficult to remove by simple shampooing. Generally speaking, the heavier waxes, grooming creams and pomades, are the *culprits* for creating this problem and men don't seem to know what to do in order to remove them properly. This can often be an issue for hair cutting as it means that the hair must have a clarifying shampoo before they have it cut. This is fine for scissor cutting but just adds unexpected extra time for clipper work, particularly as clippers are used on dry hair. Fortunately, this has less impact upon styling and finishing the hair, as the hair has to be shampooed before you can start.

Being organized

Choosing and finding the correct tools is also important. For example, if you are going to finger-dry your client's hair, you need to make sure that you have found a diffuser and cleaned it ready for use. Likewise, if you need a particular set of brushes to cope with longer length hair make sure that you have those ready too.

Organizing yourself in the way that you use the available time is part of being a professional. Running around, finding things that you need when the client is sat waiting in the chair may seem amusing to the client the first time that you do it. But that novelty soon wears off if that turns out to be your normal method of working. We all want to appear to be in control, organized and in charge of the situation and you can too, by giving yourself enough time beforehand to prepare properly.

Consultation

It is unlikely that you will just be drying your client's hair, as the styling part is the finishing bit – i.e. it follows on from other services. So therefore, your initial consultation should be focused upon the haircut, or a colouring service.

BEST PRACTICE

Men may not be quite as competent at applying styling products – Make sure that you tell them how to use them correctly.

TOP TIP

You are the professional and people will listen to the advice that you give.

TOP TIP

Self organization will save you a lot of time during the service and a lot of stress too.

Go to **CHAPTER 6** Consultation for more information on all the things that you should consider before you start.

BEST PRACTICE

The client's overall satisfaction will depend on your consultation – the choices and decisions you make have a critical impact on what you do and what can be achieved.

Brief summary of things to consider

Things to look out for	Things you could ask the client	Why ask this?
Look at the hair shape	'How would you like your hair styled?'	You can see if the style is achievable from the lengths and layering patterns as you brush through the hair and what sorts of products you will need to help style it.
Look for infections or infestations that will stop you from carrying on.	'Have you had any scalp problems recently?'	If the client has had problems it gives you a lead to investigate further.
Look at the type and tendency of the hair	'Is your hair naturally wavy (or curly)?'	If there is movement in the hair you need to find out if it is natural to get an idea of which brushes you need to use and whether you will need to use other heated styling equipment too.
Look at the amount and texture of the hair.	'Does your hair take long to dry and style?'	Thicker hair and some hair textures take longer to dry. You need to find out if there are any condition issues first.
Look at the head and facial shape.	'Do you find that some styles suit you better than others?'	Find out whether the client naturally chooses and wears styles that are aesthetically correct for them.
Look at the natural partings.	'Is this the way that your hair usually falls?'	If the natural parting is not where the client wants it, you need to point out the pitfalls of working against the natural fall of the hair.
Look at the quality of the hair and the way that it lies.	'Do you normally use a finishing or defining product on your hair?'	Will the final look be improved by definition, serums or other finishing products?
Likes and dislikes, visual aids/pictures.	'Would you like something along these lines or do you prefer a simpler style?'	You must get the client to confirm the desired effect before you start.

Dry and finish hair

BEST PRACTICE

If you use a particular product explain why you are using it.

Men's hairstyles tend to rely upon simpler effects. Admittedly, some men do dry their hair in a more formal blow-dried way but the vast majority tend to create their desired effects from finger-drying or **scrunch drying**, with the backup of products to achieve the effects they want.

After making your choices about styles and products, you should think about the sorts of tools equipment that you could use.

Tools and equipment

- Denman Classic Styling brush
- Vented brush
- Paddle (flat) brush

- Radial brushes
- Diffuser

Styling hair – Blow-drying

Believe it or not, the blow-drying technique of styling hair with a hand-held dryer started in the barber's shop. It's only since the 60s that the ladies hairdresser has *hijacked* the technique and made it the most popular way of styling hair.

Historically, the barber's styling tools were limited to a range of combs and a couple of brushes, so when in the ladies salon, the hairdresser found that with one hand free, they could create volume, curl, lift and movement by using brushes. The styling technique has become the core service to finishing hair.

Blow-drying enables the stylist to control the direction of the airflow, over a brush or comb, so that the heat generated does not burn the client.

Blow-drying dos and don'ts

Dos	Don'ts
✓ Make sure that you have everything that you need at hand before you start.	✗ Use dirty tools or equipment. Check them all before you need them.
✓ Unravel the lead before you start so that you don't end up 'lassoing' the client.	✗ Forget to visually check the leads and plug before you plug it in.
✓ Remove excess moisture from saturated hair.	✗ Direct the flow of hot air near to the client's scalp, it will burn very quickly.
✓ Take small sections of damp hair so that the hair will dry evenly and quickly.	✗ Over dry the sections of the hair as it will make the hair unmanageable and damage it.
✓ Try to use lower heat settings/speeds as this provides far more control in the quality of your work.	✗ Forget to use a 'cold-shot' to fix movement or volume into the hair.
✓ Use a diffuser for finger-drying as this disperses the heat evenly and allows you to manipulate the hair with your hands, pressing it into shape.	✗ Forget to ask your client to move their head to enable you to dry all the hair properly and evenly.

BEST PRACTICE

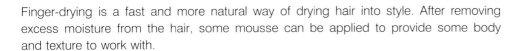

Often men's appointments tend to be short – make the most of the time available, give good advice and the reasons why you do things in certain ways.

Finger-drying is a fast and more natural way of drying hair into style. After removing excess moisture from the hair, some mousse can be applied to provide some body and texture to work with.

STEP-BY-STEP: FINGER-DRYING AND STRAIGHTENING

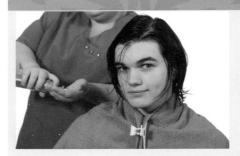

1 After shampooing and conditioning the hair, towel-dry any excess moisture before detangling.

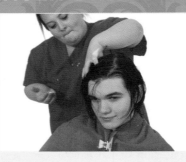

2 Then add your styling product evenly into the hair.

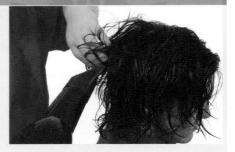

3 Rough-dry the excess moisture first to cut down drying time.

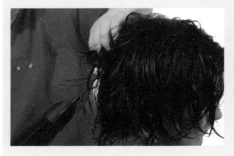

4 If you want to encourage movement into the hair, it will scrunch dry better if it is dryer rather than wetter.

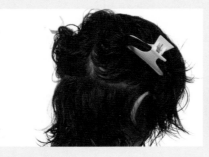

5 Now with the hair rough-dried, you can start at the back and section the hair off so that you work on smaller areas of hair.

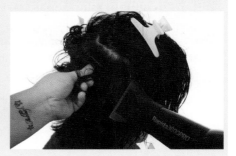

6 Rub the hair between the fingers and hold in a scrunch until dry.

As an alternative you could use a diffuser.

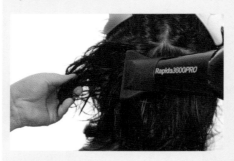

7 As the hair dries the movement will fix into place.

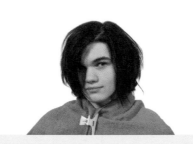

8 A very natural and casual finish.

Alternatively, and for a straight finish you could use straightening irons.

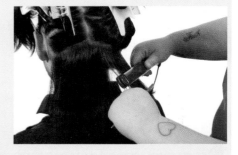

9 Re-section the hair and start at the bottom to pass the heated plates over each held mesh of hair.

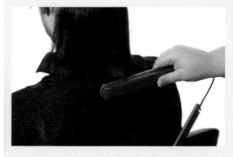

10 Take care to straighten the hair with one smooth motion without grabbing or jerking.

Be careful not to damage the hair. Heat protection is recommended.

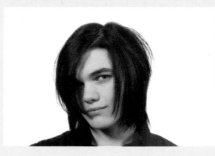

11 Same hairstyle but with a straightened effect. This provides more definition and can be textured further with wax or moulding paste.

The main idea of finger-drying is to use a blow-dryer with the fingers in a directional drying method, on generally shorter hair. Using the fingers to produce the effect provides three main benefits for this technique:

◆ It allows a style to be moulded on hair that would normally be too short to dry with brushes.

◆ It enables the stylist/barber to keep a check on the dryer heat as the fingers act as a temperature gauge for the client's head.

◆ It provides the stylist/barber with a non-fussy styling option for the male client.

The checklist below covers the main considerations for finger-drying men's hair.

✓ Always work with damp and not saturated hair – rough-dry if necessary.

✓ Work on small areas/sections of hair.

✓ Try to dry the hair in the direction of roots to points – it will dry more quickly and keep the cuticle layer smoother, making it look healthier and shinier.

✓ Avoid burning the scalp – angle your dryer away from the head.

✓ Move the position of your client's head in order to get around and cover all areas of the head.

✓ Use both hands to dry the hair, so swap the dryer around: this allows you to work on both sides of the head effectively.

Not as popular now as in the past, blow comb styling is a way of creating lift or movement within a hairstyle to emphasize partings, particularly in difficult or unruly hair. The effect created produces strong movement that a brush and blow-dryer could not achieve.

STEP-BY-STEP: BLOW COMB STYLING

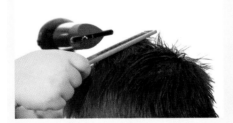

1 The blow comb is a drying technique that is really useful for adding lots of lift into men's short hair.

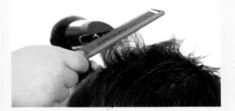

2 The hair is lifted with a cutting comb and the hot stream of air is introduced to the surface of the comb.

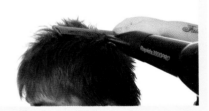

3 This is done all over the hair at any point where lift is needed.

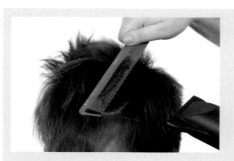

4 As the style progresses, you can see that a randomized form of lift and texture is created.

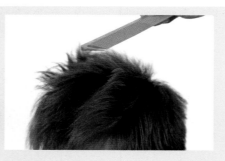

5 This close-up shows you the amount of lift that can be achieved.

The final effect can be enhanced with wax or hair putty products.

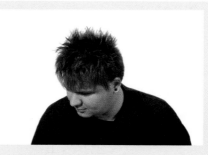

6 Final effect.

Provide aftercare advice

Men are not usually as adept at handling hair or being as *hair-aware* as women and that means more work for you as this particular segment of your market will need better advice if they are going to be able to manage their own hair between visits.

When you use a particular product on their hair, don't expect them to know:

◆ What it is that you are using.

◆ What it will do for them as a benefit in handling their hair.

You need to tell them what it is that you are using and why you have chosen to use it. Believe it or not, men are generally far easier to sell to than women. Quite simply, if they can be given a logical reason for doing or using something, they will accept what they have been told and take up that advice. They will then carry on using that product or item, until such a time that it no longer provides them with the same benefits.

SUMMARY

As a final reflection on what you have covered in this chapter, you should now have a clearer picture of all the essential aspects for styling men's hair. In particular, you should now have a basic understanding of the key principles of:

1 Why preparation is essential to the service.

2 The science aspects relating to styling and finishing men's hair.

3 The styling products available for men and the tools and equipment used within men's styling services.

4 The techniques involved to create the finished effects.

5 How to use and maintain the tools and equipment associated with the different styling services.

6 Providing advice to the clients about styling and maintaining their hair.

And collectively, how these principles will enable you to provide a comprehensive range of styling services to your clients.

ASSESSMENT OF KNOWLEDGE AND UNDERSTANDING

Project

For this project you will need to select two of your clients.

1 Client 1 should have short hair.

2 Client 2 should have longer hair.

For each of these clients:

1 Describe what your client's hair was like before you started.

2 Describe what techniques and tools were used to complete the look.

3 Explain what products you used and how they helped to achieve the look.

4 Take a photograph (perhaps with your mobile) of the finished effect.

Revision questions

A selection of different types of questions to check your men's styling knowledge.

Q1 The common name for drying hair with just the hands is _____ drying.   Fill in the blank

Q2 Humidity in the atmosphere will cause a finished style to drop.   True or false

Q3 Which of the following are finishing products?   Multi selection

Mousse	☐ 1
Wax	☐ 2
Gel	☐ 3
Setting lotion	☐ 4
Hairspray	☐ 5
Conditioner	☐ 6

Q4 The keratin bonds of stretched hair are said to be in the beta keratin state.   True or false

Q5 Which of the following is the odd one out?   Multi choice

Vented brush	O a
Denman brush	O b
Round brush	O c
Paddle brush	O d

Q6 Finger-drying is similar to scrunch drying.   True or false

Q7 Which of the following are better sterilized in a UV cabinet rather than in Barbicide®?   Multi selection

Cutting comb	☐ 1
Conditioning comb	☐ 2
A Denman brush	☐ 3
A vented brush	☐ 4
Plastic sectioning clips	☐ 5
Metal sectioning clips	☐ 6

Q8 A _____ is an attachment for a blow-dryer which reduces the hot hair blast.   Fill in the blank

Q9 Which item of equipment is best for smoothing and flattening frizzy, unruly hair?   Multi choice

Curling tongs	O a
Ceramic straighteners	O b
Crimping irons	O c
Blow-dryer	O d

Q10 Hair should be rough-dried before styling.   True or false

10 Cutting

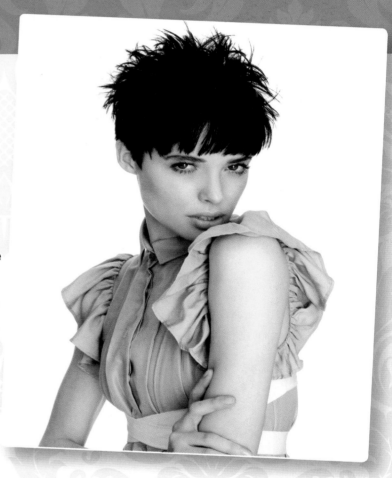

LEARNING OBJECTIVES

◆ Be able to maintain safe methods of working

◆ Be able to cut hair to achieve a variety of looks

◆ Know how to work safely, effectively and hygienically

◆ Understand the factors that can affect the service

◆ Understand one length, graduation, reverse graduation, and uniform layering cutting techniques

◆ Understand the aftercare advice that you should provide to clients

KEY TERMS

African type hair

blending

blunt cutting

chipping

club cutting or clubbing hair

concave

contrasts

convex

cross checking

cutting angle

disconnection

feathering

freehand

graduation

holding angle

holding tension

humidity

inversion

neck brush

oblong facial shape

one-length haircut

open (cut throat) razor

point cutting

reshape/reshaping

reverse graduation

safety razor

scissor over comb

shaper razor

shaving cream

short graduations

slicing

T liner

tapered necklines

texturizing

uniform layer cut

Unit topic

Cut hair using basic techniques.

INTRODUCTION

Cutting is the most important service in hairdressing or barbering, it is the core service that we provide to clients, which they consider to be an essential part of their lives. For us, as hairdressers, it forms the basic technical service, from which we build our livelihood. Cutting is a basic service but that doesn't mean it is a simple service. Quite the contrary, for many student hairdressers or barbers, it is the most difficult thing to learn.

Cutting is a 'basic' service because it is fundamental to all the other services we provide, it forms the basis from which all other services develop. In creative colouring, it reinforces the detail within the colour effect. In styling and dressing, it controls the final shape and balance. And in perming it can reduce, or increase the amount of movement or volume that has been applied.

◆ In good times, when people do well and have a strong *'feel good factor',* people have their hair cut and spend more on their appearance.

◆ In times when things are not going so well, i.e. a recession, people **still** have their hair cut, even if they don't spend more on their appearance in other ways.

Cutting men's and women's hair

PRACTICAL SKILLS

Preparing yourself, the client and the work area correctly

Preparing and maintaining your tools and equipment

Following your cutting guidelines and maintaining the accuracy by cross checking your cut

Producing a range of effects for men by using different cutting techniques and methods

Producing a range of effects for women by using different cutting techniques and methods

Providing aftercare advice

Learn how the holding of tensions and angles maintains the accuracy of a cut

Learn about the advantages for cutting hair when wet or dry

UNDERPINNING KNOWLEDGE

Learn about the factors that influence haircutting for men and women

Learn how to assess the potential of the hair

Learn how to recognize different facial shapes and work with facial features

Learn how to recognize contra-indications and other things that can affect intended services

Learn how to recognize various contagious and non-contagious conditions

Learn how to recognize a range of hair factors and defects

Learn about a variety of cutting angles and effects and how they are achieved

---

TOP TIP

People still need to spend money on a haircut, even if they choose not to have any other services.

Preparing to cut hair

You

Your preparation for this service is equally as important as the preparations for any other hairdressing or barbering process. It is essential that you work safely and methodically throughout a cutting service and the overall effectiveness of that process, including the result, relates to the preparations that you make.

You must make sure that you work safely at all times:

◆ So that the way in which you work does not present a hazard to yourself or anyone else.

◆ Ensuring that your tools are prepared, maintained and hygienic to use.

You must be organized in the way in which you work:

◆ Get yourself ready before the client arrives.

◆ Prepare a trolley and the work area so that you can start promptly and are not wasting time.

◆ Prepare the gowns, towels, cutting collars, neck wool, etc. so that you don't keep running off during the service.

Remember, a professional service starts long before the client's appointed time, whereas an unprofessional service does not. In other words, the time that you spend **before** the client arrives, is equally as important as the time you spend **during** the service and the two things are directly linked.

One provides good customer service and efficiency, where everything runs smoothly and the client receives a professional service that they will remember and be happy to talk about. The other provides something quite different!

The client

Your salon will have its own policy (rules – their way of doing things) for preparing the clients for treatments and services and this will include a procedure for gowning and protecting the client from spillages or hair clippings. It will also include the methods for preparing tools and equipment and expectations of your personal standards in relation to technical ability and personal hygiene.

You may be still learning but you do need to remember the client's personal comfort and safety throughout the salon visit is paramount. That is, covering the client's clothes with a clean, laundered gown or cutting cape, placing a cutting collar over their shoulders and keeping clean, laundered towels close at hand along with some neck wool to 'tuck in' around the cutting collar to keep loose clippings out.

Gowning Make sure that the gown or cutting cape is on properly and fastened securely around the neck. It should cover and protect their clothes and come up high enough to cover collars and necklines. Don't make the fastening too tight, but it should be close enough at least to protect the client's clothes and help to prevent hair clippings from going down their neck. This is both uncomfortable while they are in the salon and irritating if they are returning to work or doing things for the rest of the day.

HEALTH & SAFETY

A cutting cape is a sleeveless type of gown more suited to dry cutting as it doesn't have the same protection as a full gown. The cutting cape provides cover over the shoulders and down the front whereas the gown covers all the clothes at the back as well as the arms.

The work area

Your first consideration should be the styling section. Is the mirror clean and not smeary? Nobody wants to sit in front of a dirty mirror and it will be the first impression that the client gets about the cleanliness of the salon. The following table provides a quick view of the preparations that need doing before the client arrives.

HEALTH & SAFETY

Personal hygiene is especially important to hairdressers. You work in close proximity to the client so make sure that you eliminate body odour, bad breath or dirty hands and nails by taking the appropriate action.

For more information about personal hygiene, go to **CHAPTER 11** Cutting Facial Hair, p. 327.

Work area preparation

Area	Things to look for	Things to do
Workstation	**Mirror** – Is it clean and free from smears?	Use a cloth and a spray glass cleaner to remove traces of dust, hairspray and grease. Then using a second, DRY cloth, polish off the smears to produce a sparkling finish.
	Shelving – Is it clean and clear?	Remove any magazines, cups and styling tools, then using a cloth and a spray detergent cleaner, remove any traces of dust, hairspray and grease from the laminated surface. Never use scouring pads on these surfaces as it may scratch them and dull the shiny surfaces.
	Styling chair – Is the chair the right way round and is the chair base and seating clean?	Brush out any debris or trapped hair clippings, letting them fall to the floor. Make sure that the chair hydraulic lift is rear facing. Then dust off the metal base and feet and polish up the chrome finish. Finally, using a cloth and a spray polish remove traces of dust and hairspray from the upholstered areas, including the back of the chair too.
	Foot rest – Is there any mud or dirt left on it from the shoes of the last client?	Use a cloth and a spray polish cleaner to remove traces of dust, hairspray and grease. Then using a second, DRY cloth, polish off the smears to produce a sparkling finish.
	Barbicide® – Does the sterilizer need to be changed?	If the fluid hasn't been changed or replaced for some time, empty out old Barbicide® at the sink and rinse away with plenty of cold water. Then, following the manufacturer's instructions, produce the right dilution with water and top the jar back up.
Trolley	**Drawers and surfaces** – are they clean and free of debris?	Brush out any fragments of hair. Use a cloth and a spray glass cleaner to remove traces of dust, hairspray and grease.
	Tools and equipment – are all the tools clean, hygienic and safe to use?	Combs should be clean and placed in the Barbicide® between clients, then before use they can be rinsed and dried, ready for use. Scissors and clipper blades can be placed in the UV cabinet – remember to turn over after 15 minutes. Electrical items like clippers and blow-dryers should be visually checked for damage or loose blades or cables and any suspect items should be removed from the trolley and notified to a senior member of staff.
Floor	Is all the work area clean?	Sweep away all loose clippings, ensuring that you get into all the difficult edges and parts in front of chair that don't get swept throughout the working day. If you need to mop up any areas, make sure that you dry the damp areas after with a used towel from the laundry bins.

Your working position and posture

The client's position and height from the floor will have a direct effect on your posture too. You must be able to work in a position where you do not have to bend 'doubled up' to do your work. Cutting involves a lot of arm and hand movements and you need to be able to get your hands and fingers into positions where you can cut the hair unencumbered, without bad posture.

◆ You should adjust the seated client's chair height to a position where you can work upright without having to overreach on the top sections of their head.

◆ You should never have to work in a position where your arms are above shoulder height for more than a few moments – this will quickly cause fatigue and muscular pain, so adjust the seat height to suit your needs during the haircut.

◆ You should clear trolleys or equipment out of the way, so that you get good all-round access (300°) around the client.

Hairdressing, as you already know, involves a lot of standing and because of this, you need to be comfortable in your work. You should always adopt a comfortable but safe work position.

Working efficiently, safely and effectively

Working efficiently means working in a way that maximizes your time and uses the salon's resources without wastefulness, but not at the cost of working unsafely. It is essential that you make the most of your time. Always treat the salon's materials in the same way that you would look after your own equipment: always try to minimize waste, being careful of how much shampoo, conditioner, styling aids, hot water, electricity, in fact all the products, you use.

As already addressed earlier: the salon's cleanliness is of paramount importance – the work area should be clean and free from clutter or waste items. Any used materials should be disposed of and not left out on the side; failure to do so is:

◆ unprofessional; and

◆ presents a health hazard to others.

You need to work in an orderly environment: you need to have the materials that you need at hand and the equipment that you want to use in position and ready for action. This is a good exercise in self-organization and shows others that you are a true professional.

You will also need to keep an eye on the clock: remember you need to keep 'on-time' and that means providing the service in a commercially acceptable time.

TOP TIP

Always remember that clients have busy lives too, they may be making an appointment within their lunch hour or before going in to work.

BEST PRACTICE

Always dry the client's hair well to remove the excess water before cutting, blow-drying or finger-drying.

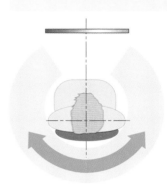

Cutting access

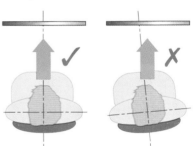

Chair/client angle to mirror

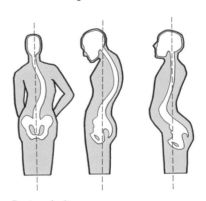

Posture faults

To read more about preventing infection, go to **CHAPTER 5** Health and safety, pp. 127–130.

To find out more about methods of sterilization, go to **CHAPTER 5** Health and Safety, pp. 127–130.

Tools and equipment

Tool preparation

All of your tools, scissors, combs, brushes and electrical items like clippers must be hygienic and safe to use.

Scissors

Scissors are for cutting wet or dry hair and they are the most important piece of hairdressing equipment that you will ever own. Their quality, precision and durability, like anything else in life, is related to their cost. You can pay as little as £20.00 for a college training pair, up to several hundred pounds for the best that technology can provide. If you own a pair of reasonable quality and look after them you will be surprised how long they will last. Scissors vary greatly in their design, size and price. There isn't any single way of choosing the correct pair for you. However, there are things that you should consider.

Scissors vary in type; for both left and right handed people, and in length ranging from very tiny four inches up to 'American type' shears at around seven inches. They should never be too heavy or too long to control. Heavy scissors become awkward to use and if their blades are too long you may not be able to manipulate them properly for smaller sections of hair, particularly if they involve precision angles. There are pros and cons for all length scissors – long blades are good for cutting solid baselines on longer hair, but a real nuisance for precise work around hairlines and behind ears!

You can check the suitability of a pair of scissors for you by assessing their balance and length. This is done by putting your fingers in the handles as if you were about to use them; when the scissors are held correctly, the pivotal point should extend just beyond the first finger. This allows the blades to open easily and means that the thumb is in an ideal position to open and close them easily.

The more expensive the scissors, the higher the specification and quality. Top quality scissors will often have one single lower cutting blade that has small serrations throughout the length. This is beneficial as this lower blade grips the hair as the blades close, without pushing the hair away. This provides a higher accuracy in the haircut and is ideal for precision type work. However, the sharpening of this type of scissor blade is not recommended, as normal sharpening processes will remove this feature immediately by grinding the serrations flat.

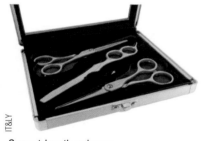

IT&LY

Correct length scissors

Serrated scissor blades

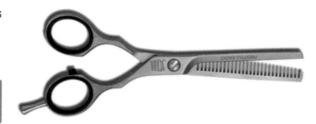

HEALTH & SAFETY

Take care with your scissors – the precision finish on the blades is easily damaged if they are dropped.

Cutting combs

Get into the habit of only using good-quality cutting combs. You will find that by spending only a little more you will get so much more out of them. The design of a cutting comb for hairdressing is different to that of barbering. The ladies' hairdressing cutting comb is rigid and parallel throughout its length, whereas the barbering comb is flexible and tapered, i.e. narrows towards one end.

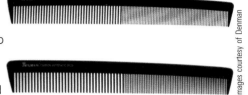

Cutting comb and barbering comb

There are two teeth patterns for cutting combs:

◆ The first and most popular type has two differing sets of coarseness, one end (up to the middle) has fine, closer teeth and the other end has wider, coarser teeth that are further apart. This provides more control with taking small sections for fine hair and combing and detangling the remaining hair before that is sectioned and cut.

◆ The second type of cutting comb has one set of uniform teeth throughout the length of the comb.

The length of cutting combs varies greatly. Again, what's best for you will depend on the size of your hands and what you can manage and manipulate quite easily. The normal length of a cutting comb is around 15cm but long ones are now very popular and provide a better aid when cutting **freehand** baselines and visualizing layer patterning.

Modern technology in plastics has produced a variety in combs and their quality. The best quality combs are made from plastics that have the following properties:

Quality combs are:

◆ Very strong but flexible – the teeth do not chip or break in regular use.

◆ Straight in regular use and do not end up looking like a banana after a couple of weeks!

◆ Constructed by injection moulding and do not have sharp or poorly formed edges – as opposed to combs that are made from pressings and have flawed seams and tend to scratch the client's ears and scalp.

◆ Resistant to chemicals, making them ideal for cleaning, sterilization and colouring as they will not stain.

◆ Constructed with anti-static – non-flyaway – finishes that help to control finer hair when dry cutting, reducing the hair's tendency to become flyaway.

Thinning scissors

Thinning scissors will reduce bulk and thickness of hair within a held section. They can be used on dry or wet hair and can have either one or both blades with serrated teeth. The classic thinning scissor has two, opposing rows of serrated teeth and because of their uniformity, they need to be used with thought and care. There is a drawback with using them on certain hairstyles. On layered shapes they will produce a tapering effect at the ends of the section, and this doesn't present any problems. However, when they are

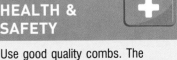

HEALTH & SAFETY

Use good quality combs. The comfort of good-quality combs is noticeable by the client, it doesn't scratch their scalp or catch on their ears while you are sectioning.

Images courtesy of Denman

used on **one-length haircuts**, thinning is not advisable on the outer lying sections of the hair as this will produce many shorter ends that can stick out and be difficult to handle or style.

Thinning does have some very useful applications for cutting:

◆ When the tips of thinning scissors are used for profiling the edges of layered shapes, it will provide a quick way for **feathering** the hair.

◆ When the whole blades are used for removing weight from sections of layered hair, but closer to the head.

◆ On short cut, straighter hair that tends to show all the cutting marks. The effect can be minimized by trimming the very ends of the hair using thinning **scissor over comb** technique – particularly useful in men's barbering when **blending** clipper cut, graded levels together.

Images	Tools	Method of cleaning/sterilization
Images courtesy of Denman	**Neck brush**	Wash in hot soapy water, dry the bristles with a blow-dryer and then place in ultraviolet cabinet for 15 minutes remembering to turn over half way through.
IT&LY	**Sectioning clips**	Wash in hot soapy water and dry, then place in ultraviolet cabinet for 15 minutes remembering to turn over half way through.
Images courtesy of Denman	**Cutting comb**	Wash in hot soapy water and dry, then immerse in Barbicide® jar for 30 minutes.

(Continued)

(Continued)

Images	Tools	Method of cleaning/sterilization
IT&LY	**Scissors**	Brush away hair fragments from pivot area and blades with a colouring brush. Carefully wipe the blades with sterile wipes and then place them in an open position in the ultra-violet cabinet for 15 minutes each side.
IT&LY	**Thinning scissors**	Brush away hair fragments from pivot area and blades with a colouring brush. Carefully wipe the blades with sterile wipes and then place them in an open position in the ultra-violet cabinet for 15 minutes each side.

BEST PRACTICE

When new scissors are bought they come in a protective case, so get into the habit of keeping them in it. This will make them easy to identify when there are plenty of other pairs about and will also provide useful protection when they are carried around.

BEST PRACTICE

Maintain your scissors. Carefully wipe over the blades at the end of the working day to remove any fragments of hair and then apply a little clipper oil to the pivot point to prevent any corrosion around the fastening screw. This will prolong their life and stop them from binding or getting stiffer to use.

HEALTH & SAFETY

Never keep scissors in your pockets: it is unhygienic but, more importantly, it is a dangerous thing to do.

Electric clippers and clipper grades

Clippers are and have been an essential item of equipment for men's styling. They have been invaluable for the popularity of short hairstyles, but are equally important for the shaping and trimming of necklines and facial hair shapes.

Clipper types The **'classic' electric clippers** are mains voltage and plug in at the styling section just before they are used. As this type of clipper have a trailing lead, it is often (incorrectly) ravelled around the clipper body when not in use. They must be checked visually before they are used to see if there is any looseness in the cables or the plug. There are a number of different profiles for the blades, some of which are narrow and parallel, which are used in basic clippering, clipper over comb and with clipper grades.

Another form of electric clipper for men's detailing is the **T liner** – this is a clipper with extended *shoulders* on the clipper blades. This extended blade area makes it far simpler to work near and around areas such as the ears, where the body of the more conventional clippers get in the way.

A more popular and arguably, safer type of clipper is the 'cordless' **rechargeable** type. These are not as heavy as the classic clipper, but without any leads to worry about, they can be handled very easily without trailing a lead across a client during use. When the rechargeable clipper has been finished with it must be put back into the charger unit, otherwise it may run out of electrical charge before it can be used again. Typically, a charger unit will need at least 30 minutes to top-up the clipper when it is not being used, so that it is in peak performance, next time it is used.

Trimmer, shaper and detailer – the final category of clippers are the small, battery operated trimmers and detailers. These small clippers are lightweight and are easily manipulated to trim necklines, ear hair and nostrils. The detailer is a special clipper that produces the patterned designs over the head on shorter cut hair.

Clipper maintenance
The electric clippers cut hair by oscillation. That is, the side-to-side movement of an upper metal blade passing over a lower rigid or fixed one. On each pass of the upper blade, the hair caught between the teeth of the lower blade is cut and falls away. Regular cleaning and lubrication is essential maintenance and will prolong the blades' useful life and keep the cutting edges sharp. Without this care, the constant friction of one blade passing over another will affect their ability to work properly. Electric clippers generate quite a lot of heat and, if they have not been maintained properly, their cutting ability deteriorates quickly. New replacement blades are relatively expensive, and may cost over half the price of a new pair of clippers, so look after them. If the clipper blades are 'dulled', i.e. blunt, you will not be able to trim, shape and style neck or facial hair shapes accurately.

You should always take care not to drop them, as this can easily cause damage to the cutting teeth or even break them! Any missing areas of teeth along the blades will be extremely dangerous and, if they were used, could easily cut the client. So when they are not in use, hang them up out of the way or replace them back in the charger unit.

Clipper blades must always be checked for alignment; each time, *before* use. The fixed lower blade is adjustable and this allows for small adjustments to be made backwards, forwards or even side-to-side, and in constant use the vibration may put the blades out of alignment.

Loosening the small retaining screws underneath allows the blades to be adjusted. This also provides access to the upper blade, for removal and cleaning out the fragments of hair and essential oiling/lubrication. When the blades are replaced the retaining screws must be retightened properly. If this is not done, the vibration will dislodge the alignment and this could easily take a chunk out of your client's hair, or worse, even cut them!

Clippers are used on dry hair and this enables the stylist to cut the client's hair first, and then wash it after, which removes all the small, loose fragments, and make any final checks.

Clipper grades

Clipper attachment size	Length of cut hair
No attachment	Very close to skin, almost as close as shaving.
Grade 1 = 3mm (⅛ inch)	Very short, on darker hair it will only leave a stubbly shadowing effect.
Grade 2 = 6mm (¼ inch)	Close cut, will see some skin on finer hair types but short enough for the hair to appear straight even if it is naturally curly.
Grade 3 = 9mm (⅜ inch)	Popular length grade for short groomed effects. Typically cuts to that of short scissor over comb lengths.
Grade 4 = 13mm (½ inch)	Popular length which has a similar effect to longer scissor over comb type effects.
Grades 6–8 = 16–25mm (½–1 inch)	Popular longer length used for beard shaping.

Avoiding in-growing hairs

You need to be aware of one problem caused by the continual close cutting of very curly hair.

In-growing hair can occur when hair is cut into **short graduations** or hairstyles that have faded hairlines techniques using clippers, or particularly, when men shave with a razor. When hair is cut very close to the skin, the blade tends to slightly pull the hair within the follicle before the blade severs the hair shaft. When the tension is released the hair retracts into the follicle and the curl direction of the hair can pierce the sides of the follicle – particularly if the opening of the follicle becomes blocked, say by using **shaving cream** and is not cleansed properly – to produce a 'diverted' growth direction within the skin. This can result in small lumps forming which can become infected, causing irritation and swelling.

'Backed-off' clipper blades This term relates to the blade position on electric clippers. Normal 'classic' clippers have a blade adjustment lever on one side of the clipper body. This lever makes the lower, fixed cutting blade go forwards or backwards by a small amount (5–10mm). But as the blades are slightly bevelled in profile, this movement brings the upper, cutting blade 'closer' or 'further away' from the front cutting edge and ultimately, the skin. This enables the stylist or barber to create closer cut tapered or faded edges to the perimeter shape quite safely, without having to use a razor. Hence, a 'backed-off' blade moves the cutting edge further away from the front, so it provides the longer cutting option when using clippers without grades.

Razors

The **open or 'cut-throat' style razor** used in men's shaving is made out of a single steel blade which is hinged and closed into a protective handle. The modern counterpart has disposable blades which can be removed and safely disposed of in a 'sharps box' after use.

The razor used for styling and **texturizing** women's or men's hair is called a shaper. It too has disposable blades which are fitted into a hinged sheath that provides a handy, safe to use styling tool. Razor cutting is always carried out on wet hair and with sharp blades. This is because of the way in which razors are used and the angle at which they cut through the hair. Razoring should never be done on dry hair as this will be painful for the client and pull and tear the hair, possibly causing it to split, even if the blades are new.

TOP TIP

In-growing hair:

◆ Hair grows under the skin and the follicle becomes blocked.

◆ Common in **African type or curly hair**.

◆ Particularly affecting dark skin – Asian, African and Mediterranean skin types.

Types of razors	
Open (cut-throat) razor	This barbering razor is used for shaving and has a fixed/rigid blade that folds into its handle for safety. The blade is kept keen by regular stropping and honing and must be sterilized on each use between clients.
Safety razor	This razor simulates the shape and feel of the open razor with disposable blades which make it more hygienic, as blades can be replaced for each client.
Shaper razor	This is a popular razor with disposable blades that is used for cutting and styling hair, but not for shaving. It therefore has uses for both women's and men's hairstyling.

Neck brushes, water sprays and sectioning clips

Neck brushes are used to remove loose hair clippings from around the neck and face, during and after finishing the haircut. Get used to passing the neck brush to your client when you are cutting dry hair as the small fragments are irritating when they fall onto the face. Neck brushes usually have soft artificial bristles and these are easily washed and dried before they are sterilized in a UV cabinet. Historically, the best neck brushes (like men's shaving brushes) were made from 'natural' bristles and these were far more durable then their modern counterpart. However, you can prolong the life of artificial brushes if you make sure that the bristles are either, allowed to dry, or dried, flat and straight. If they are allowed to dry on the side, the bristles will lose their shape and bend.

Water sprays are used for damping down dry or dried hair to assist you in controlling the haircut. Make sure that the spray nozzle is adjusted so that it produces a fine mist when used. This will prevent you being embarrassed at some other time, when you accidently squirt the client with a '*super soaker*'.

Another thing to remember is regarding the water's freshness: stale water is unhygienic, so make sure that the water is emptied out and the spray is refilled on a daily basis.

◆ *Sectioning clips* are made from plastics or lightweight metals, they are used to divide the hair and keep bulk out of the way while you work on other areas.

◆ *Flat clips* are ideal for securing longer hair and in many ways they are better for the hair as they don't tend to tangle in the client's hair in use. Unfortunately, they don't cope with short layered hair.

So this is where:

◆ '*Jawed' crocodile clips* are better suited. They can be sterilized by immersing them into Barbicide®, but because of their tiny metal springs, they would be better being sterilized in a UV cabinet.

Cutting techniques

Overview of cutting techniques

Cutting tools	Techniques that can be achieved	Explanation of technique
Scissors	Club cutting (blunt cutting)	The most basic and most popular way, cutting sections of hair straight across, parallel to the index and middle finger. The blunt, straight sections of cut hair that it produces are ideal for precise lines. The different angles that the hair can be held will produce one-length, square layers, **uniform layers**, **graduation** and **reverse graduation**.
	Freehand cutting	Cutting without holding with the fingers is known as freehand cutting. It is a technique that allows for cutting with natural fall and without tension. Its main uses are at the perimeter edges around ears, fringes and trimming awkward growth patterns.
Thinning scissors	Thinning/texturizing	Thinning scissors will remove uniform bulk from any point between the root area and ends. However, they have more creative uses when they are used to 'feather' the perimeter edges of hair styles (which is often more difficult with conventional scissors).

(Continued)

(*Continued*)

Cutting tools	Techniques that can be achieved	Explanation of technique
Electric clippers	Clippering with grade attachments	Clipper grades (the attachments that provide uniform cutting lengths) are made in a range of sizes for different purposes, and are numbered accordingly. They will provide closely cut uniform layering, or if differing grades are used they can provide graduation on hair that is too short to hold between the fingers.
	Fading	A way of blending short hair at the nape or edges of a hairstyle down or 'out' to the skin. It is achieved by using the clippers with the blade 'backed off', creating a very short, tapered effect with a smooth blended effect without any lines.
	Clipper-over-comb and scissor over comb	Both techniques are a popular way of layering or fading very short hair into styles that can't be held between the fingers. The hair is held and supported by a comb and the free edges protruding through are removed.
Razors	**Slicing**, tapering texturizing	A variety of techniques that are collectively called texturizing can be achieved by using a shaper razor. The angle and position of the blade in relation to the hair will produce either thinning, tapering or feathering effects.

Club cutting

This is the method of cutting hair bluntly straight across. It systematically cuts all the hair, at an angle parallel to the first and middle finger, to the same length. It is the most popular technique and often forms the basis or first part of a haircut, before other techniques are used. Club cutting will produce both one-length haircuts and the layering techniques.

The majority of our clients have fine to medium hair textures so this technique is ideal for them as it makes their hair fuller or more bodied. Club cutting is produced by holding the hair out, away from the head, and using the fingers to form a guiding line, beyond which the cut is made. This is repeated throughout the cut, providing an organized, step-by-step approach to creating the final effect.

Cutting faults can occur if:

◆ You don't maintain the correct tension throughout the cut.

◆ You twist the cutting meshes while you are holding and cutting them.

◆ You over-direct the hair, allowing parts of the cut meshes to be longer than needs be.

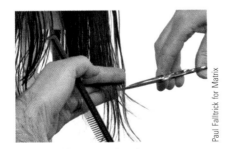
Holding with an even tension

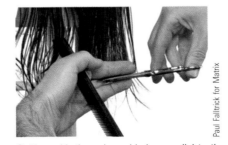
Cutting with the scissor blades parallel to the fingers

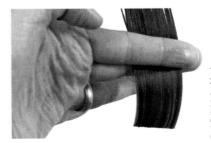
A completed 'club cut' section

Freehand cutting

As the name suggests, freehand cutting relies upon one hand holding and combing the hair into position, and the other controlling the scissors to make the cut. More often than not, when cutting longer, one-length hair, the comb is used to create the guide for making the cut. This technique is often used on straighter hair because curlier hair needs more control, through holding and tensioning.

This technique is widely used in cutting fringes. Adults with fringes are particularly cautious about where the exact finished length should be. Therefore, it is easier to comb the length into position and create a profile shape that both suits the client and follows or covers the eyebrows. This would be guesswork if the hair were held between the fingers and cut because the width of your fingers would obscure the exact length and position you are trying to cut.

Therefore, the freehand cut is made with the scissors very close to the skin, head or neck, as this gives you a clearer idea of what needs to be cut off to achieve the exact, final length required by the client. Obviously, you need to be particularly careful in cutting your profiles as it would be easy to snip an eyebrow or an ear! One thing that you can do to minimize any risk to the client is to use your comb behind the hair you want to cut as this has a couple of benefits.

◆ The comb can be held in parallel to the angle of the scissor blades, giving you a useful back-up guideline.

◆ The comb keeps eyebrows, ears and lined or 'sagging', skin back away from the cutting edges/points of the scissors.

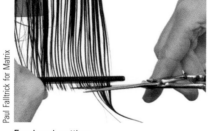

Paul Falltrick for Matrix

Freehand cutting

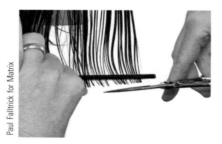

Paul Falltrick for Matrix

Freehand cutting

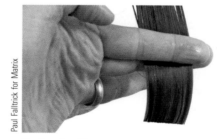

Paul Falltrick for Matrix

Freehand cutting

What do you do if you accidently cut a client?

If you do accidently cut a client put on a pair of disposable gloves and apply a small amount of pressure with a hygienic swab or pad to the area to constrict the wound and stem the blood flow. Keep yourself calm and the client reassured.

Ask someone to call for the first-aider and stay with the client until they arrive and take over. Immediately after the client has been attended to, you can create an accident report form setting out a record of what has taken place.

HEALTH & SAFETY

If an accident does occur and a client has been harmed in some way you must inform the salon manager.

Scissor over comb

This technique has been traditionally a barbering technique. In recent years there has been a move in hairdressing generally towards easier-to-manage hairstyles, so therefore this technique is widely used in hairdressing for cutting short styles on both men and women.

Scissor over comb cutting is ideal for producing:

◆ Tapered layering shapes with close-cut, 'fade-out' perimeters – faded or graduated perimeters have no set baselines: they rely upon the hairline profile and are graduated out from that into the rest of the hairstyle.

◆ Uniform layered shapes with layers of equal lengths.

The technique is used with either wet or dry hair and uses the comb as a guide to hold the hair and maintain an even lift or tension away from the head, while you cut.

Scissor over comb is ideal for very short hair that cannot be held between your fingers, it is best started at the lower nape area providing that the hair isn't too long. The hair is lifted away from the head and the comb mirrors the contour of the back of the head so that the upper edge is tilted away and not inwards, towards the back of the head. If the angle of the comb leans towards the head your finished cut length will gradually get shorter as you work upwards.

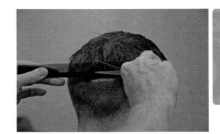

Correct angle of scissor over comb

Reverse graduation/graduation

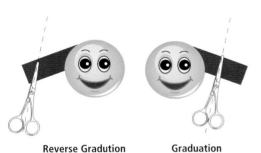

Reverse Gradution   **Graduation**

Thinning

Thinning can be done with scissors or a razor and can be used for reducing or tapering bulk from thicker hair without reducing the overall length. It is also used as a way of texturizing the edges of hairstyles to remove solid lines from profile shapes to create softer, faded or 'shattered' effects.

When thinning is done to remove bulk and weight in short or long layered hair, the hair sections should be held in vertical meshes and the thinners should be introduced to the hair at an angle so that the longest parts of the thinned hair are nearer to the base-lines or perimeter. This helps the hair to remain smoother without 'bunching' when it is dried. When longer thinned hair overlies shorter thinned hair an unflattering result occurs, producing width with fluffy, unruly edges.

Cutting technique	Description of technique
Club cutting	**Club cutting** Cutting by holding the hair between the first and second finger and cutting across bluntly.

(Continued)

Cutting technique	Description of technique
Point cutting	**Point cutting** Holding a section of hair between the first and second finger but leaving enough length to cut downwards at an angle to create angular points of hair. Adds movement and texture to hair.
Chipping	**Chipping** Holding a section of hair between the first and second finger but leaving enough length to cut inwards from the side to remove small sections at the ends to add light texture or to get rid of cutting marks.
Deep pointing	**Deep pointing** Holding a section of hair between the first and second finger but leaving enough length to cut deep sections from the hair to add lots of texture.
Scissor over comb	**Scissor over comb** The hair is held and lifted by the comb and this creates the cutting line for the scissors.
Razoring	**Razoring** The hair is held by the first and second finger while the razor is introduced to the section of hair and unwanted areas are sculptured by slicing through with the razor held at a narrow angle to the hair.

Controlling the haircut

Good cutting is a skill derived from applying knowledge to a sequence of events. In other words it matches some technical know-how to a methodical process. The process is the step-by-step actions, done in an order that will reach the desired outcome. The technical know-how is the controls covered below that maintain your accuracy while you work.

Accurate sectioning

Bearing in mind what has just been covered in relation to controlling a haircut, the only other considerations which are going to affect that are the amounts of hair that you are dealing with. Short hair doesn't present the same problems as long hair and sparse hair creates challenges that thicker hair doesn't. The main thing to remember is that you need to approach the hair in an organized way and any hair not being cut, needs to be sectioned up and out of the way so you can see what you need to be doing.

In order for you to be able to manage sizeable amounts of hair at any one time, you must organize and plan the haircut. The planning bit becomes automatic – it's the few moments that you spend thinking:

◆ How do I go about this?

◆ Where do I start?

◆ What is the finish going to be like?

Quite simply, being organized is about working in a logical way, it is the way in which you routinely start at one point, divide all the rest of the hair out of the way, finish that bit, and then take down the next part to work on and so on. Each part or section that you work on should be small enough for you to cope with without losing your way, or more importantly, your guideline! If the sections are too deep, or too wide, you will not be able to see the cutting guideline that you originally created. Accurate sectioning guarantees that every section combed and divided is handled and held to the same length every time.

Cutting hair and working with natural fall

There will be occasions when you are cutting clients' hair dry, and other times, wet. When cutting hair dry – and as long as the hair is clean – the growth patterns should be fairly obvious. So you should be able to compensate for the obstacles by leaving extra length or by removing hair to diminish the effect.

Unfortunately, seeing the natural lie and fall of the hair when it's wet, isn't quite so simple. True, you will have done a consultation, but sometimes that doesn't reveal all the issues. You will need to get into the habit of thoroughly drying the hair, before you start cutting, so that it is still damp but not saturated. That way you will be able to see the natural tendencies of the hair and work with them. Better that, than cutting hair that is soaking wet, then having a shock later when it starts to dry and you find that it is sticking out in all sorts of directions!

Cutting with the natural fall of the hair is extremely important. Looking for the directions of growth within the hair is an essential part of consultation as it is within the execution of

BEST PRACTICE

The finished hairstyle always looks better if it is cut wet. Try to get your clients to book in for a wet cut; at the very least:

◆ It will be easier for you to create new effects.

◆ They will be able to see a better, more professional result.

◆ You will generate a better professional service with your clients.

◆ You will break the habits of men expecting a quick, cheap haircut.

◆ It is more hygienic for everyone concerned.

the haircut. If you work with the natural fall, i.e. partings, nape hair growth, double crowns, etc. you will be compensating for these features and be able to produce an easier to manage result. If however, you ignore these factors you and your client will have a hard job in styling it.

Cutting baselines/perimeter outlines A baseline is a cut section of hair which is used as a cutting guide for following sections of hair. There may be one or more baseline cut: for example, a graduated nape baseline may be cut and another may be cut into the middle of the hair at the back of the head. Other baselines may be cut at the sides and the front of the head. The baselines will determine the perimeter of the hair style, or part of the style and may take different shapes according to the effects required:

- ◆ **Symmetrical** – The baseline for evenly balanced hair shapes in which the hair is equally divided on both sides of the head. Examples are hairstyles with central partings or with the hair swept backwards or forwards.

- ◆ **Asymmetrical** – The baseline to be used where the hair is unevenly balanced, for example where there is a side parting and a larger volume of hair on one side of the head, or where the hair is swept off the face at one side with fullness of volume on the other.

- ◆ **Concave** – The baseline may be cut curving inwards or downwards. The nape baseline, for example, may curve downwards.

- ◆ **Convex** – The baseline may be cut curving upwards and outwards – the nape baseline, for instance, may be cut curving upwards.

- ◆ **Straight** – The baseline may be cut straight across, for example where you wish to produce a hard, square effect.

Controlling the shape

There are three aspects of a haircut that you must get right every time:

- ◆ **Holding angle** – the angle at which the hair is held out, away from the head.

- ◆ **Cutting angle** – the angle at which the scissors, razor, etc. cuts the hair in relation to the position in which it is held.

- ◆ **Holding tension** – the even tension applied to the hair within a held section, so that all of the hair remains taught.

That doesn't seem much to guarantee success, but it does take a lot of practise and concentration. Even if you start well, you cannot afford to lose any of these controls in the closing stages.

Cutting outlines Cutting outlines, or perimeter shapes, are the outline shape that is created when layered hair is held directly out with tension (perpendicular) from the head. The curves and the angle in relation to the head, determines the shape of the cut style. The main ones are the:

- ◆ Contour of the shape from top to bottom.

- ◆ Contour of the shape around the head, side to side.

Cutting guidelines Cutting guidelines are prepared sections of hair that control the uniform quality of the haircut. When the cutting guide is first sectioned and then cut, it is to this length and shape that all the other following sections relate. In preparing this cutting guide you need to take all the client's physical features and attributes into consideration, i.e. eyes, eyebrows, nose, bone structure, head shape, neck length, hair-lines, etc.

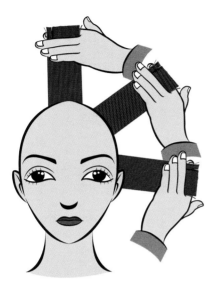

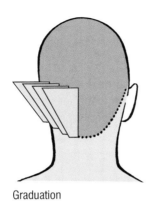

Graduation

Uniform layers

Creating guidelines

The guideline is the initial cutting line that creates a template for all the following sections.

As a general rule the simpler or more basic the hairstyle the fewer guidelines there will be. On the other hand, the more complex the hairstyle, the more guidelines will be involved.

◆   A uniform layered haircut has one guideline.

◆   A one-length haircut has one guideline too.

A uniform layered haircut has layers of equal length all around the head, so the first cutting guideline dictates the overall length for the rest of the haircut.

For simplicity, the guideline should always start at the back of the head: this way the majority of the client's hair is tackled first and cross checked before moving onto the sides and top. So after dividing the hair vertically and centrally, down the back of the head from the crown to the nape, take a horizontal section from the centre out to each side, about 2cm above the hairline. Secure the remaining hair out of the way with sectioning clips. Start at the centre below the vertical division and cut this baseline to the required length. After checking the accuracy, take down the next section 2cm above this first one and again, secure the remaining hair out of the way.

At the point beneath the vertical division in the hair, take and hold a vertical section, as shown below, without twisting and with an even tension. Cut this perpendicularly (at a vertical angle) to the head. (The client's head should be horizontal and not chin down or head back.)

With the guideline cut, you take the next section – parallel to the guideline – with the same even tension, so that you can see the lengths of the previously cut guideline through the held mesh. Cut this to the same length as the guideline. Continue this throughout each section until the complete horizontal area has been cut. Then take down another 2cm on either side and repeat the process, slowly working up the back to the crown.

With the back done, you take a horizontal section above the ears through to the front. Cut your perimeter baseline and follow the guideline through from behind the ear, working towards the front hairline. Repeat up to the top and cut the other side in the same way.

Finish the haircut over the top, working forwards from the known guidelines at the top. Finally, trim the front hairline perimeter shape to complete the hairline profile shape and cross check to see that the sides, back and top are all in balance.

The graduated haircut uses a similar guideline process to that of uniform layering. The only difference is that the hair is held out at an angle from the head as opposed to perpendicular. The steeper the angle is held away from the head, the lower the bulk line will be and the greater the weight distribution for the overlying lengths. Conversely, the shallower the angle of the cut, the higher the bulk line will be and the less weight distribution for the overlying lengths.

Rear view layering

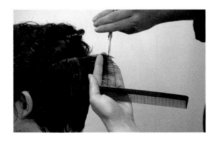

Maintaining accuracy – cross checking

As each horizontal section moves up the head, you will need to recheck the accuracy and balance of what you have already done. Do this by taking and holding sections at an angle which is at right angles (90°) to the original cut sections. In other words, if you originally cut the hair in vertical meshes, your cross check will be done with horizontal meshes.

Cross checking provides a final technique for checking the continuity and accuracy of the haircut. Where you find an imbalance in weight, or extra length that still needs to be removed, it provides you with the opportunity to remove it in order to create the perfect finish.

TOP TIP

Many men have shorter hairstyles, so their nape hair growth patterns will have far more impact on what hairstyle you choose.

Outlines – Men's perimeter shapes

Many short men's layered cuts are graduated at the sides and into the nape sometimes by clipper over comb or, when left slightly longer, by scissor over comb techniques. On shorter hair styles the neck- and hairlines become the main focal perimeters of the hairstyle and, in emphasizing these, you will need to give them careful attention as it is very easy to infringe into the hairline and remove hair that is needed for the outline shape.

Where possible always use the natural hairlines as the limit for the hairstyle. This produces a smoother effect on the eye and produces styles that look balanced and right. If you ignore the natural hairlines and cut above them, you will find that the hair below will grow back very quickly and produce a stubbly, spiky effect within a few days. Or, if done on dark hair, it will produce a 'shadowed' effect within 24 hours.

However, natural necklines often lack consistency; the growth is often uneven, intermittent or sparse. Therefore the outline shapes for these men wearing shorter hair need to be defined. The more natural the nape line, the softer and less severe will be the look.

Round

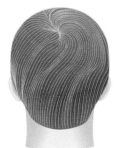

Round neckline

Tapered

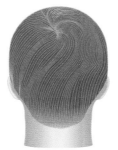

Tapered/faded neckline

Square

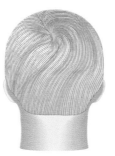

Square neckline

Hair perimeter shapes

The shaping of front hair into a fringe can produce a variety of facial frames and the focal point it creates changes the overall effect dramatically. In many men the front hairline recedes and this is often a sign of male pattern baldness. This influences the choice and positioning of perimeter fringe shapes. Always give this some thought before cutting the hair.

In men, the side hairlines, sideburns or sideboards 'bridge' the hairstyle and beard shape. These need to be balanced and fit the overall effect, so use the mirror to check your balance, it is far easier and more accurate than rushing around the chair from side to side. Also, take your time when creating an outline profile on short hair, stand directly behind the client so that you can see that your work is balanced. You can then finish off the outline with the scissor points or carefully held, inverted clippers with the blades 'backed off'.

BEST PRACTICE

In order to create clean lines around the ears on shorter hairstyles, you will need to hold the tops of the ears down so you can see what you are doing and ensure that you are working safely.

Common cutting problems

A lack of attention during the cut or a missed detail or aspect during the consultation can lead to cutting mistakes. The variety of mistakes is too varied to cover, but usually, it's an imbalance in weight proportions or a difference in perimeter lengths.

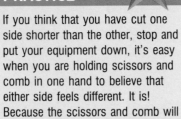

If, on finishing a symmetrical cut, you feel that one side seems to be slightly longer than the other; you need to stop before taking anything off the apparently longer side. If it is obviously longer and the client has commented too, you need to *put your comb and scissors down* and recheck through the fingers.

Standing behind the client, you take a small piece of hair from the same position on the head at either side with your forefingers and thumbs. Then slowly slide your fingers down either side until you get to the ends. Looking at the length through the mirror, see if the ends terminate at the same lengths either side, if they do, the cut is fine. Often a cut can seem wrong and the more you look at it the worse it seems. By putting the scissors and comb down you break the *fixation* of blind panic and have a chance to review it again calmly, with your hands empty. Most hairdressers make the fatal mistake of immediately taking some off the apparently longer side, only to find that the other side then seems wrong and then as they continue, each side gets shorter and shorter! If, however, there is a difference in both lengths then you now have the chance to redress the balance.

Clients are particularly attached to their fringes (pardon the pun): if a fringe is taken too short the client generally feels very conspicuous. So how can you replace hair that is already too short? Well you can't replace the hair but you can lessen the effect by reducing a solid fringe line by slightly point cutting to 'break up' the density and reveal a little skin of the forehead through.

What really bothers people is the stark contrast created between the solid line created by the fringe against the skin – this focuses even more attention on the area. Therefore, the solution is to reduce this contrast by softening this *demarcation line* between the two areas. This technique of reducing obvious mistakes can be used throughout the perimeter of hairstyles as it works in most cases.

Finally, another popular cutting fault is caused by an imbalance of weight in layering on one side to the other. Again if you get to a cross check situation and find that the layer pattern on one side seems different to the other side, stop!

You need to find out if it is due to:

◆ one side being longer than the other; or

◆ a greater reduction in weight by texturizing on one side rather than the other.

If it is length then you can easily re-cut the longer side to match. But if it is due to weight reduction, you will see a 'collapse' in the overall style shape on the side that has had the greater amount of texturizing. You can then remedy the fault by further texturizing the hair from the thicker side.

Very short necklines All of the classic perimeter neckline shapes above can easily be ruined if a lack of care and attention occurs. Careless layering or clippering can easily spoil the detail of the outline of very short hair. Every millimetre counts. You need to make sure that your outlining with the clippers is even and smooth throughout. If you do make a mistake and find that you have encroached on the outline shape you would be better off re-cutting the outline slightly shorter to eliminate the fault.

Blending men's clipper lengths to scissor length Another common problem on short hair is found at the blend area between different clippered grades, or between the clippered and hand-held cut lengths. If a careful blending hasn't been made cutting marks will show at the point where the two areas combine.

There are two ways of tackling this problem:

- If the hair is still too long on the hand-cut/held side, you can re-fade the two zones together by scissor over comb methods. Be careful not to undercut the longer lengths as this will mean that you will have to re-cut all the clippered area.

- If the lengths of hair between the two areas are slightly uneven it will definitely show unless you correct it. In any area where clippers fade out to club-cut lengths you can resurface the hair by using thinning scissors over comb just on the very tips of the hair. A light blending of thinned hair produces an optical illusion that cheats the eye by softening the two hard cut edges and the final effect appears correct.

Ears Nature does not guarantee symmetry, and this is particularly true with faces. One side of the face is not exactly the same as the other and this applies to ears too. One may be larger than the other, they may be irregular in shape or at different heights, so you need to make sure that you have considered this before you start. Unevenness on long hair doesn't matter, but when it's on short hair the imperfections will be made clear.

You need to find out how your client feels about his facial features. Sometimes these natural imperfections are not a concern, they are merely a characteristic of the client's personality. Don't forget to check on whether your client wears glasses or a hearing aid – take all of these factors into your assessment.

Finally you and your client will be able to agree exactly what look is required and you will then have a basis on which to decide how the work is to be carried out.

Hair type If your client's hair is very curly, do remember that it will coil back after stretching and cutting. Similarly, wavy hair, when cut too close to the wave crest, can be awkward to style as it tends to spring out from the head. Very fine straight hair will easily show cutting marks or can disclose unwanted lines from clippering if you take too large sections. Make sure that the sections you take are accurately divided and sectioned.

Consultation

Effective communication with the client, as in any service, is an essential part of cutting hair. Consultation is not just a process that takes place before a service, it is a continual process of reconfirming what is taking place while it is taking place. So, during your discussions, you must determine what the client wants and weigh this against the limiting factors that will influence what you need to do.

You need to understand your client fully and be able to negotiate and seek agreement with him or her throughout the service.

Be sure to listen to your client's requests. Many mistakes can be avoided if you achieve a clear understanding of what the client is asking for.

The haircutting style that you choose with your client should take into account each of the following points about the client's:

- face and head shape;

- physical features and body shape, size and proportion;

TOP TIP

The thinning over comb technique can be used as a corrective method on most clipper-cut or scissor-cut lengths to 'join' areas of differing grades/lengths or to remove cutting marks on fine, medium and coarse hair textures.

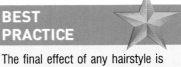

BEST PRACTICE

The final effect of any hairstyle is based on the information that you get during the consultation. Be thorough: the time spent in discussion before styling can save you lots of time later, particularly if the result is not what the client expected!

◆ hair quality, abundance, growth and distribution;

◆ age, lifestyle and suitability;

◆ purpose for the hairstyle;

◆ hair texture, condition, contra-indications;

◆ piercings;

◆ ability or time to recreate the effect themselves.

Face and head shapes

Facial considerations – general styling factors in relation to facial features	
Physical feature	**You need to consider**
Square and oblong facial shapes 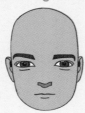	**Females** – These features are accentuated by hair that is smoothed, scraped back or sleek at the sides and top. The lines and angles are made less conspicuous by fullness and softer movement. **Males** – More angular features may have less impact on hairstyle options for male clients. Square and oblong are typically masculine and provide a perfect base for traditional classic, well groomed looks on shorter hair. These facial shapes have less impact on longer men's hairstyles.
Round faces	**Females** – Are made more conspicuous if the side and front perimeter (the longest outline hair) lengths are short or finish near to the widest part of the face. This is made worse if width is added at these positions too. Generally this facial shape is complimented by length beyond the chin and/or height on the top. **Males** – If shorter, more classic styles are required, the round face is improved by the introduction of angular or linear perimeters. On the other hand, if the hair is to be worn longer the roundness of the face will be reduced, as more will be covered.
Square angular features, jaw, forehead, etc. 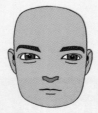	**Females** – Are improved with softer perimeter shapes, so avoid solid, linear effects around the face. Shattered edges and texturizing will help to mask these features. **Males** – Again these are traditionally accepted as a feature of masculinity. They do not really pose any limitations for classic type work. They also work well with longer hair too. Squarer more angular features are softened with beards and moustaches. **Males and Females** – Are improved by graduation, creating contour and shape that is missing from having a flatter occipital bone, particularly noticeable on male clients who have clippered effects.

(Continued)

(Continued)

Facial considerations – general styling factors in relation to facial features	
Physical feature	**You need to consider**
Flatter heads at the back 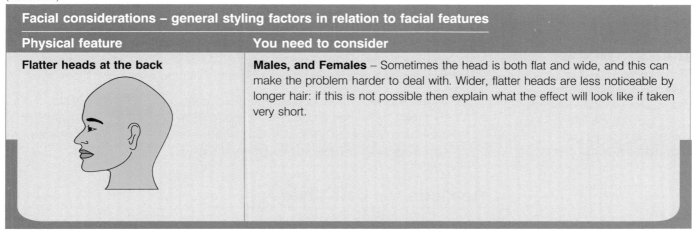	**Males, and Females** – Sometimes the head is both flat and wide, and this can make the problem harder to deal with. Wider, flatter heads are less noticeable by longer hair: if this is not possible then explain what the effect will look like if taken very short.

Hair growth patterns

Hair doesn't just grow out of the scalp and downwards – it would be very easy to deal with if it did. Unfortunately, people's hair grows in all sorts of ways and you need to consider this and the impacts that it will have on your haircut.

Some hair growth patterns provide useful aspects to work with and can enhance what you are trying to do. Here are some helpful ones:

Working with natural fall

◆ **Low hairlines** – A client with a low front hairline will naturally have hair that falls as a fringe. Don't ignore this as a fringe is a good choice for this client: it hides their narrow forehead.

◆ **Nape hairlines** – Some nape hair growth tends to grow inwards towards the centre of the neck and not straight down. Now this is not really noticeable on long hair, but if it is cut short and tightly graduated onto the neck, you can make a feature of this as the finished effect will always look really neat and tidy, even if after washing it doesn't always get blow-dried.

◆ **Natural partings** – This should always be noticed. If a client with longer hair tends to have a definite split in hair directions around the parting at the front, then you can safely suggest shorter styles as options too. The hair around the face, even if it is cut shorter, will always lie well as it won't fall across the face when it is finished. Needless to say if you ignore a strong natural parting and try to create a new one somewhere else, it just won't work.

◆ **Double crowns** – The client with a double crown will benefit from leaving sufficient length in the hair to over-fall the whole area. If it is cut too short, the hair will stick up and will not lie flat.

◆ **Nape whorls** – A nape whorl can occur at either or both sides of the nape. It can make the hair difficult to cut into a straight neckline or tight 'head-hugging' graduations. Often the hair naturally forms a V-shape. Tapered neckline shapes may be more suitable, but sometimes the hair is best left long so that the weight of the hair over-falls the nape whorl directions.

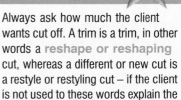

BEST PRACTICE

Always ask how much the client wants cut off. A trim is a trim, in other words a reshape or reshaping cut, whereas a different or new cut is a restyle or restyling cut – if the client is not used to these words explain the difference.

◆ **Cowlick** – A cowlick appears at the hairline at the front of the head. It makes cutting a straight fringe difficult, particularly on fine hair, because the hair often forms a natural parting. The strong movement is improved by moving the parting over so that the weight over-falls the growth pattern. Sometimes a fringe is achieved when leaving the layers longer so that they weigh down the hair.

◆ **Widow's peak** – The widow's peak growth pattern appears at the centre of the front hairline. The hair grows upward and forward, forming a strong peak. It is often better to cut the hair into styles that are dressed back from the face, as any 'light fringes' will be likely to separate and stick up.

Reasons for hair style

A style suitable for a special occasion will differ from one that is selected for work. The requirements for competition or show work are quite different from those for general daily wear. But versatility needs to be considered for everyone: people want styles that they can dress up or down. Modern hairdressing has parallels with modern lives: both are about flexibility and choice. People like options, so build this into your plans. The majority of clients need hairstyles that are easy-to-manage and that can be dressed up with styling products or accessories for social events. Versatility is definitely the key: while people like simple, easy-to-manage effects, they also like the opportunity to look different now and again.

Some jobs have special conditions about hair lengths and styles – for example, people working in the armed services or police have to wear their hair above the collar while at work. Men have easily accommodated this by using clippers for very short styles. Women have either had to have short layered styles or hair that is long enough to wear up and out of the way.

How quality, quantity and distribution of hair affect styling

Good hair condition is essential for great hairstyling. It doesn't matter how much work has gone into the thought and design of a hairstyle, if the hair is in poor condition to start with, it still will be after. Some aspects cannot be altered by cutting alone: for instance, if the hair is dry, dull and porous when the client enters the salon, it still will be when they leave.

Regular salon clients in the UK – the ones you tend to see more often than the others – tend to have something in common.

Difficult hair It can be difficult for a number of reasons: it can be fine or unmanageable, lank and lacking volume or just not responsive to styling without force. Thin, sparsely distributed hair is always a problem: if there isn't enough hair to get coverage over the scalp, then there is not a lot you can do about it. One thing that you should remember though is not to put too much texturizing into it – this will only make the problem more noticeable. Fine hair presents many problems too. Very fine hair is affected by **humidity**, i.e. dampness in the air, and quickly loses its shape. This type of hair always benefits from moisture repelling styling products so get your client used to using them.

Dry, frizzy hair Dry and frizzy hair can also be a problem, as the more heat styling it receives, the more moisture is lost and the less it responds to staying in shape – in other words, the harder it is to style. The problem just keeps going on like a merry-go-around. Dry, unruly thick hair needs to be tamed and most clients with this problem would like their hair to look smoother and shinier. Again this is a conditioning issue and you need to attack the problem before tackling the style. Sometimes this type of hair benefits from finishing products so put them on as you finish and define the hairstyle.

Very tight curly hair Tight curly hair can be difficult to cut too. Is it possible to smooth or straighten out the hair first so that you can see more clearly what you have to work with?

Wavy hair Cutting wavy hair presents some problems but not if it is looked at carefully before it is wet. Avoid cutting across the crests of the waves – you can't change the natural movement in the hair so try to work with it.

Straight hair Particularly if it is fine textured, straight hair can be difficult to cut. Cutting marks or lines can easily form if the cutting sections and angles are not right. Make sure that you only take small sections of hair and remember to crosscheck after, at 90° to the angle in which you first cut, to avoid this happening to you.

Hair growth rate Hair tends to grow at a steady, regular rate of about 1.25cm per month, so you need to consider this as a factor for how long a hairstyle will last. For example, a one-length classic bob may look really good if it is cut so that it creates a continuous line just above the shoulders. But how long will it last like that? When it gets to the point of touching the shoulders, the clean sharp line to which it was originally cut to will now be broken up by falling in front and behind the shoulder line. Always consider the impact that a small amount cut off will make and more importantly how long a style will last.

Male pattern baldness

Your consultation will cover a wide variety of factors that influence what happens next and male pattern baldness or the early signs of it should be high upon your list of things to look for.

Male pattern baldness (MPB) is a balding or thinning condition the cause of which, regardless of claims, is still eluding the scientists. It may be due to high levels of the male hormone testosterone within the body. Many treatments have been developed with little or no long-term remedial effects. Hair transplants have been a possible option in the past, but this type of treatment is expensive and needs a lot of upkeep.

Depending at what stage the MPB is, you need to find out how your client feels about it. If the hair loss is relatively slow, there is no need to rush immediately for the clippers and a Grade 2. There could be some considerable time before the condition requires a focused attention and, therefore, you need to provide advice and reassurance with a range of styling alternatives.

If however, the MPB is in a progressed state then it is obviously going to impact on what styles are achievable. For example, if there is a significant general thinning or hair loss on top (MPB type 1) then your styling options are far more limited than if MPB is only apparent in the receding area around the forehead (MPB type 2).

If your client has lost their hair and wears a toupee, you must account for this in your styling. Obviously, there has to be some blending between the natural, remaining hair and the added hair. Be careful not to leave the hair either too long or too short around the blend area. If there is any imbalance in lengths between the two, it is definitely going to show.

BEST PRACTICE

Many men choose to go very short when they are faced with thinning or bald areas on the scalp. If you can, provide them with alternatives – let them see the benefits of styling their hair in different ways if at all possible.

If, however, the client wears a full hairpiece then they might just prefer to keep whatever remaining hair very short beneath it. This makes fitting and positioning of the hairpiece easier and will be more comfortable to wear over long periods of time.

Male pattern baldness

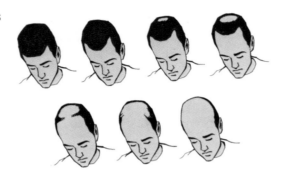

Style suitability

Style suitability refers to the effect of the hair shape on the face, and on the features of the head and body. A hairstyle is, quite simply, suitable when it 'looks right'. But this is a difficult or certainly a subjective thing to quantify.

Aesthetically and artistically speaking, the client's hair will 'look right' when the hairstyle does one of two things. It either harmonizes – i.e. fits the shape of the face and head – and is therefore a backdrop to an overall image, or **contrasts** – i.e. accentuates features of the face and head – creating a prominent frame for the overall image.

Age

As much as you would like to demonstrate your creative ability on everyone who walks through the salon door, bear in mind that some styles are inappropriate for certain clients. Beyond the physical aspects of style design, age does create some barriers to suitability.

Younger children Children aged 7–11 are better suited to simpler hairstyles that don't require too much maintenance. More often than not – and certainly from a hair health and hygiene point of view – they are better off with shorter hairstyles. The next age banding – 12–16-year-olds – want to have fashionable looks and many want colours too!

Unfortunately, these are still minors and the paying parent and educational establishments must have the last say.

Young men and women When they are young, both men and women can get away with almost anything. However, fashion will always dictate, and, more often than not, even if there are reasons for not doing a particular style, they will insist on it. This group can enjoy more extreme and dramatic effects and what's more they can get away with it. There are more styles applicable to the 16–25 year old age group than to any other. This is because of social cultures and the diversity of music and TV. These people are influenced by the music they buy, the celebrities they follow on TV and the people they mix with.

Professional men and women Professional people tend to go for watered-down versions of young fashion. Thinking about this in another way: in the clothing fashion world the designs that are seen on catwalks in Paris, London and New York are always the catalysts and precursors for what the high street shops will sell. Dozens of the haute couture fashion houses demonstrate their season's offerings at the pre-season shows. But not all designs are picked up by the buyers of commercial high street fashion chains – they usually go for the lesser extremes. People want to appear to be trendy and in touch, but not look ridiculous.

Older clients Greater consideration needs to be given to the older clients. Often the signs of ageing in the skin show quite clearly and therefore they must influence the way in which you select only appropriate and suitable effects.

Checklist before cutting

◆ Prepare the client and your working area.

◆ Find out what the client wants.

◆ Ask the client if they have brought any pictures of their ideas. Use pictures to look at options.

◆ Examine the hair – its type, length, quality, quantity and condition. Look for factors that influence the choice of style and cutting methods.

◆ Explain if there are any limitations that will affect the result.

◆ After your analysis, tell the client their options and provide suitable courses of action.

◆ Show the hair length to be removed with your fingers. Get agreement from the client.

◆ Discuss the time that will be taken and the price that you will charge.

◆ Summarize everything that you are about to do for the client before you start.

Starting the cut

Make sure that the hair is clean

You can't cut hair well if it is loaded with hairspray or it has product build-up. If the client uses a lot of finishing products on their hair you will need to make sure that this has been thoroughly washed out before you start. The quality of the finish that you can achieve upon the hair is directly related to the freedom needed to complete the job without the hair locking together with grease or gum. The hair should comb easily and freely during sectioning so that you achieve the correct holding angles and cutting angles without tangles or binding.

Adjust the working position and height

Client positioning has a lot to do with your safety too. If a client is slouched in the chair, they are a danger not only to themselves but to you too as they will put unnecessary pressure on the spine and you will not be able to stand up properly, causing fatigue or risk of injury from poor posture.

Client comfort should extend to the point where it makes the salon visit a welcome and pleasurable experience. They shouldn't clutter the floor around the styling chair with bags, magazines and shopping. Anything that can safely be stored away should be. It is not only a distraction, it's a safety hazard too.

Salon chairs are designed with comfort and safety in mind. Your client should be seated with their back flat against the back of the chair, their legs uncrossed, and their feet resting on the footrest.

You need to be able to get to all parts of the head, so the chair's height should be adjusted to suit the particular height of the client. Don't be afraid of asking the client to sit up: it is in their best interest too!

Position in relation to mirror The positioning of the client in front of the mirror is very important. Any angle of the head other than perpendicular to the mirror and the angle of the head to the seated position will affect the line and balance of the haircut.

Many salon workstations have built-in foot rests and there are good reasons for this.

The foot rest:

◆ is there to improve the comfort for the seated client at any cutting height;

◆ helps balance the client and encourages them to sit squarely in front of the mirror;

◆ tries to discourage the client from sitting cross legged;

◆ promotes better posture by making the client sit back properly with their back flat against the back of the chair.

All of the above factors are critical for you and the client in ensuring their comfort throughout, and that you are not hindered in doing your task. For example, if your client sits with crossed legs, it will alter the horizontal plane of their shoulders and this will make your job of trying to get even and level baselines more difficult.

Rough-dry the hair so that you work only with damp hair throughout the cut. Dry off the client's hair so that they are not sitting with saturated hair, it is uncomfortable for them, as wet hair soon feels cold even if it doesn't drip onto the gown and their clothes. During cutting, having the hair pre-dried allows the natural tendencies, movements and growth directions of the hair to be seen. This is extremely important for cutting, as the wave movement and hair growth patterns are all being considered as the style develops and starts to emerge.

Step-by-step cutting

STEP-BY-STEP: UNIFORM LAYERS

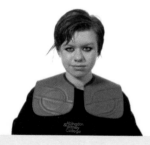

1 A uniform layered haircut is cut to the same length all over. When it is done on short hair, it creates a 'head hugging' shape.

Gown and prepare your client.

Check hairlines and growth patterns before you start.

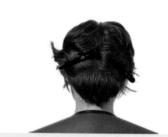

2 Start at the back, section off an area so that you can work without hair falling in the way.

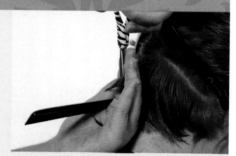

3 Take a central, vertical section to create your guideline and cut your first section.

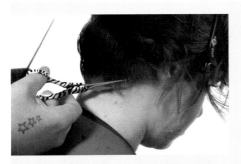

4 Continue the same layer pattern length to either side.

Tidy up the perimeter shape now and it will save time later on.

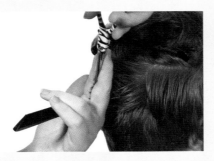

5 Moving up further, take another central section and cut it to the same length as the guideline below.

Again, extend this to both sides of the head.

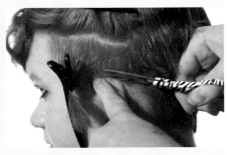

6 If, on short hair, you intend to take it around the ears, you need to do this before cutting your layered length.

Remember to hold the ears out of the way.

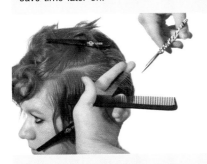

7 Now blend the side length to the same previously cut hair at the back.

Work forward to the front hairline.

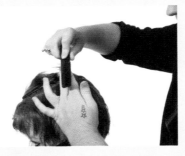

8 With the back and sides done, you now need to connect the side and back length into the top area.

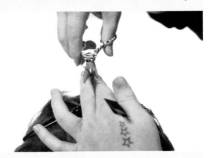

9 Working forwards, make sure that your lengths are even by **cross checking**, i.e. holding the hair in the opposite plane to which it was cut.

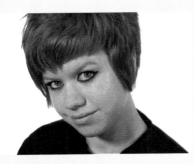

10 The final effect.

CourseMate video: Uniform Layer

STEP-BY-STEP: UNIFORM LONG LAYERS

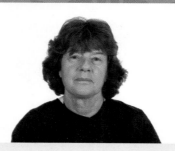

1 Uniform layering can be quite a versatile styling option, although it is a basic cutting technique. Here we see it used on longer hair.

Gown and protect your client.

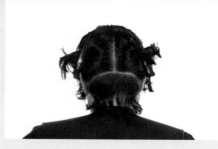

2 Section off the lower part of the hair and secure out of the way.

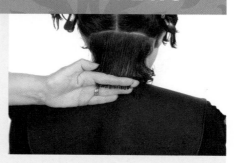

3 Choose your guideline length and cut all the perimeter.

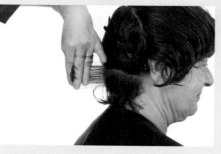

4 The first vertical layer section is critical, as this dictates the length of all the layers within the cut.

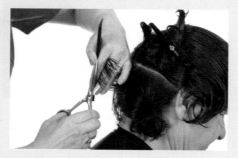

5 Cut your guideline vertically at 90°, without graduation or reverse graduation.

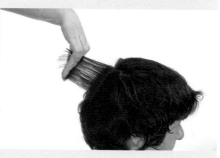

6 As you can see, in order for the layers to be uniform, they must follow the curvature of the head.

So extend your guideline up to the crown on the next section to reflect this.

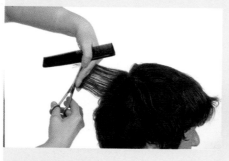

7 Cut to the guideline.

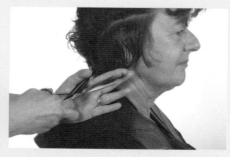

8 With the back done you can move to the sides and extend the perimeter back length to fit in with the sides.

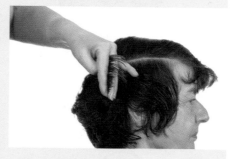

9 Now holding a previously cut section from the back, use the guideline to extend through to the front.

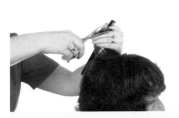

10 Sides and back done, continue layering through the top to the front hairline.

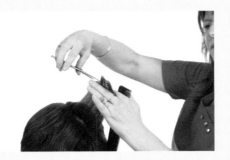

11 Be careful near the fringe even if it means leaving it slightly longer.

Cross check your work.

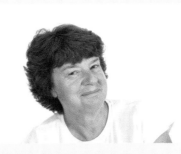

12 Final effect.

STEP-BY-STEP: ONE LENGTH CUTTING

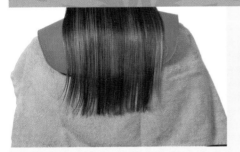

1 Very long one length hair can be very difficult to cut.

People that have one length long hair often have quite a lot of damage and this needs to be looked for before you start.

One of the main areas is the underlying lengths around the nape. These can often get caught in clothes and over time will start to break.

CHECK FIRST to see if there is any missing hair as it may prevent you from cutting too much off.

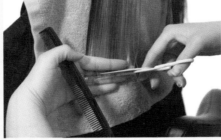

2 If the hair is quite thin, you may not need to section so far down as the nape. In this situation you could take your first section below the occipital and secure the remainder out of the way.

Start in the centre of the back and work outwards to the shoulders.

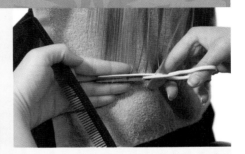

3 Check your balance, before taking down another section. Then use the previously cut guideline to act as a template for this section.

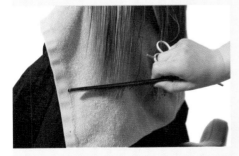

4 Check with the client if they want the same amount off all around and if there is an area that is still growing down, ask them if they want it trimmed or not.

Don't just go ahead and think that they need it cut.

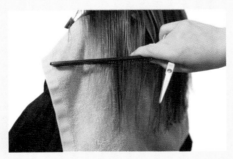

5 When you move around to the sides, section off the lower hair and comb down the length to see where it fits with the back.

Damaged hair will look frayed or tapered, so if you are permitted to tidy the ends up, carefully trim the profile shape.

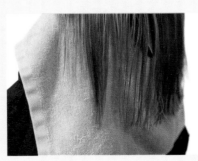

6 Take down subsequent sections and trim the same length.

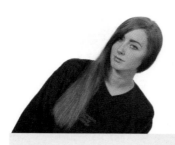

7 You can check your final balance and shape when the hair is dry.

CourseMate video: Long Length Cut

STEP-BY-STEP: GRADUATION

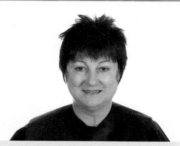

1 Before.

Prepare your client with a clean fresh gown and a cutting collar to stop fragments of hair going down the client's neck.

Make sure you check the growth patterns before you start.

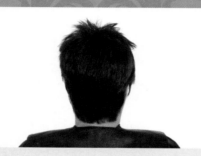

2 Haircuts are easier if started at the back because it enables you to ensure that the balance is correct, whether it is perimeter length or layer patterning.

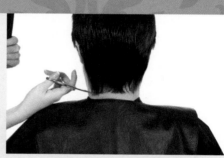

3 Tidy the perimeter shape first.

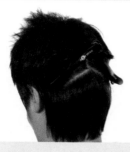

4 Section off the back so that you have a clear area to work with.

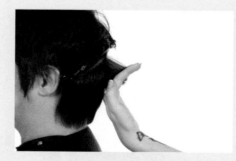

5 A graduation is where the lower perimeter length hair is shorter than the overlying, upper and inner length hair.

The cutting angle is held like this.

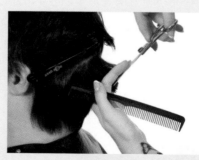

6 Take a section of hair from the centre and hold it vertically and create your cutting guideline.

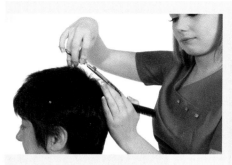

7 Follow the guideline out to either side and the graduated part is complete.

Now determine the overall length for the top and cut this guideline over the crown.

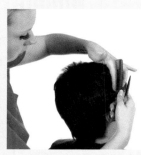

8 Follow the graduated lines from the back into either side and work forwards.

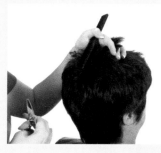

9 The length cut at the crown should now be continued forwards to the fringe area.

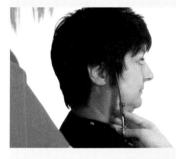

10 Profile the perimeter edges around the sides taking care around the ears.

Follow this length to finish the fringe.

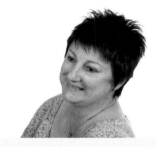

11 Finished effect.

CourseMate video: Graduated Layer

STEP-BY-STEP: REVERSE GRADUATION

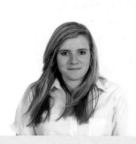 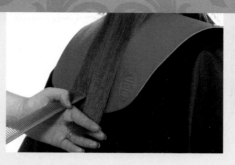 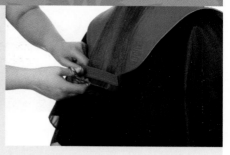

1 A reverse graduation is probably the most difficult to grasp at Level 2. It is all too easy to take too much hair away (especially on longer hair) and leave the hair with little density.

Prepare your client with a clean fresh gown and a cutting collar to stop fragments of hair going down the client's neck.

Make sure you check the growth patterns before you start.

2 Haircuts are easier if started at the back because it enables you to ensure that the balance is correct, whether it is perimeter length or layer patterning.

3 After sectioning off the lower nape section of the hair, start at the centre and create your first guideline.

Cut the perimeter to the same length and do the same with subsequent sections, up to the occipital.

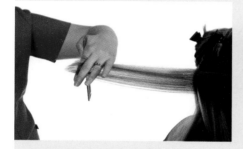 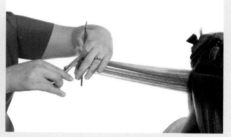 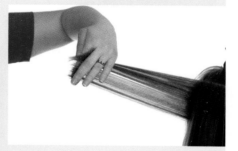

4 The first reverse graduation guideline is taken at the occipital bone area and is held out away from the head.

The reverse graduation cut creates a cut line that is longer towards the perimeter length and runs to a shorter length towards the crown.

5 Use this reverse graduation cut line to create your guideline.

Continue this at either side.

6 On the next section towards the crown we can clearly see the guideline and the hair that needs cutting to continue the style line.

Cut this through to the crown and at either side.

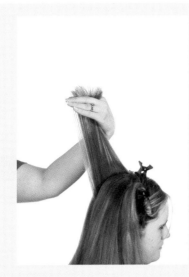

7 With the back done, you now need to hold and cut the hair over the top.

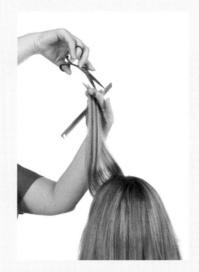

8 You can see from the guideline that had been created that the angle inverts downwards towards the parting.

Use this **inversion** as your guideline towards the parting at both sides of the head.

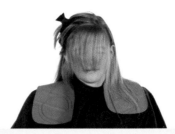

9 With the reverse graduation completed, you now need to profile the fringe and sides.

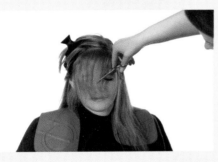

10 When hair is worn in a side parting, you have to create a fringe somewhere, and this is the most daunting aspect of the haircut.

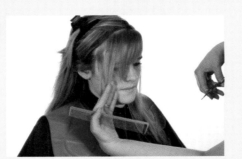

11 Take time to choose your shortest point and take the plunge. Start at this point and graduate downwards and into the side length.

Finally, check the balance and tidy where needed.

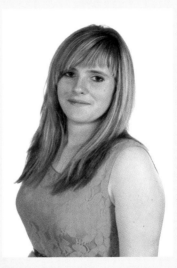

12 Final effect.

STEP-BY-STEP: SQUARE LAYERS

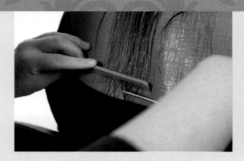

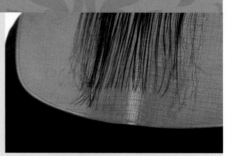

1 Gown and prepare your client. Square layers are ideal for someone who wants to retain density and weight in the perimeter, but also wants to add some varying lengths in the side for movement or volume.

2 Most of the work starts in a similar way to a one length cut.

Start by sectioning off the back so that you can work on the perimeter length first.

3 Start your guideline centrally at the back.

Then as you take down further sections, you can cut each subsequent layer to the same length.

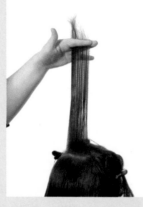

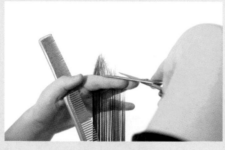

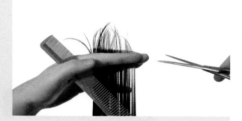

4 With the density retained at the bottom, take a vertical section at the crown up and hold it horizontally with your fingers.

5 Club cut straight across, as this now creates a guideline for the top square layering.

6 Continue to work forwards, cutting the hair to the same length.

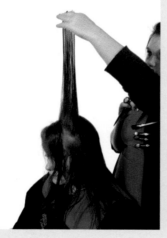

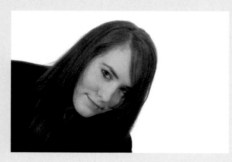

7 Work all the way forwards to the front hairline.

Finally shape the side fringe to angle downwards, so it doesn't cause a step or **disconnection**.

8 Final effect.

STEP-BY-STEP: CLIPPER GRADUATION

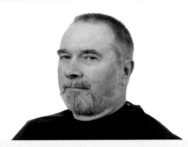

1 This sequence shows a typical men's graduated clipper cut. However there is another sequence that focuses upon the beard shaping.

CHECK THE BLADE ALIGNMENT FIRST!

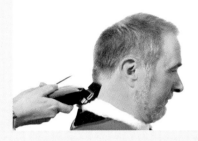

2 When hair is too short to section, you need to start at the bottom with the longest grade attachment first.

This enables you to work up the head, cutting the longest hair first and then working down to the shortest required grade and fading through from the shortest to the longest.

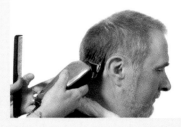

3 Cut all the back hair in direct vertical movements first.

Make sure at this stage that you don't go around the occipital bone as this can often need blending into the top with scissors – but not in this case.

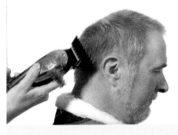

4 After cutting vertically, you can sweep across at an angle to ensure that the clippers have picked up all the hair that needs to be cut.

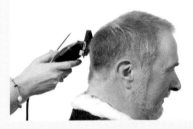

5 Here we see the exit point at the occipital and the hand position which enables the clippers to leave the cutting line at the back of the head – IN ONE COMPLETE MOVEMENT.

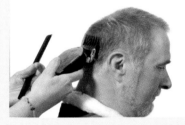

6 Change down to a shorter length grade and re-cut the back, fading out into the longer length grade below the occipital.

Continue with shorter grades depending on the client's wishes. Remember to fade the short grade into the longer grade above AT A LOWER POINT EACH TIME.

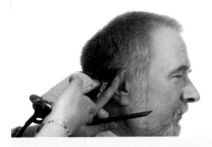

7 When working on the sides, make sure that you hold the ear out of the way.

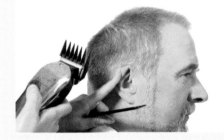

8 Also make sure you cut upwards, away from the ears.

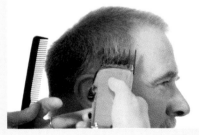

9 Continue around the sides to the frontal area, blending the shorter grades into the longer one at the top.

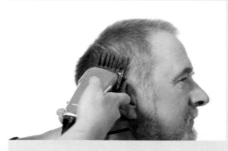

10 Fade out to the longer grade above.

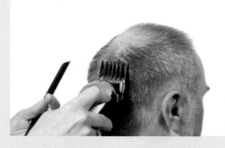

11 Finish blending the clippered area with a longer length grade for the top.

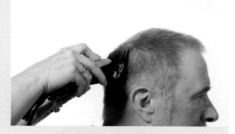

12 Or you could finish blending with a scissor over comb technique.

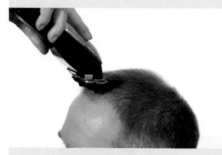

13 With back and side done, work through the top area to the crown – depending on whether the client wants clippers that will give a scissor-cut length effect.

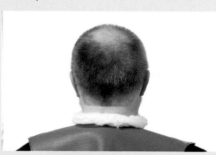

14 Finally, remove the attachments and recheck the blade alignment. You can now profile the back hair by turning the clippers over and cutting 'edge' onwards to create the U, V or square outline required.

TOP TIP

Far more customers are dissatisfied as a result of the stylist not listening and taking too much off than because of poor or inaccurate haircuts.

Aftercare advice

Good service is supported through good advice and recommendation. The work that you do in the salon needs to be cared for at home by the client too. What would be the point of creating something if the client doesn't know how to achieve and maintain the same effects at home?

Style durability

Hair grows at a steady rate of around 1.25cm per month, so at the six to eight week point the hair will be considerably longer than when it was first cut. If the hair is thick and coarse, the first thing that the client will notice is an increase in the width of the hairstyle on both sides. Similarly, if a client has a shoulder-length cut, then it will now be beyond the shoulders and separating in front and behind. In other words whatever the client selected for a style at the beginning, it will now have taken on a different look.

Make a point of outlining the benefits of having a regular cut: give your client an idea of how long the style will last and, ideally, because you know how long that will be, get them to re-book their style re-shape before they leave the salon. People who don't make appointments before they leave the salon often tend to drift beyond the normal interval times. Then, when they do realize that their hair needs doing, they find that they can't get an appointment at a time that suits them. So by the time you get to work on it again the hair really needs a sort out.

Aftercare checklist

◆ Talk through the style as you work – that way the client sees how you handle different aspects of the look.

◆ Show and recommend the products/equipment that you use so that the client gets the right things to enable them to get the same effects.

◆ Tell the client how long the style can be expected to last and when they need to return for re-shaping.

◆ Demonstrate the techniques that you use so they can achieve that salon hair look too.

Talk through the style as you work

Make a point of talking through your styling techniques as you go as:

◆ it eliminates long periods of silence while you are working and, more importantly;

◆ it is really useful to the client as they get useful advice on how to recreate a similar effect at home.

Show and recommend the products/ equipment that you use

As you talk about the ways in which you have styled the hair, make a point of talking through the products that you have used as well.

This way they will be able to see a direct link between the effects that you are achieving on their hair, with the added benefits of buying those particular products that will help them to recreate a similar effect.

Explain how routine styling tools can have detrimental effects

Only hair in good condition is easy to maintain. You know how difficult it is to make dry, damaged hair look good. With these known facts, you would be doing an injustice to your clients if you didn't warn them of the pitfalls of repeatedly using hot styling equipment, so make a point in asking them if they use them at home too. If they say that they use straighteners or tongs on a daily basis then tell them about the benefits of using heat protection.

Demonstrate the techniques that you use

Clients want to be able to recreate the effects that you achieve in the salon and this is your chance to show them how to do it. Clients haven't had the benefit of your training and they don't know the little tricks and techniques that make it seem so simple. Show them how to do things – correct combing, blow-drying or positioning of brushes. We have all seen the effects when these are not done properly, so make a point of giving them a few tips on how they can achieve a similar result themselves and how long they can expect it to last.

SUMMARY

As a final reflection on what you have covered in this chapter, you should now have a clearer picture of all the essential aspects for cutting hair. In particular, you should now have a basic understanding of the key principles of:

1 Why preparation is essential to the service.

2 The theoretical aspects relating to cutting hair.

3 The techniques of graduation, reverse graduation, uniform layering and one length cutting.

4 How to use and maintain the tools and equipment associated with the different cutting services.

5 Providing advice to the clients about maintaining their hair.

And collectively, how these principles will enable you to provide a basic range of cutting services and effects to your clients.

ASSESSMENT OF KNOWLEDGE AND UNDERSTANDING

Project

For this project you will need to gather information from a variety of sources.

Close observation of your senior colleagues while they work is an invaluable means of learning. At first, cutting hair can be slow and difficult, but with practise this soon changes.

To gather together information on cutting and styling you will need to visit hairdressing demonstrations, exhibitions and competitions. Using photography and video recording is ideal. Practising first cuts, or experimenting with the various techniques, can be carried out on modelling blocks, slip-ons and models.

You need to record as much as you can, including the following:

1 Carefully list the movements and techniques that you see and outline the effects produced. Try to capture the positions of the sections taken, the angles of cut, the direction of cutting lines, etc.

2 Outline the plan of the cut and list the important factors to consider.

3 How do the different growth patterns affect your cutting? Describe these and try to illustrate them in your notes.

4 Try to describe the different cutting procedures and refer particularly to the different parts of the head – the fringe, sides, nape, top and back. Explain how these parts are blended or fit together.

Investigate other sources of haircutting information – magazines, DVDs, TV. The information you collect could include these items:

1 How to choose suitable cutting tools.

2 The effects produced by the different tools.

3 How metal cutting tools are maintained and cleaned.

4 How to select the right tool for the effect required.

5 The difference between wet and dry cutting, and the tools used for each.

6 How tools should be used safely.

Revision questions

A selection of different types of questions to check your cutting knowledge.

Q1   Accuracy is achieved by _____ and cutting the hair at the correct angle.   Fill in the blank

Q2   Scissors should be sterilized in Barbicide®.   True or false

Q3   Select from the following list those that are *not* texturizing techniques: Multi selection

Club cutting	☐ 1
Graduation	☐ 2
Slice cutting	☐ 3
Layering	☐ 4
Point cutting	☐ 5
Chipping	☐ 6

Q4   Symmetrical shapes produce equally balanced hairstyles.   True or false

Q5   Which of the following is not a cutting term?   Multi choice

Cross checking	○ a
Thinning	○ b
Free hand	○ c
Free style	○ d

Q6   Precision cutting is dependent upon cutting angles and even tension.   True or False

Q7   Which of the following hair growth patterns will affect the natural fall and way that a fringe lies after it is cut?   Multi selection

Nape whorl	☐ 1
Double crown	☐ 2
Widow's peak	☐ 3
Low hairline	☐ 4
Cow's lick	☐ 5
High hairline	☐ 6

Q8   A _____ is the perimeter shape produced by cutting.   Fill in the blank

Q9   Which of the following cuts would easily describe a disconnection?   Multi choice

Graduation in a long hairstyle	○ a
Reverse graduation in a long hairstyle	○ b
A fringe in a shoulder-length bob style	○ c
Texturizing in a short cropped style	○ d

Q10   Clubbing is a technique of cutting that maximizes the hair density.   True or false

11 Cutting facial hair

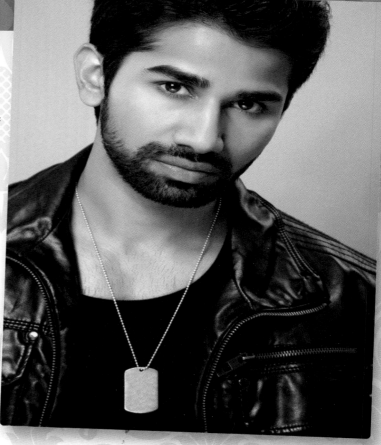

LEARNING OBJECTIVES

- ◆ Be able to maintain effective and safe methods of working

- ◆ Be able to cut beards and moustaches to maintain their shape

- ◆ Be able to provide aftercare advice

- ◆ Know how to work safely, effectively and hygienically when cutting

- ◆ Know how to use cutting tools and equipment

- ◆ Understand the cutting techniques used for trimming and shaping facial hair

KEY TERMS

anchor

barber's itch

beard and moustache shaping

curtain rail

dermatologist

epilation

exfoliation

furunculosis

folliculitis

goatee

halitosis

ingrown hair

lip line moustache

Male Pattern Baldness MPB

Mexican moustache

pencil moustache

pharaoh

rooftop moustache

whorls

Unit topic

Cut facial hair.

INTRODUCTION

This chapter extends beyond the previous one for cutting and looks more closely at a specific area of styling and shaping that only affects men. This chapter addresses the skills of trimming and shaping men's beards and moustaches. The cutting techniques involved in this aspect of barbering use the free hand, scissor over comb and clipper over comb techniques covered elsewhere, but now apply them for a different purpose.

The tools used in this area of work are the same as those used before, so to save duplication, go to CHAPTER 10 Cutting, where much of this information is cross-referenced.

Shaping beards and moustaches

PRACTICAL SKILLS

Preparing yourself, the client and the work area safely and correctly

Preparing and maintaining your tools and equipment

Learn how to create different facial hair shapes for men

Producing a range of effects for men by using different cutting techniques and methods

Trimming and shaping beards, moustaches and sideburns

Providing aftercare advice

Learn how to apply a different range of barbering techniques and when they should be used

UNDERPINNING KNOWLEDGE

Learn about the factors that influence cutting men's facial hair

Learn how to recognize different facial shapes and work with facial features

Learn how to recognize contra-indications and other things that can affect intended services

Learn when you need to adapt your service to cater for different needs

Preparing the client

Your attention to personal and client safety is just as important in this area of work as it is in any other area in hairdressing or barbering and you must ensure that you prepare yourself and the client correctly before you start.

Gowning the client

Always use freshly clean, laundered protective equipment:

◆ Fasten a gown at the back, or secure the cutting square with a clip ensuring that the covering is close fitting around the neck and protects the client from any clippings or spillages.

◆ Place a towel around the front of the client so that the free edges are fastened at the back.

◆ Tuck a strip of neck wool (or neck tissue) into the top edge of the towel to stop hair fragments from falling inside the client's clothes.

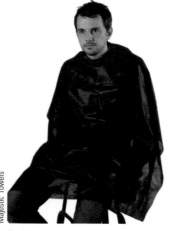

Majestic Towels

Cutting cape

TOP TIP

Remember you need to prepare all the things that you need before the client arrives.

BEST PRACTICE

Depending on what you are about to do and the type and texture of the client's hair you are working with, you may consider covering the client's eyes with a cotton wool pad to prevent sharp hair fragments and clippings from entering their eyes.

Positioning the client

Facial hair cutting requires the client to tilt their head back so that you can work at an angle that enables you to work safely and carefully. The barbering chair is designed for this with its inbuilt headrest and reclining ability.

Your working position and posture

Barbering involves a lot of standing and because of this you need to be comfortable in your work. You should always adopt a comfortable but safe work position, and sometimes comfortable and safe are not necessarily the same thing.

Cutting involves a lot of arm and hand movements and you need to be able to get close enough so that your hands and fingers are in a position where you can cut the hair unencumbered, without bad posture.

Your personal hygiene

Personal hygiene can't be stressed enough, it is vitally important for anyone working in personal services. Your personal hygiene, or lack of it, will be immediately noticeable to everyone you meet. You may have overslept, but if you haven't showered, it will be very uncomfortable for you, your colleagues and the clients, as BO is unpleasant in any situation. Other strong smells are offensive too. The smells of nicotine or smoking are very off-putting to the client, particularly if they are a non-smoker.

Be organized

You must be organized in your work – and in any work situation – in order to be organized, you must have a plan. That plan has been prepared for you – it's called the

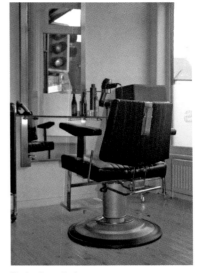

Barbering chair

TOP TIP

If you need to recline the chair do it before the client is seated.

TOP TIP

If you need to make any adjustments to working height or angle do this too.

HEALTH & SAFETY

Bad breath is offensive to clients too. Bad breath – halitosis – is the result of leaving particles to decay within the spaces between the teeth. You need to brush your teeth after every meal.

appointment book.

So always start your day by:

◆ Checking the appointment book – to see when clients are due.

◆ Preparing client records – to see what equipment and products you need.

◆ Prepare the work area – so that you are ready to receive the clients.

Always use your time effectively – making the most of your time is part of your job and it is something that everyone does to a different level of ability. If you really want to impress the people you work with as well as your clients, then this should be your goal. People always notice when others are efficient; *or go the extra mile,* as this is the difference between being a professional, or being part of the wallpaper. So stand out! Get noticed and most of all, be good at what you do.

Go to **CHAPTER 10** Cutting, for more information about posture.

Go to **CHAPTER 5** Health and safety, for more information about preventing infection.

Go to **CHAPTER 10** Cutting, for more information about working effectively.

Consultation

Check the client's requirements

If the main aim of hairdressing and barbering is about delivering a satisfactory repeated service that our clients are happy to pay for, then we can only satisfy the clients if we find out what they want and act upon those instructions.

When we do this it:

◆ Ensures that we only do things that the clients want.

◆ Makes the client more confident about what we are doing.

◆ Removes any misunderstanding or confusion.

◆ Gives us more confidence in what we are doing for the client.

◆ Involves the client and helps us to establish a professional relationship.

Pros and cons for cutting wet and dry

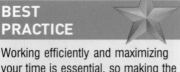

BEST PRACTICE

Working efficiently and maximizing your time is essential, so making the most of the resources available should occur naturally. Always treat the salon's materials in the same way that you would look after your own equipment and always try to minimize waste, being careful about how much product you use.

Cutting	Advantages	Disadvantages	Tool suitability
Wet	◆ Better accuracy for club cutting technique ◆ Cleaner sections, better holding tension ◆ Better accuracy, cleaner cut lines ◆ Easier to control and section out of the way ◆ Hair will cut easier with less pressure	◆ Harder to see natural growth patterns ◆ Can easily lead to taking too much hair off	◆ Scissors ◆ Thinning scissors ◆ Razor/shaper
Dry	◆ Better accuracy for scissor over comb technique ◆ Easier to work with natural fall and growth patterns ◆ Easier to see final perimeter length without 'shrinkage' ◆ Easier to see overall shape and the impact that cutting will have upon that shape ◆ Better for finishing off profile features, i.e. fringes, necklines, sideburns, beards, moustaches, etc.	◆ Easy to hold, but harder to maintain an even, holding tension ◆ Hair may not be clean enough to achieve a satisfactory result ◆ Clippings/fragments fly everywhere – particularly clippering.	◆ Scissors ◆ Thinning scissors ◆ Clippers

Look for contra-indications

When you are preparing to trim and shape facial hair, the contra-indications to the service are not going to be necessarily as obvious as those in other services. For example, if you had a client that wanted highlights and their hair was already lightened, or severely damaged, you wouldn't need to touch the hair to know that further lightening is not an option.

So when it comes to facial hair services, you are going to need to comb and brush the hair, partly to detangle it, but more importantly, to take a closer look.

The table below looks at some of the common contra-indications affecting **beard and moustache shaping**.

Identify factors that influence the service When you are unsure or need more information, don't be afraid to ask questions. Listen to your client's responses as many simple mistakes can be avoided if you have a clear understanding of what your client wants.

Facial hair shaping for beards and moustaches needs to be suitable for the client. You will need to consider:

◆ Their face and head shape/size.

◆ Working with facial physical features such as piercings, earrings, etc.

◆ Disguising unwanted physical features such as scars, blemishes or birthmarks.

◆ The hair quality, abundance, growth and distribution.

HEALTH & SAFETY

Used razor blades and similar items should be placed into a safe container – sharps box.

TOP TIP

You can't do a consultation without doing an inspection.

Typical infections/contra-indications

Disorder	Symptoms	Cause	Treatment
Sycosis barbae – common name **Barber's itch** *Prof. Andrew Wright, Dermatologist Bradford*	A reddened rash appearing within the beard of facial hair areas, often with small pimples or pustules. Causes discomfort and itching.	Bacterial infection – infection of the hair follicles in the bearded area of the face, usually the upper lip. Shaving aggravates the condition.	Referral to Pharmacist – condition treated with antiseptic ointment/creams.
Folliculitis *Courtesy of Mediscan*	Inflamed hair follicles resulting in a tender red spot, usually superficial, but may be deeper, often with a surface pustule and hair growing in the centre.	Usually bacterial – but can be fungal or viral – an infection caused by: ◆ The friction/rubbing of the skin by clothing. ◆ Insect bites. ◆ Regrown hair – after shaving or plucking.	Referral to Pharmacist – sometimes treated with antiseptic ointments/creams. **More severe cases** – referral to GP. Condition is treated by prescribed antibiotic medication.

(Continued)

(Continued)

Disorder	Symptoms	Cause	Treatment
Boils (Furunculosis) *Prof. Andrew Wright, Dermatologist Bradford*	A boil is a deeper form of bacterial folliculitis and has similar surface symptoms.	Bacterial infection caused by: ◆ Nicking the skin when shaving. ◆ The friction/rubbing of the skin by clothing.	Referral to GP. Condition is treated by prescribed antibiotic medication.
Ingrown hair common name (Razor bumps)	The surface symptoms can easily be misdiagnosed as folliculitis – includes rash, itching skin, hair which remains in spite of shaving, and infection and pus collecting under skin.	Prevalent on people with curly hair, it is a condition where the hair curls back or grows sideways into the skin. It occurs due to continual close cutting, e.g. shaving, plucking, **epilation**, etc.	Ideally, the ingrown hair should be removed using tweezers, but this can make problems worse causing a secondary infection. For this reason referral to GP/**dermatologist** for specialist treatment.

Go to **CHAPTER 6** Consultation, For more information on other contra-indications.

HEALTH & SAFETY

Always make sure that the clippers are cleaned before they are used. Any hair caught between the blades will limit their ability to work, and is unhygienic for the client.

Facial features

Facial features	How best to work with it
Square and oblong faces	Square and oblong are typically masculine and provide a perfect base for traditional, classic, well groomed looks. The angular features of the face can be augmented with closer, shorter beards or moustaches and would probably benefit from fewer curves and more angular, linear effects.
Round faces	The effect of a round face can be lessened or increased: it depends what the client wants. If the plan is to reduce the effects, then choose beard designs that lengthen the jawline and incorporate lines and angles rather than curves. If the round features suit the personality and image of the client then work with it by cutting uniform length shapes.

(Continued)

(*Continued*)

Facial features	How best to work with it
Square angular features, jaw, forehead, etc.	Again these are traditionally accepted as a feature of masculinity. These can be handled in a similar way to that of the squarer features above. Squarer, more angular features can also be easily softened with beards and moustaches.
Wider heads	These wide features will be increased with full, long beards. Create beard designs that are closer cut at the sides and extend to more length at the chin.
Scars, birthmarks and blemishes	If the client has any scars, birthmarks or blemishes, this may be the reason for growing a beard or moustache in the first place. You need to ask if there are any features that the client wants to disguise. Always make a point of looking for these during your consultation.
Facial piercings	Facial piercings around the mouth and ears do need to be considered during your consultation as well. It is unlikely that the client will want to remove them/it so you have to be very careful in combing, detangling and cutting anywhere near to the area(s) of the piercing(s).
Earrings, studs, etc.	Not normally a problem, but make sure that you are careful when working on sideburns or full beards as you will be particularly close to the ears and it is very easy to catch studs/earrings in a comb or if you are clumsy with the clippering.

Quick reference – suitability guide	
Feature to work with	**Suitability**
A prominent nose	◆ Is diminished by a larger moustache. ◆ Is more obvious with a smaller moustache.
Longer narrow nose	◆ Looks balanced with a narrower, thinner moustache.
Larger, wider mouth	◆ Is diminished by a chevron or triangular shaped moustache. ◆ Is more obvious with a straighter lined moustache.
Small, narrow mouth	◆ Looks in balance with a narrower, shorter moustache. ◆ Looks out of balance with a larger, or wider moustache.
Smaller, narrower faces	◆ Look balanced by smaller, neat edged beards and/or moustaches.
Wider faces – wide mouths	◆ Look in balance with wider, fuller moustaches. ◆ Look out of balance with wider, short but full beards. ◆ Are diminished with longer beards.

BEST PRACTICE

ALWAYS check the blades on the clippers before you use them, check for looseness, check the alignment of the cutting edges.

(*Continued*)

(Continued)

Quick reference – suitability guide	
Feature to work with	**Suitability**
Rounder faces	◆ Are diminished with squarer cut beards/moustaches.
Squarer faces	◆ Are diminished with moustaches with downward curving edges.

Other influencing factors

Hair growth patterns If you have already read the consultation or the main cutting chapter, you will have seen the typical growth patterns that affect the client's options for hair styling and style maintenance. In facial hair, these growth patterns aren't so prominent, in fact in many ways they are hidden by the:

◆ Length of the facial hair.

◆ Density of the facial hair growth.

However, there is one feature that does cause problems and it can affect the direction of the 'lay' of the hair on one side of a beard or moustache to the other. This has implications when you try to finish the hair shape as it does affect the visual balance.

When you do your consultation with your client, you will as a matter of course be combing through the facial growth in order to detangle the hair and to see the overall length. While you are doing this look out for 'swirls' within the hair. These denote *mini crown-like* patterns, and when you cut near these, the hair directions will be opposite on either side. If you don't notice these features before you start, it may cause you problems later on, as you will not be able to *camouflage* them with clever cutting.

Swirl patterns in beards

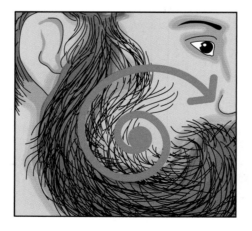
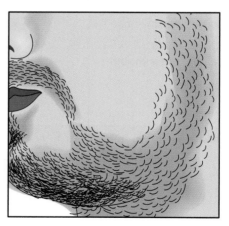

Hair density Apart from clients who have some form of alopecia like **male pattern baldness**, the distribution of hair over the client's head is usually uniform. In other words, you don't normally find that as you cut one area, the amount of hair density changes dramatically to the next area to it.

This isn't the same in men's facial hair. It is quite normal to find that the hair coverage and therefore the density, changes from heavy, thick, coarse parts to that which is thin, or finer and shows the skin through it quite easily. You need to be aware of this from the outset, as it will affect what you are trying to do and the overall effect that you are trying to achieve.

5-o'clock shadow Some men have a heavy, daily growth of facial hair and they find that they need to shave every day. This heavy growth can be obvious for a range of reasons.

◆ The growth appears heavy because the contrast of hair colour against the skin looks dark.

◆ The hair seems to grow particularly fast.

◆ The density of hair distributed on the face is particularly thick.

◆ The density of hair distributed on the face in comparison to the hair on their head is particularly thick.

So with these factors in mind – males that are most likely to choose to grow beards and/or moustaches will have ticked two or more of the above. But they are not the only ones who choose to do this, as many others with a poorer growth or definition will grow facial hair for other reasons.

Mouth and width of upper lip to base of nose The size and width of the mouth forms the basis for any moustache. The distance between the upper lip and the base of the nose creates a sort of *canvas* for the moustache. If the distance between the two areas is quite deep, it will provide more outline shape options for the wearer rather than if it were narrow.

Similarly, the width of the face at the cheeks will also determine the best suited effect. Someone with a wide face will be able to wear a fuller moustache, whereas someone with a narrow face could be swamped by this much hair.

Bone structure and facial contours You should take particular care for clients who have a well-defined bone structure, i.e. cheekbones, jaws and facial contour. If they have a particularly angular/linear aspect to their facial features then it would be wiser to retain that similar effect with the overall shapes and outlines. That is unless they want to disguise themselves or have physical features they want to cover up.

On the other hand, the man who has a rounder, fuller face can benefit from a shape that defines the face with a more structured effect. Remember that these people can wear beards with fuller effects than those men with narrower facial features.

Width of chin and depth of jawline Facial hair growth forms a *frame* for the physical features of the face, and therefore the width of the chin and the depth down to the bottom of the jaw that become the focal point of any facial hair shaping. The outlines of the shapes created here are more noticeable than any others. Historically, beards were left relatively full, which meant that there was very little upkeep for the wearer, apart from keeping the beard from getting too bushy. Latterly, the fashion for wearing more chiselled effects has meant that not only thickness but an outline shape (i.e. outlining) is equally important to the overall effect.

HEALTH & SAFETY

Always make sure that the clippers are cleaned before they are used. Any hair caught between the blades will limit their ability to work, and is unhygienic for the client.

Preparing the client's facial hair

Many men with longer beards never comb them out because they don't want to lose the shape they naturally take on, or they simply don't see the benefits of doing so. Obviously, this is a mistake, as regular grooming keeps them free from debris and reduces the chance of infections, e.g.:

◆ *Sycosis barbae*

◆ *Folliculitis*

◆ *boils*

◆ *ingrowing hair*

You should always make a point of giving the clients advice on this or at least tell them how they can manage their own facial hair between visits.

Moustaches and beards get matted as they get longer because the bristles tend to get curlier and 'lock' together. So these tangles have to be removed so that the longer hair is revealed. This allows you to style all of the hair and not just part of it.

Clean hair is important too. A beard with debris or grease cannot be styled until it has been cleaned. If you are shampooing the hair as part of another service, then the beard can be done at the same time. Or alternatively, you can ask the client to wash their face and beard in the front wash basin, or cleanse with facial wipes.

Tools and equipment

The tools used for trimming beards and moustaches and the maintenance and preparations needed are the same that you would use in any other barbering techniques.

Cutting techniques

Most of the techniques that you will use for trimming facial hair have already been covered in the main cutting chapter. However, there are ways of using those techniques that specifically apply to this type of work.

For all of these techniques, you must make the following preparations before you start:

1 Look for the growth directions within the hair.

2 Look for differing densities of growth within the hair, i.e. areas that may be thinner with weaker growth.

3 Look for growth directions within the hair that may affect your overall plan.

4 Disentangle the beard or moustache to remove any debris or knots and to see the true length of the facial hair.

And during the cutting make sure that you:

5 Frequently brush the cut hair fragments away from the client's face and neck.

6 Check your shaping for balance and accuracy.

7 Use damp cotton wool pads to protect the client's eyes from hair clippings.

If you do cut the client:

◆ Put on a pair of disposable, non-latex gloves.

◆ Use a medical sterilized wipe to clean the area and remove any hair or bristle.

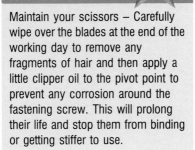

BEST PRACTICE

Maintain your scissors – Carefully wipe over the blades at the end of the working day to remove any fragments of hair and then apply a little clipper oil to the pivot point to prevent any corrosion around the fastening screw. This will prolong their life and stop them from binding or getting stiffer to use.

Go to **CHAPTER 10** Cutting pp. 286–292, for more information on tools and equipment.

Go to **CHAPTER 10** Cutting pp. 292–297, for more information on cutting techniques.

◆ Apply pressure to the cut to stem the flow of blood.

◆ When the wound has stopped bleeding finish the service and give the client a clean, dry tissue for any minor seepage.

Scissor over comb This technique is used more often than any other in this type of work. So in addition to the above, make sure that you do the following:

Scissor over comb techniques: At-a-glance

The way that the hair is lifted with the comb, before it is cut with the scissors will allow you to:

◆ Follow the comb with the scissors in the same direction – matching the movement of the one hand – which holds the comb: to that of the other hand – which holds the scissors.

◆ Keep the comb moving upwards within the shaping – enabling you to start at the lower point of the cut and to work upwards in a consistent methodical approach.

◆ Hold the comb horizontally and to cut the hair using the comb as a guide and a guard – the normal holding angle for cutting scissor over comb.

◆ Hold the comb at other angles – enabling you to work around physical features, i.e. ears, lips, nose, head contours, sideburns and facial piercings, etc.

◆ Comb the hair towards you – checking the density of the hair before choosing the point at where to cut.

◆ Hold the comb parallel to the facial contour – enabling you to match shaping and trimming to physical proportions. Or:

◆ Angle the comb outwards – away from the face to apply a small amount of graduation in the scissor over comb effect. Or:

◆ Angle the comb inwards – towards the face, to apply a small amount of reverse graduation in the shaping.

◆ Use damp cotton wool pads to protect the client's eyes from hair clippings.

Clipper over comb This technique is also particularly useful in this type of work, so before you start, make sure that you also remember that clippers:

◆ Cut hair far quicker than scissors, so you have to be more careful when using them.

◆ Are relatively heavy and this can affect the way that you cut the hair.

Clipper over comb techniques: At-a-glance

The way that the hair is lifted with the comb, before it is cut with the electric clippers will allow you to:

◆ Work more quickly than scissor over comb – because the electric clippers are faster, enabling you to cut hair by just 'sweeping' across the face of the comb in a sideways action, cutting away all that protrudes through the teeth.

◆ Cut closer to the body of the comb than using scissor over comb techniques – often providing a higher degree of accuracy.

◆ Keep the comb moving upwards within the shaping – enabling you to start at the lower point of the cut and to work upwards in a consistent methodical approach.

◆ Hold the comb horizontally and to cut the hair using the comb as a guide and a guard – the normal holding angle for cutting clipper over comb.

◆ Hold the comb at other angles – enabling you to work around physical features, i.e. ears, lips, nose, head contours, sideburns and facial piercings, etc.

◆ Use damp cotton wool pads to protect the client's eyes from hair clippings.

(Continued)

(Continued)

Clipper over comb techniques: At-a-glance

◆ Comb the hair towards you – checking the density of the hair before choosing the point at where to cut.

◆ Hold the comb parallel to the facial contour – enabling you to match shaping and trimming to physical proportions. Or

◆ Angle the comb outwards – away from the face to apply a small amount of graduation in the clipper over comb effect. Or

◆ Angle the comb inwards – towards the face, to apply a small amount of reverse graduation in the shaping.

Go to p. 292 for detailed information about routine maintenance and safety checks.

Clippers with attachments (grades) This technique provides an easier way to ensure the overall finished length of the cut because the clipper grades keep an even distance between the contours of the face and the cutting edge of the clippers.

This, however, has positive and negative impacts on the final effect, because it:

◆ Provides better accuracy within the cut as it removes the risk of holding a comb at different depths while you work.

◆ Controls the cutting depth (and effectively the layering depth) between the skin and the cutting edge of the clipper blades.

◆ Can create other problems because the cutting depth is indiscriminate, i.e. will cut all areas: either thinner, or thicker, heavier hair growth to the same length – and this *will* expose the thinner areas.

Clippering with attachments: At-a-glance

The way that the hair is lifted by the attachment before the clippers cut away the hair will allow you to:

◆ Back-off the blades of the clippers so that the edge of the plastic attachments don't impede the moving, cutting edge of the upper blade.

◆ Work more quickly than scissor over comb – because the electric clippers are faster, enabling you to cut hair by just '*sweeping*' across the contour of the face.

◆ Use two hands on the clippers while you work, producing a more controlled and safer method of working.

◆ Use a neck brush to brush away the cut hair fragments more easily and frequently during the cutting, which will be more comfortable for the client and enable you to see the shape emerge more quickly.

◆ Use damp cotton wool pads to protect the client's eyes from hair clippings.

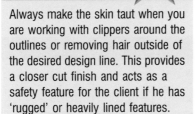

BEST PRACTICE

Always make the skin taut when you are working with clippers around the outlines or removing hair outside of the desired design line. This provides a closer cut finish and acts as a safety feature for the client if he has 'rugged' or heavily lined features.

Freehand cutting This technique provides the final touches to your work as it enables you to finish off edges without holding them with a comb.

Freehand cutting: At-a-glance

The freehand cutting technique enables you to profile the facial hair by cutting:

◆ Hair that still protrudes from a moustache over a lip, or sticks out at a different angle, that could not be cut any other way.

◆ Longer hair beneath the nose in a moustache that could be uncomfortable if cut with clippers.

◆ Stiff, protruding hairs within a beard or moustache that have a different texture or tendency to the surrounding hair, which may look odd if left and spoil the overall finished effect.

◆ Odd hairs outside the defined outlines to finish the overall look and desired effect.

◆ Curving perimeter outlines of moustaches and beards that could look odd, if cut with the straight, indiscriminate lines of the clipper blades.

Fading – Faded outlines Language is continually developing and new words like hairstyles, are created all the time. Each year new terms or expressions find a place in common language and a place in the *Oxford English Dictionary*.

Fading – which is a form of graduation – isn't a true cutting technique, but it is a commonly used term by clients and barbers, for *describing* how a perimeter outline will appear.

In principle there are only two types of perimeter outlining in hair styling:

◆ *Club cut outline* – where hair is cut bluntly to create *punctuation* in a hairstyle as a solid, continuous, curved or straight line.

◆ *Faded outline* – where hair is graduated from longer down to the skin in a smooth, blended, layering pattern that doesn't create a solid, continuous line. That is, working with the natural hairlines to show contour in the outline perimeter shape.

Shapes of beards and moustaches

Beard and moustache shapes	
Full-beard	Downward flowing beard with either styled or integrated moustache.
Anchor	A beard shaped like an anchor from the centre of the bottom lip and around and up the chin.
Circle beard	Commonly mistaken for the goatee, the circle beard is a small chin beard that connects around the mouth to a moustache. Also called a 'doorknocker'.
Sideburns	Patches of facial hair grown on the sides of the face, extending from the hairline to below the ears and worn with an unbearded chin.
Chinstrap	Facial hair that extends from the hairline of one side of the face to the other, following the jawline, much like the chin curtain. Unlike the chin curtain though, it does not cover the entire chin.
Curtain rail	A particular style of facial hair that grows along the jawline and covers the chin completely.
Garibaldi	A wide, full beard with rounded bottom and integrated moustache.
Goatee	A tuft of hair grown on the chin, sometimes resembling a billy goat's beard.
Junco	A goatee which extends upward and connects to the corners of the mouth but does not include a moustache, like the circle beard.

(Continued)

(Continued)

Beard and moustache shapes	
Hollywoodian	A beard with integrated moustache that is worn on the lower part of the chin and jaw area, without connecting sideburns.
Reed	A beard with integrated moustache that is worn on the lower part of the chin and jaw area that tapers towards the ears without connecting sideburns.
Royale	A narrow, pointed beard extending from the chin. The style was popular in France during the period of the Second Empire, from which it gets its alternative name, the 'Imperial'.
Stubble	A very short beard of only one to a few days growth.
Five o'clock shadow	Stubble that is visible late in the day on men who have shaved their faces that morning.
Van Dyke	A 'goatee' accompanied by a moustache.
Verdi	A short beard with rounded bottom and slightly shaven cheeks with prominent moustache.
Soul patch	A small beard just below the lower lip and above the chin.
Monkey Tail	A 'Van Dyke' as viewed from one side, and a 'Chinstrap' and moustache as viewed from the other, giving the impression that a monkey's tail stretches from an ear down to the chin and around one's mouth.
Pharaoh	A beard of any length, starting from the base of the chin.
Lip Line moustache	A narrow moustache following the natural line of the upper lip.
Mexican moustache	A moustache following the natural line of the upper lip and extending down towards the chin.
Pencil moustache	A horizontal moustache about the width of a pencil.
Rooftop moustache	A moustache that extends from under the nose to form a straight 'chevron' shape.

Work with the facial contours
Always work to and with the natural facial hairlines. It's OK to leave length longer and cover the feature, but encroaching over this natural division will cause problems.

Because taking your outlines shorter over facial hairlines will make:

◆ the results look strange, unnatural and out of balance;

◆ the bristles show quickly and would need razoring to remove;

◆ it difficult for the client to maintain the style, as he would need to change his shaving technique to keep the lines clean,

work with the natural growth patterns too.

You can't change the direction of the bristles as they grow out from the face. You have to accommodate them within the shaping and trimming. Remember, no two heads of hair are the same and this goes for the positioning and natural shapes of beards and moustaches on faces too.

Make allowances for any particular anomalies such as:

◆ Strong directional movements, say to one side – this will limit the wearer to a particular length before it is very noticeable.

◆ Whorls or circulatory growth patterns – the effects of these are lessened by more length.

◆ Missing or thinning areas – again the effects of these areas are reduced if you leave extra length, but it will be more obvious when cut short.

You need to remember that facial hair is bristle. It is stiffer than hair on the head and this is partly due to the frequency that it is cut in relation to hairstyles. This creates its own problems, as it is more difficult to cut by the scissor over comb method. This leads stylists and barbers to choose clipper over comb, as the mechanical advantage makes the job far easier. But as you need to use one hand to steady and position the comb, you can only use one to hold the *relatively* heavy clippers. This technique is more complex than using clippers held with two hands and clipper-grade attachments.

When the interior of the facial hair shape has been cut, you can then concentrate on defining the shape by creating the outside perimeter line. Hair growth can often be uneven across the head, let alone the face. Even if the client is a regular visitor to the salon, you will need to check for balance throughout the shaping, to make sure that the growth doesn't occur thicker and deeper on one side than the other.

Although comfort is always a major concern, for beard trimming it may be easier to start your outlining with the clippers, centrally up the neck, to the point below the chin to start the perimeter shape. By doing this, you can define the exact position where you stop and you will find that you can then work on either side of the client to create an even, symmetrical finish. After this you can complete the shape behind or over the jaw, and finally from the cheek area down to the desired top profile of the beard.

On the other hand, most moustaches are trimmed at or above the upper lip using scissors, which are easier to handle and it stops the vibration of the clippers tickling the client and causing him to pull back.

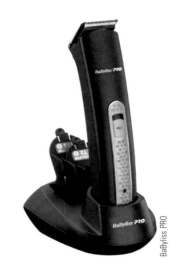

BaByliss PRO

Removing unwanted hair from outside the defined perimeter shape
After completing the finished beard or moustache shape, there only remains one task to finish the service. Your final tidying-up will be in the remaining hair or stubble that exists outside of the perimeter line that you have created.

It's always better to leave this until last as it is like *the icing on the cake*. If you don't do this correctly then you will spoil the whole effect, as the eye is always drawn to disorder, rather than order – i.e. things that are out-of-place. That may seem hard to follow, but it is true in most aspects of life, and in hairdressing and barbering, it is the difference between a professional finish and something else.

The time that you take in finishing the look by removing the untidy hair outside of the perimeter shape will create a focus to the work you have already done. If you don't remove this hair, the definition in your work will be lost and the facial hair shape will not have any particular style.

If you have created your final outline shape say for a beard, then the last thing that you need to do is get the client to sit back in a position so that you can work with the clippers 'edge-on' to carefully remove any untidy bristles that remain on the neck or face. Remember to ask the client to close their eyes, or you can cover them with cotton pads, particularly as the fragments can *fly* everywhere. You may find that you need to stretch the skin around the neck and face to get a cleaner, straighter cut close to the skin. Then, working back from the design (perimeter) line, draw the clippers away over the neck/cheek or jaw to create a clean finish. Take a neck brush and carefully brush away any fragments. A final brush and the cutting is over.

HEALTH & SAFETY

Always look for any contra-indications before you start any facial hair shaping. Look carefully for any suspected infestations or viral or bacterial infections.

HEALTH & SAFETY

Ask the client to close their eyes as tiny fragments of bristle are very strong and can enter their eyes.

◆ Use damp cotton wool pads to protect the client's eyes from hair clippings.

Trimming and shaping beards, moustaches and eyebrows

STEP-BY-STEP: BEARD TRIMMING AND SHAPING

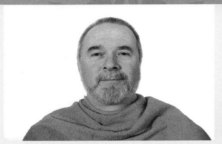

1 Prepare the client by placing neck wool around the cutting collar and then cover this with a clean fresh towel.

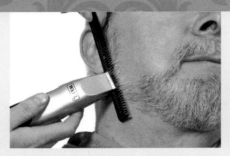

2 With lighter facial growth, a normal set of clippers may be too aggressive, so a cordless profiler/trimmer may be better.

Use your cutting comb to detangle the facial hair and cut a guideline length for the shaping.

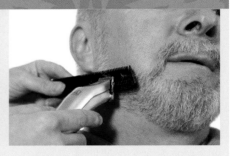

3 With the guideline cut you can cut clipper over comb up that guide.

Keep your comb (and subsequently the trimmers) angled away from the face

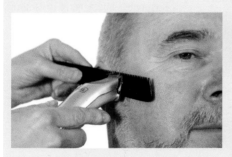

4 Check around the face on both sides to ensure evenness.

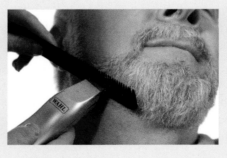

5 Work underneath the neck, ensuring that all the loose hair is removed by combing away or brushing.

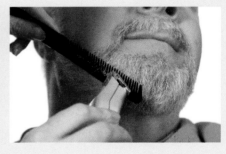

6 Work forwards up and around the chin to trim and shape the front beard shape to the required length.

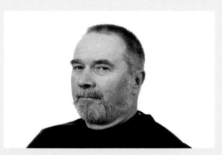

7 Hair and beard final effect.

STEP-BY-STEP: MOUSTACHE TRIMMING AND SHAPING

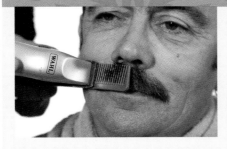

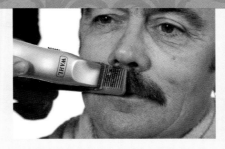

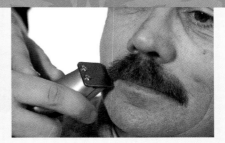

1 Some men prefer a moustache that has longer top length without any layering, these moustaches only require lip lining as in step 4/5.

For shaped moustaches, remove any tangles by light combing, then using cordless trimmers over comb and remove the longer bristles.

CHECK THE BLADE ALIGNMENT FIRST.

2 Take care around the nose as the edge of the clippers are still very sharp. Also ask the client if they want to wear eye protection to avoid hair fragments entering the eyes.

3 With the length of the moustache cut to the required length, you can now start at the outer edges to trim the lower profile shape.

Do not cut above the natural hairlines as this will make it very difficult for the client to maintain, and it will look very odd.

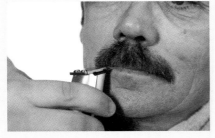

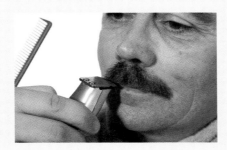

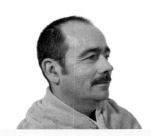

4 Continue the lip lining on both sides working from the outer edges towards the centre.

5 Remove any loose hairs and brush the client's face. (They may want to use a towel.)

Final effect.

STEP-BY-STEP: SHAPING AND TRIMMING SIDEBURNS

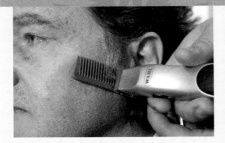

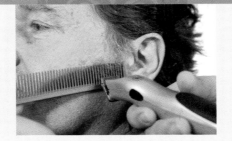

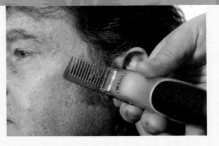

1 Sideburns can be cut scissor over comb, but it is far easier cutting bristly, coarse hairs with electric trimmers, but remember to check the blade alignment before you start.

If the client has longer hair, clip it out of the away, as electric clippers will quickly take it away!

Comb through to detangle.

2 Lift the sideburns to trim the length within the sideburn before any shaping or profiling.

3 Work through the areas from the lower part, up to the upper parts.

Remember, the growth may be uneven, and you will need to check this before you start. Here we see some white hair in and among the darker growth. This is often different in texture and will need to be taken into consideration.

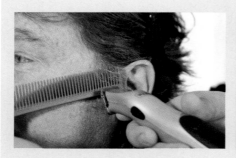

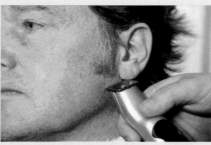

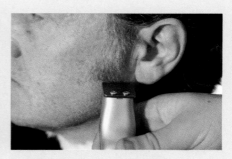

4 As you work through you may find that because of thickness, the effect and balance in the mirror is disproportionate for the client and you may have to take the complete sideburn even closer and shorter.

5 When you are satisfied with the length, you can then tidy the outline shape.

6 For lining and profiling, you will need to turn the trimmer over to create a neater edge.

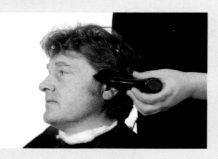

7 Finally, when you have done both sides, brush away any loose hair and check the final shape with the client in the mirror.

STEP-BY-STEP: EYEBROW TRIMMING

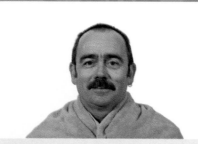

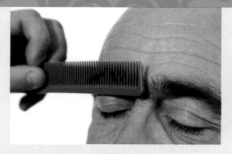

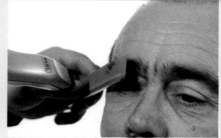

1 Before

As a barbering technique, eyebrow shaping can be carried out by either trimming with scissors over comb or by small battery operated trimmers.

Note: Eyebrows seldom grow evenly and from a shaping point of view you need to even out the lengths to make them appear tidier.

2 Scissor over comb method.

Comb through the eyebrows to remove tangles and to find the longer lengths that need trimming.

Note: If your client prefers to not wear cotton pads ask them to close their eyes to prevent fragments entering them.

3 Scissor over comb method.

Repeat over the other eye

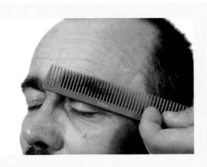

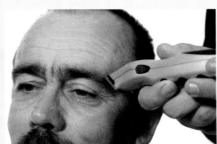

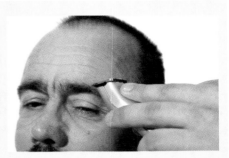

4 Electric trimmers method.

Comb through the eyebrows to remove tangles and to find the longer lengths that need trimming and glide the trimmers over the comb's surface to remove the longer hairs.

5 Electric trimmers method.

Repeat over the other eye.

6 Electric trimmers method

If the final outline eyebrow shape needs attention too, this should be done with trimmers not scissors.

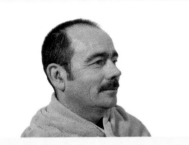

7 Final effect.

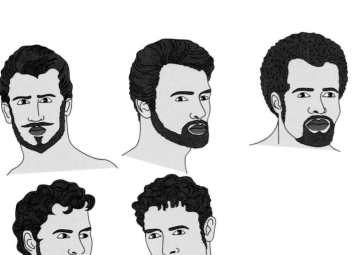

Examples of beard shapes

Provide aftercare advice

No service is complete unless the client leaves in the knowledge that he can achieve the same result as that done in the salon. If he can't achieve a similar effect, he is unlikely to return. You can make sure that he does and the real sign of client satisfaction is the booking of his next visit before he leaves the salon.

You can help to achieve this by making sure you tell him:

◆ How long the effect will last and when he needs to come back.

◆ Which products and equipment you have used and how they might benefit the client at home.

◆ How to maintain the effect himself.

How long will it last?

Facial hair grows at an average 1.25cm (12.5mm) per month, so a shorter, closer styled beard or moustache will have grown out within a month, whereas longer facial designs will last longer. Or, more to the point, the growth won't be quite as noticeable and therefore the client will tend to go longer in-between visits. Remember, if the effect incorporates a moustache, then it will need trimming anyway, as it will over-fall the upper lip fairly quickly.

Whatever the length or effect created, you need to tell your client from the outset how long they can expect it to last, so that they don't have any unrealistic expectations.

Products and skin care

Explain to the client how they can manage the effect themselves. You need to provide advice on cleansing:

◆ What to use, in relation to their hair and skin types.

◆ How often to use it.

◆ What products wouldn't suit them and therefore should be avoided and your reasons why.

Professional and younger males pay more attention and take more care with their skin than their counterparts used to, so skin care for men is a very popular and growing business area. It is as important to men as it is for women and the only difference is the range of products that are available. Men who shave regularly will already know that blunt razors and shaving creams are a contributing factor for skin infections or blocking pores and follicles and starting inward-growing hairs. When this occurs, a spot forms on the surface of the skin and the bacteria will have started a small infection such as 'barber's itch'. This, like ingrowing hairs, is uncomfortable and itchy and can easily be avoided if you give the client the correct advice.

Exfoliation is beneficial to the client. It removes dead skin cells from the epidermis and stimulates blood circulation, which will generally improve the skin's condition. There are many different products now available for men and these can be bought as grains that are mixed with water and applied as a paste or, alternatively, a wide range of ready-to-use products with a variety of bases such as fruit acids or herbals with essential oils.

Home maintenance

Finally, no complete service can end without the professional advice on how a look or effect can be maintained between visits. You need to give your client tips and advice on how he can keep the beard and moustache tidy. The hair will continue to grow between visits and the first thing that the client will be aware of is longer perimeter hair over-falling an upper lip, or a beard that is getting rather bushy.

We don't expect the client to try and maintain the denser, inner parts of facial hair shapes, but he will want to tidy edges if they become an irritation or look wild!

A few suggestions on what tools he can use – such as trimmer edges on electric shavers or nail scissors for slight trimming – and some advice on how to use them will suffice. You can sort the rest of it out when he returns.

SUMMARY

As a final reflection on what you have covered in this chapter, you should now have a clearer picture of all the essential aspects for shaping and trimming men's facial hair. In particular, you should now have a basic understanding of the key principles of:

1. Why preparation is essential to the service.

2. The contra-indications that are specific to shaping and trimming facial hair.

3. The range of different facial hair shapes that can be created.

4. The techniques involved in creating the effects.

5. How to use and maintain the tools and equipment associated with shaping and trimming men's facial hair.

6. Providing advice to the clients about maintaining their moustache and/or beard.

And collectively, how these principles will enable you to provide a basic range of cutting services and effects to your clients.

ASSESSMENT OF KNOWLEDGE AND UNDERSTANDING

Project

For this project you will need to collect historical examples of different beard and moustache shapes.

Use the Internet to find your examples, giving:

1. A brief description for each of the styles.

2. The following details for each look:

   ◆ the source for the style/shape;

   ◆ its historical time point in history; and

   ◆ either an image or sketch of the selected looks.

Revision questions

A selection of different types of questions to check your knowledge of cutting facial hair.

Q1 Closer cutting is achieved by using the clippers without the_____ attached.

Fill in the blank

Q2 Razors should be sterilized in Barbicide®.

True or false

Q3 Select from the following those tools that need sterilizing in a UV cabinet:

Multi selection

Cutting collar	☐ 1
Cutting square	☐ 2
Scissors	☐ 3
Clippers	☐ 4
Thinning scissors	☐ 5
Clipper grades	☐ 6

Q4 Outline shapes for beards are best cut with clippers.

True or false

Q5 Which of the following is not a cutting term?

Multi choice

Cross-checking	○ a
Fading	○ b
Freehand	○ c
Free style	○ d

Q6 Close accurate cutting is dependent upon cutting angles and tensioning on the skin.

True or false

Q7 Which of the following is not a facial hair term?

Multi selection

Goatee	☐ 1
Side burns	☐ 2
Handlebar moustache	☐ 3
Mohawk	☐ 4
Full beard	☐ 5
Mullet	☐ 6

Q8 The pre-application of hot_____ will soften facial hair, making it easier to cut.

Fill in the blank

Q9 Which of the following should not be used for trimming facial hair?

Multi choice

Clippers	○ a
Shaper	○ b
Scissors	○ c
Razor	○ d

Q10 Thinning is a technique of cutting that maximizes the hair density.

True or false

12 Colouring and Lightening

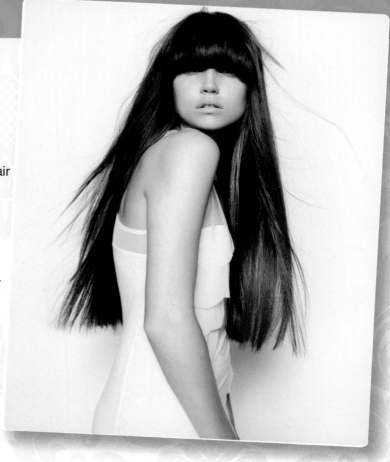

LEARNING OBJECTIVES

- Be able to maintain effective and safe methods of working
- Be able to prepare for colouring and lightening hair
- Be able to colour and lighten hair to create a variety of effects
- Understand how to work safely, effectively and hygienically
- Know and understand the tests for colouring hair
- Understand the basic science of colouring and lightening
- Understand colouring products, equipment and their uses
- Know and understand different colouring techniques
- Know how to give aftercare advice to clients

KEY TERMS

activator
ammonia
booster
chemically treated hair
colour stripper
colour wheel
compound henna
depth
discolouration
emulsify
eumelanin
fading (colour reference)

full head application (of colour lightener)
highlight cap
high lift colour
hydrogen peroxide
International Colour Chart system (ICC)
incompatible
irritant
lacquer
melanin
metallic dye

oil lightening product
para-phenylenediamine (PPD)
permanent colour
pigments
pheomelanin
pre-pigmentation
pre-soften
Quasi-permanent colour

regrowth
slicing (colouring)
synthetic colour
T-Section highlights
temporary colours
warmth

Unit topic

Colour and lighten hair.

INTRODUCTION

Colouring is probably the most difficult aspect of hairdressing for any student to grasp, there is so much to *learn* at level two and there is so much to do. Moreover, with the ever-increasing expectations of our clients, it has made colouring an essential skill for hairdressers and barbers, and particularly rewarding for those who eventually master it.

With the amount of people who colour their hair from products bought at the chemists and the disasters it creates, the stylists involved in colour work can look forward to a challenging, but in the longer term, very successful and fulfilling career.

Colouring and lightening hair

PRACTICAL SKILLS

Carrying out the necessary tests for colouring and lightening services

Carrying out consultation and evaluate the suitability of colour for clients

Using a variety of colouring and lightening products

Using different methods for colouring and lightening hair

Providing aftercare advice

UNDERPINNING KNOWLEDGE

Learn how to prepare for colouring and lightening services

Learn about the principles and effects of colour and colouring

Learn about the factors that influence and affect colour selection for clients

Learn about the hazards and problems involved with colouring and lightening services

Learn about the International Colour Chart system (ICC)

Learn about the types of colouring products and equipment available and their applications

Learn how to use, select and dilute hydrogen peroxide

Learn about different problems that can occur during processing and the remedial action you should take

The principles of colour and colouring

What is colour anyway?

We see colour because of light, however, light waves are not in themselves coloured. Our perception or *recognition* of colour arises in the human eye and brain. A particular light ray (of electromagnetic energy) defines each hue, or pure colour.

The human eye sees visible light, falling between wavelengths of 400 and 700 nanometres (nm). We are not able to see (perceive) other forms of light rays, such as infrared or ultraviolet light, without the use of other equipment.

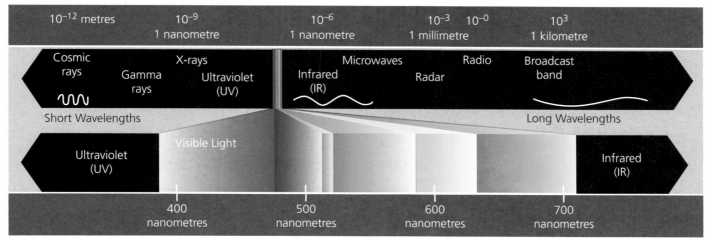

10^{-12} metres	10^{-9} 1 nanometre	10^{-6} 1 nanometre	10^{-3} 1 millimetre	10^{-0}	10^{3} 1 kilometre

The electromagnetic wave spectrum

Daylight (white light) is made up of numerous waves or impulses each having different dimensions or wavelengths. When separated, any single wavelength will produce a specific colour impression to the human eye. What we actually see as colour is known as its *colour effect*. When light rays illuminate an object, the object absorbs certain waves and reflects others. This determines the colour effect.

The coloured light in the visible spectrum ranges from violet to red. We can see this process by passing sunlight (white light) through a prism. Upon entering the prism, white light refracts – is bent, causing light waves of different lengths to be revealed, red having the longest wave length and violet having the shortest – into the visible spectrum. This splitting of white light creates what we see as seven different colours: red, orange, yellow, green, blue, indigo and violet.

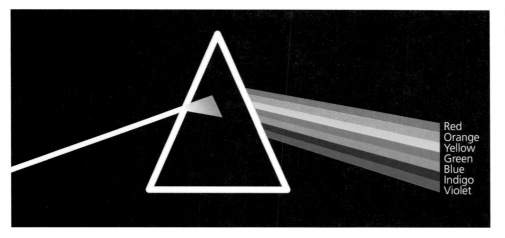

Red
Orange
Yellow
Green
Blue
Indigo
Violet

White light refracted through a prism into colours of the rainbow

A white object reflects most of the white light that falls upon it, whereas a black object absorbs most of the light falling on it. A red object reflects the red light and absorbs everything else.

TOP TIP

This rhyme reminds us of the colours of the rainbow: *Richard Of York Gave Battle In Vain* – Red, Orange, Yellow, Green, Blue, Indigo and Violet.

Light reflecting on a coloured object

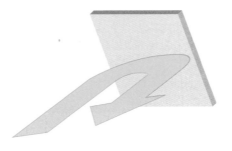 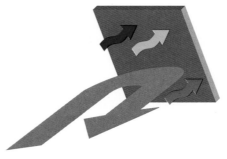

(1) A White Object   **(2) A Black Object**

The colour white: If *all* light waves are *reflected* from a surface the surface will appear to be white.

The colour black: Similarly, when *all* light waves are *absorbed* by a surface the surface will appear to be black.

Colour addition

If we take the three primary colours of Red, Yellow and Blue – then pairs of these give the secondary colours – i.e. red and blue mixed together creates violet, yellow and blue creates green and yellow and red creates orange. White and black can be added to vary the tone of the colour.

Adding further colours together, secondary colours can be added to primary colours to give further variations of tertiary (third level) colours.

Mixing primary and secondary colours

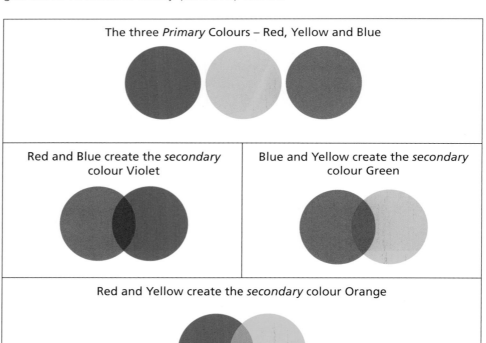

The three *Primary* Colours – Red, Yellow and Blue

Red and Blue create the *secondary* colour Violet

Blue and Yellow create the *secondary* colour Green

Red and Yellow create the *secondary* colour Orange

The colour wheel

You are probably wondering how knowing the basic principles of colour will benefit your appreciation of colour. Well, by understanding the relationship colours have to one another, you learn which clash and which work harmoniously in your personal colour choices.

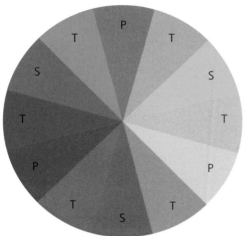

The Primary, secondary and tertiary colour wheel

Another way to look at colour would be the **colour wheel**. This illustration provides a quick reference guide to how colours harmonize with others or contrast against one another.

The primary and secondary colours sit an equal distance away from each other, and this forms a relationship with other colours on the wheel.

P = Primary Colours

S = Secondary Colours

T = Tertiary Colours

A colour wheel provides a fast visual guide to how colours interact. The colours on opposite sides of the wheel contrast against one another, whereas colours next to each other harmonize.

Contrasting colours   In colour *parlance,* these are known as complementary colours and they are positioned on opposite sides of the wheel. When they are included in the same colour theming, they will clash (and neutralize each other), adding impact to the resulting colour effect.

For example. If a client's hair is looking *green*, a colourist will use *red* tones to balance out and cancel the unwanted effect. Similarly, if a client has had a lightening service and their hair is looking *yellow*, they will use a *violet* toner to neutralize the unwanted tones.

TOP TIP

This neutralizing or cancelling-out effect is used in advanced colouring to balance out unwanted tones within the hair.

TOP TIP

The colour directly opposite on the colour wheel when used together will neutralize its effect.

Unwanted *Green* tones are neutralized by adding *Red* tones and vice versa

Unwanted *Yellow* (golden) tones are neutralized by adding *Violet* tones and vice versa

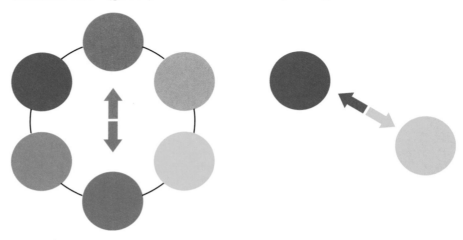

Depth and tones

Dominant and recessive colours (warm tones and cool tones)

When choosing colours for hair, (let alone for clothes, fashions or for home decoration) it's important to remember that some have more impact than others. *Warm tones*, like red, yellow and orange, stand out more and are therefore regarded as *dominant* or advancing colours.

In contrast, *Cool tones*, like shades of blue and green, are said to recede and are commonly known as recessive colours.

The choice and use of colour is often an instinctive, intuitive skill. If you were taking a photograph, it is best to include receding colours in the background and advancing ones in the foreground. Objects of a dominant colour make eye-catching and bold foreground interest, so take full advantage of them by making them prominent in the frame. For instance in an image, a red sign or vibrant yellow flower will look striking against a recessive colour, like blue sky or green foliage.

The same principles here in photography, apply in hair colour selection too. The same advancing colours will make hair look vibrant and bold, or sometimes inappropriate and too dramatic! Conversely, recessive colours in hair tend to *sink* backwards and have far less visual impact. Choosing the correct colours for clients, and getting it right, is the difference between a novice and an expert.

How colour is used in life			
Red	**Yellow**	**Blue**	**Green**
Red is a strong, intense colour, especially when contrasted against a dark background. It is a colour universally used for warning or danger and is hard to ignore. Red is the most powerful and attention-grabbing colour in	Yellow is another bold, advancing colour, often used to represent happiness or brightness. It will add warmth to fashion images and colour schemes and works particularly well	Blue is a cool, recessive, retiring colour, which can convey a mixture of emotions. In photography, it is commonly used to convey coldness, restfulness, sadness and tranquillity, which works especially well when com-	Green is often used to signify health and life. Obviously, green is the predominant colour of vegetation and therefore it is dominant in many scenic images, but it is seldom wanted in hair.

(Continued)

(Continued)

How colour is used in life

hair, fashion, decoration and photography and should really be used with care!

It can overwhelm weaker colours, which, unless intentional, can undermine the overall impact.

Red can be used to add eye catching colour when used as partial hair colouring or in fashion accessories: as hats, belts, shoes and bags, but can prove distracting in photography if included small within the landscape, for instance, a distant car, boat or letterbox.

when combined or contrasted with blue.

Yellow, along with rich colours, like gold and orange, conveys feelings of autumn.

It can prove a good background in photographic effects for still-life images, and close-ups of bright yellow flowers like corn, marigolds or sunflowers will burst with impact.

bined with water and wintry scenes.

In fashion blue is a very popular colour for fabrics and prints for both men and women.

It creates classic effects that last and last, creating flattering images for a variety of subjects and purposes.

Green is easily overwhelmed by bright advancing colours like red, and generally (and scientifically) speaking, the impact is neutralized.

However, when isolated, say within a decor colour scheme, green can still create strong, interesting effects.

As a photographic subject, fresh vibrant leaves can look striking, especially when backlit, or light through green glass, say from a stained glass window.

The effects of light and lighting upon hair

Hair colour depends chiefly on the **pigments** in the hair, which absorb some of the light and reflect the rest. The colour that we see is also affected by the light in which it is seen, and (to a lesser extent) by the colours of clothes worn with it.

◆ *White light* from halogen bulbs and full daylight will show the hair's natural colour.

◆ *Yellow light* emitted from standard electric light bulbs adds **warmth** to hair colour, but neutralizes blue, ash or ashen effects.

◆ *Blue or green light* from fluorescent tubes and *long-life* energy saving bulbs, reduces the warmth of red/gold tones in hair.

BEST PRACTICE

Hair colours viewed in different lighting will look very different, you should always explain this to your clients.

Naturally occurring pigments – natural hair colour

When we look at the natural colour of hair, what we are really seeing are microscopic pigments scattered about like grains of sand within the hair's cortex. This naturally occurring colouration is created when nutrients in the blood supply are converted to form the pigment melanin. This pigmentation is then added into the newly formed keratin at the germinal matrix.

The natural hair pigments are collectively called **melanin**, and different quantities of these pigments; (**eumelanin**, **pheomelanin** and trichosiderin) vary between individuals, giving us all the colour of our hair.

Facts about colour pigments and their effects

Pigment	Facts	Effects
White hair (Grey hair) has lost all natural pigments and therefore appears colourless.		
Eumelanin	◆ Produces cool tones. ◆ Brown or black in colour.	◆ Dark hair/base – have high levels of eumelanin, but little pheomelanin.
Pheomelanin	◆ Produces warm tones. ◆ Yellow or red in colour.	◆ Light hair/base – have high levels of pheomelanin, but little eumelanin.
Trichosiderin	◆ Are very rare. ◆ Produces warm tones. ◆ Golden red or red in colour.	◆ Red, Celtic hair – have high levels of trichosiderin and also high levels of pheomelanin.

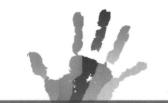

ANATOMY & PHYSIOLOGY
Pheomelanin pigments are larger than eumelanin and are harder to remove from hair during lightening.

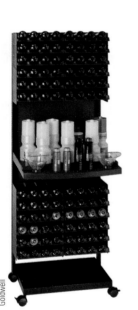

Goldwell

Colour trolley

The hair colour you actually see is affected by the amount and proportion of the pigments present. But remember, the type/amount of light/lighting also affects how it is seen.

With age, or after periods of stress, the production of natural pigments may be reduced. The hairs already on the head will not be affected, but the new ones will. As hairs fall out and are replaced, the proportion that have the original pigmentation reduces and the hair's overall colour changes. It may become lighter. If no pigment is produced at all, then the new hairs will be white/grey.

The proportion of white hairs among the naturally coloured ones, causes the hair to appear grey. Grey hair or greyness (Canites) is often referred to as a percentage: for example, 50 per cent grey, means that half of the hairs on the head are white and the rest are pigmented.

It is not uncommon for young people to exhibit some grey hairs – however, this does not necessarily mean that they will go grey, or completely white, at an early age.

Types of synthetic or artificial hair colour

Natural hair colour is made up from melanin, but these pigments, or the appearance of these pigments, can be changed or modified. Hair colour can be changed by the *addition* of artificial pigments, i.e. colour application, or the *reduction*, i.e. the removal, of artificial or natural pigments, through lightening colouring techniques.

Different effects and the colouring products linked with it

Effect that can be achieved	Colouring product
You can *add* artificial colour pigments to hair on a temporary basis.	◆ **Temporary colour.**
You can *add* artificial colour pigments to hair that last for several washes.	◆ **Semi – permanent colour.**

(Continued)

(Continued)

Different effects and the colouring products linked with it	
Effect that can be achieved	**Colouring product**
You can *add* artificial colour pigments to hair so that they fade over time or stay there permanently.	◆ **Quasi – permanent colour.** ◆ **Permanent colour.**
You can *remove* natural colour pigments permanently.	◆ **Lightening product.** ◆ **High lift colour.**
You can *remove* artificial colour pigments permanently.	◆ **Colour strippers.**

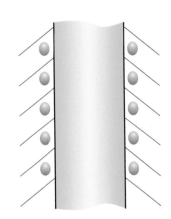

Colour chart

Temporary colour – uses, applications and facts

Temporary colours are available in the form of lotions, creams, mousses, gels, **lacquers**, sprays, hair mascara, crayons, paints and glitter dust. If the hair is in good condition, they will not penetrate the hair cuticle, nor do they directly affect the natural hair colour: they simply remain on the hair until washed off.

Temporary colours are ideal for a client who has not had colour before, as they can be easily removed. They can be used to produce subtle colour effects, or bright, bold, options without any adverse effects to the quality and condition of the hair.

However, if they are used on badly damaged or very porous hair, the temporary colour may quickly be absorbed into the cortex, producing unwanted, long lasting, uneven, patchy results.

Features and benefits of temporary colour	
Features	**Benefits**
Have large pigments/molecules and sit on the surface of the hair.	Easy to remove as they are washed away during the next shampoo.
Come in a variety of types as mousses, setting lotions, gels, creams, colour sprays and colour shampoos.	Easy to apply as they can either be applied during the shampoo process or alternatively as a styling or finishing product.
Come in a variety of shades and colours.	Can be used as a fashion statement or alternatively to enhance natural tones by either adding **depth** to faded hair or neutralizing unwanted tones from hair.

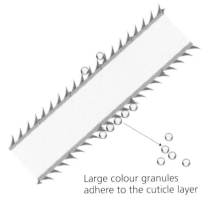

Large colour granules adhere to the cuticle layer

Facts to remember

Temporary colours have large colour molecules that sit on the outside of the hair and get trapped in the cuticle layers.

Facts about temporary colours:

- Temporary colours only last for one wash in good conditioned hair.

- They are often difficult to remove from hair that is damaged, porous or lightened.

- You cannot lighten hair with temporary colours.

- You cannot achieve a specific target shade in the same way as you can with longer-lasting or permanent colours.

- They may not give you an even coverage on the hair.

Semi-permanent colour – uses, applications and facts

Semi-permanent colours are made in a variety of forms – some are used as shampoos or conditioning rinses, which make them easier to apply, others are applied directly from the bottle on to dry hair.

Semi-permanent colours have pigments which deposit into the hair cuticle and outer cortex. This type of colour gradually fades each time the hair is shampooed. Some colour will last through six washes, others longer.

These colours are not intended to cover white/grey hair – they will only produce translucent effects, masking some of the grey.

Features and benefits of semi-permanent colours
Semi-permanent colours are ideal for those people who want to try colour but are not ready yet to take a big step forward into the maintenance of permanent colour effects. They generally last up to six or eight shampoos and do not produce any **regrowth** – the hair loses the colour on each shampoo so the effect lessens each time.

Semi-permanents also provide an ideal solution for livening up faded mid-lengths and ends for clients who have permanent colours – this is particularly useful if the hair is not really ready yet for further permanent processing.

TOP TIP

Compound henna is incompatible with hairdressing materials. It should not be confused with natural (vegetable) henna which is compatible with other hairdressing services.

Semi-permanents will colour white/grey hair to *some* extent, although the penetration doesn't extend beyond the cuticle layer, so colour density is relatively poor. This is because white hair tends to have a very smooth cuticle, so there are fewer spaces for the pigments to bond on to. The colour range is varied, ranging from fashion effects to many of the shades you would expect to see in a standard shade chart. They are simple to use and require no developer and hence no mixing.

Features and benefits of semi-permanent colour

Features	Benefits
Have large molecules that sit on the surface of the hair while other smaller ones penetrate deeper into the hair.	Good for introducing clients to colour without any long-term commitments. Fairly easy to remove as they are washed away in six or eight shampoos.
Come in a variety of types as mousses, liquids, gels, creams.	Easy to apply, normally requires no mixing, take a short time and leave no regrowth.
Come in a variety of colours as fashion effects or as standard shade chart references.	Can be used as a fashion statement or alternatively as a trial for a permanent colour effect.
Can be used in colour correction work and add tone to white/grey hair.	A simple and quick pre-filler and **pre-pigmentation** shade. Provide some masking/coverage for unwanted greys.
Provide an alternative to permanent colour.	Can provide a colour choice for those people who, because of sensitivity or allergy, may not be able to have permanent colours.

Facts to remember

Semi-permanent colours have large colour molecules (but smaller than temporary colour) that get trapped in the cuticle layer and penetrate just to the outer cortex.

Facts about semi-permanent colours:

◆ Semi-permanent colours only last for up to six or eight washes.

◆ They are often difficult to remove totally from hair that is extremely porous or lightened.

◆ You cannot lighten hair with semi-permanent colour.

◆ They will not cover white/grey hair.

◆ They cover with far better results than temporary colours.

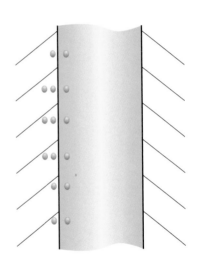

Quasi-permanent colour — uses, applications and facts

Quasi-permanent colours have large ranges that provide plenty of choice. The effects are long lasting and they are mixed with lower strengths of **hydrogen peroxide** than permanents. However, because of this, they do produce a regrowth and the colour effect fades over time. They have a larger colour molecule than permanent colours and are ideal for colour matching and refreshing worn, tired hair.

Features and benefits of quasi-permanent colour Quasi-colours make up the *bulk* of hair colour bought by people from shops, for use at home. They are not true permanent colours but do require mixing; they last for at least 12 washes and anything up to 24, but they do leave a regrowth. These types of colours do have a better ability to cover white/grey hair and this is the main reason why they are popular for home colouring.

HEALTH & SAFETY

Quasi-colour should be treated like a permanent colour or lightener – they do require a skin test 24–48 hours beforehand.

Features and benefits of quasi-permanent colour

Features	Benefits
They are processed with a developer and have molecules that swell inside the hair.	Easy solution for all-over colouring – last a long time, generally up to 12–24 shampoos.
Come as gels or creams.	Require mixing with developer and have been made easy to apply for home use.
Come in a variety of colours as fashion effects or as standard shade chart references.	Can be used for a fashion effect or as an alternative to more permanent-based colour.
Can be used in colour correction work.	Are an alternative longer-lasting pre-pigmentation shade.
Add depth and tone to white/grey hair.	Provide up to 80 per cent coverage for unwanted greys.
Provide a different alternative to permanent para-dyes.	Tend to be used regularly and more often than salon-provided treatments.
Good conditioning properties, add shine and improve manageability.	Leave hair in good condition, manageable and with added shine.

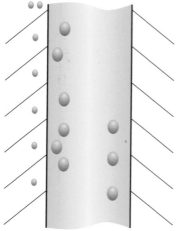

Facts to remember

Quasi-permanent colours have smaller colour molecules and are mixed with lower strength hydrogen peroxide. They enter the cortex of the hair and are oxidized during the processing. This makes them swell and then they are trapped inside the cortex.

Facts about quasi-permanent colours:

◆ Quasi-permanent colours always require a skin test.

◆ They last for 12 washes, leaving a regrowth.

◆ They can only be removed by colour strippers, not by colour lightening products.

◆ They often provide the basis for colour correction work if wrongly used at home.

◆ They offer good coverage – colour white/grey with better saturation than semis.

◆ They have similar effects to permanent colours.

Permanent colour – uses, applications and facts

Permanent colours have the largest variety of shades and tones. They can cover white and natural-coloured hair to produce a range of natural, fashion and fantasy shades.

Hydrogen peroxide is mixed with permanent colour, this oxidizes the hair's natural pigments and joins the artificial pigments together. The hair will then retain the colour permanently in the cortex. Hair in poor condition, however, may not hold the colour and colouring could result in patchy areas and colour **fading**.

HEALTH & SAFETY

When mixing colouring products, never add colour or developer together by guesswork. The amounts that have to be added together are critical to a successful outcome. Don't take unnecessary risks!

HEALTH & SAFETY

Hair products and the under 16s
All chemicals that are used within hair and beauty products are controlled under European laws (EU Directives). Some chemicals found in **permanent** and **quasi colours, bleach lighteners, permanent waving, relaxers** and **chemical straighteners**, are restricted, and no longer permitted for use on young people under 16 years of age.
Any hair preparation that falls within this group is now prohibited and you will find that these products are clearly marked **"This product in not intended for use on persons under the age of 16"**

Facts to remember

Permanent colours have small colour molecules that are mixed with hydrogen peroxide. They enter the cortex of the hair and are oxidized during the processing. This makes them swell and then they are trapped inside the cortex.

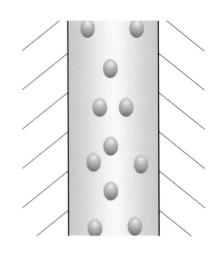

Facts about permanent colours:

◆ Permanent (para-dyes) are the only colours that cover white/grey hair with 100 per cent.

◆ Permanent colours always require a skin test.

◆ They can only be removed by colour strippers (not by colour lightening product).

◆ People can be allergic to PPD (*paraphenylenediamine)*, which is contained in all permanent colours.

◆ They are resistant to fading and have to grow out – leaving a regrowth.

◆ Have the largest choice of colours for clients.

◆ Darker colours contain more PPD than lighter shades.

Permanent colours contain a chemical compound called **para-phenylenediamine (PPD)**. This is a known **irritant** and many people are allergic to it. For this reason, it is essential that you follow the manufacturer's instructions in carrying out a skin test 24–48 hours before a permanent colouring service.

There are other chemicals within permanent colours and they have different properties and effects:

◆ **Ammonia**/resorcinol is alkaline and when it comes into contact with the hair it swells the hair shaft in preparation for the pigmentation. This provides a better penetration, but will need pH balancing to return the hair to its normal state.

◆ Conditioning agents improve the hair during the colouring process, enabling it to be smoother and shinier as a result.

◆ Hydrogen peroxide oxidizes the natural pigments of the hair and this enables the artificial pigments to bond with them, creating a permanent change within the hair's cortex.

HEALTH & SAFETY

Always follow the manufacturer's instructions for mixing the correct amounts together. If the proportions are wrong, the colour will be wrong.

Vegetable-based colour

As well as being a popular source for conditioning agents, plant extracts have been used as dyeing compounds for thousands of years. These were the only sources of colour until chemists developed synthetic alternatives. Natural henna (Lawsonia) is still used widely today in many countries and is used for dyeing skin as well as the hair. Natural plant-based dyes do not present any problems for hairdressing treatments, however, these ingredients are sometimes added to other elements to form compounds, mixtures of vegetable extracts and mineral substances. One that is still available is **compound henna** – vegetable henna mixed with metallic salts. This penetrating dye is incompatible with professional products used in hairdressing salons and will react with professional salon colours and perming products.

Metallic Salt based dyes **Metallic dyes** are surface-coating colour. They are variously known as reduction, metallic, sulphide and progressive dyes. These types of dyes are also **incompatible** with chemical hairdressing services and may be found in some colour restorers.

HEALTH & SAFETY

Metallic and compound dyes are incompatible with hairdressing materials. Always carry out a test before using a lightener, colour or perm on any new clients whom you do not know, or on clients who have been recently having their hair done overseas.

Depth and tone – the way that colours are measured

When we talk about colour, we often use the words *depth* and *tone*. Depth is used to describe how light or dark the colour is and tone is used to describe the colour or hue that we see, such as brown, golden red, etc.

- ◆ Depth = how light or dark it is.
- ◆ Tone = the colour or hue – ashen, golden, mahogany, etc.

Depth and tone

Depth	Gold	Red	Violet
Very light			
Light			
Medium			
Dark			
Very dark			

Tones →

TOP TIP

In vibrant red or bright auburn hair, nearly all the melanin is present in the form of pheomelanin – however, another alpha-amino pigment is present in a complex iron compound called *trichosiderin*. (In 100g of red hair, there are 40mg of trichosiderin.) The trichosiderin changes the colour make-up of hair, giving it the rich, attractive colour of a genetically Celtic origin. Colouring this particular type of red hair is difficult because of this different pigmentation. Lightening red hair is especially hard as this compound is very difficult to remove.

BEST PRACTICE

Colouring materials are expensive. The profitability of the work relates directly to the amount of colour you use. Always mix up a small amount to work with. If you do run out you can always mix up some more.

The International Colour Chart System (ICC)

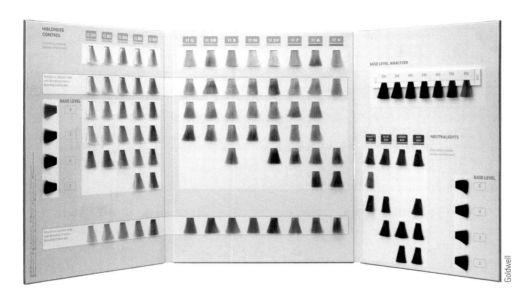

Goldwell

The ICC numbering system								
Num	Shade	Ash •1	Violet •2	Gold •3	Copper •4		Red •6	Metallic •7
10	Extra light blonde							
9	Very light blonde							
8	Light blonde							
7	Mid blonde							
6	Dark blonde							
5	Brown				5.4			
4	Dark Brown							
3	Darkest Brown							
1	Black							

The International Colour Chart system (ICC) is a system that provides a way of defining hair colours in uniform way. In this system, shades of colour are divided and numbered, with black (**1**) at one end of the scale and lightest blonde (**10**) at the other. Tones of other colours – **/1, /3**, or also shown as ● **1,** ● **3** – are combined with these, producing a huge variety of colours. The system arranges the shades in a table.

To use them, first identify the natural depth of your client's hair: then by looking along the rows, you can see the variety of tones that can be achieved.

For example, if your client has *brown* hair (**5**) and you colour with a copper tone (● **4**), the result should be a rich copper brown(**5.4** shown in the ICC table). There are many options, and the following list looks at some other possible tones:

◆ to produce ash shades, add blue or ● **1**

◆ to produce matt shades, add green ● **7**

◆ to produce gold or copper shades, add yellow or orange ● **3 or** ● **4**

◆ to produce warm shades, add red ● **6**

◆ to produce purple or violet shades, add mixtures of red and blue ● **2**

Primary and secondary tones				
Shade	**Depth**		**Primary tone**	**Secondary tone**
6.64	6	●	6	4

1 The **primary tone** denotes the range that the shade is in.

2 The **secondary tone** indicates the additional pigmentation within the shade. Like the colour wheel, this extra level of colouration provides lots of extra colour permutations.

Sometimes colour manufacturers want to increase a shade's intensity and vibrancy. This is achieved by adding double the tone to the particular shade, doubling the tonal effect.

So in the table (Primary and secondary tones) we see that we have a colour of Base 6, or dark blonde. It has a primary or initial tonal quality of ● **6** or red, it also has further colour properties as its secondary tone is ● **4** or copper.

Double strength tones				
Shade	**Depth**		**Primary tone**	**Secondary tone**
6.66	6	●	6	6

In this illustration we see that the shade has the same base and primary tones as the example above i.e. **6** ● **6** but in this scenario the secondary tone is the same as the primary i.e. **6.** These double strength hair colours mean that there is extra red in the colour, so it denotes this shade as extra bright red.

The effects of different strengths of hydrogen peroxide on hair

Hydrogen peroxide is an acidic solution used for developing both quasi and permanent colours. Its chemical make-up is hydrogen and oxygen and in a solution the elements link together to create molecules of H_2O_2, so each molecule contains two hydrogen atoms and two oxygen atoms. The only difference between the chemical compositions of hydrogen *per*-oxide and water is that hydrogen peroxide has two atoms of oxygen whereas water only has one.

This is useful in hairdressing chemistry, as oxygen is the element that does all the work. It oxidizes natural and artificial colour pigments – getting them to change their proper-

HEALTH & SAFETY

Never mix colour or put it into a bowl before you need to use it. Permanent colours will oxidize in the air – this expands the colour pigments and they will not be able to enter the hair shaft through the narrow cuticle layers, thus rendering the colour useless.

ties. So when oxygen is *given up* during processing, the hydrogen peroxide is reduced to create water as a by-product. This simple chemical reaction minimizes any damage to the hair during the process. So under normal circumstances, this acidic solution is rendered harmless, but only providing that the manufacturer's instructions are followed.

Hydrogen peroxide strength	Effect upon the hair
6 vol (1.9 per cent)	◆ Will deposit colour and tone into the hair, adding depth, making it temporarily darker when using quasi-permanent colours.
9 vol (2.7 per cent)	◆ Will deposit colour and tone into the hair, adding depth, making it darker when using quasi-permanent colours.
15 vol (4.7 per cent)	◆ Will deposit colour and tone into the hair, adding depth, making it darker when using quasi-permanent colours. ◆ Will lighten one shade when using quasi-permanent colours.
20 vol (or 6 per cent)	◆ Will deposit colour and tone into the hair, adding depth, making it darker when using permanent colours. ◆ Enables coverage of white/grey hair. ◆ Will lighten two shades above base 6 (on fine hair). ◆ Will lighten one shade below base 4.
30 vol (or 9 per cent)	◆ Will lighten hair three shades above base 6. ◆ Will lighten hair two levels below base 4.
40 vol (or 12 per cent)	◆ Will lighten hair four shades above base 6 (with **high lift colour**). ◆ Will lighten up to six shades of lift with lightener.

Diluting hydrogen peroxide Because hydrogen peroxide has different strengths based upon the amounts of *free* oxygen within it, (e.g. 6 per cent of *free* oxygen within any given amount or 12 per cent of *free* oxygen within any given amount), it can be diluted with water in times when the salon has run out of stock. The following table shows you how the strengths that you have in stock can be diluted to make a reduced strength hydrogen peroxide.

The first column refers to the strength peroxide that you have, the second refers to the peroxide you want to create. The last three columns show you how many parts of the peroxide you need and how many parts of distilled water you need to add to it.

Diluting different strengths of hydrogen peroxide				
Strength you have	Strength you want to create	Peroxide	Add	Water
40 vol (i.e. 12 per cent)	30 vol (i.e. 9 per cent)	3 parts	+	1 part
40 vol	20 vol (i.e. 6 per cent)	1	+	1
40 vol	10 vol (i.e. 3 per cent)	1	+	3

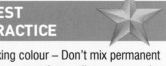

TOP TIP

When hydrogen peroxide lightens hair to any level it will remove the smaller, (eumelanin) brown/black pigments first. The larger, warmer pigments (*pheomelanin*) within the hair are more difficult to remove so unwanted golden or even orange tones are often left within the hair.

BEST PRACTICE

Mixing colour – Don't mix permanent colours together until you are ready to use them. Mix the colours carefully, making sure that you measure the amounts accurately. If the proportions are wrong the final effect will be wrong!

(Continued)

(Continued)

Diluting different strengths of hydrogen peroxide				
Strength you have	Strength you want to create	Peroxide	Add	Water
30 vol (i.e. 9 per cent)	20 vol (i.e. 6 per cent)	2	+	1
30 vol	10 vol (i.e. 3 per cent)	1	+	2
20 vol (i.e. 6 per cent)	10 vol (i.e. 3 per cent)	1	+	1

Lightening hair

Lightening products have alkaline chemicals within them that achieve lightened effects by dissolving the natural tones (pigments) within hair. Similar to para-dyes, lightening products are mixed with hydrogen peroxide to activate the oxidizing process. They are used in three main forms:

◆ High lift colour – which is a non-lightening process for lightening hair partially or whole head.

◆ Powder lightener – which is used for highlighting and partial lightening techniques.

◆ **Gel/oil lightening product** – which is suitable for on-scalp application.

The alkaline compound acts upon the hair by swelling and opening up the cuticle. This enables the peroxide at 6 per cent or 9 per cent to release oxygen and oxidize the natural pigments of melanin from within the cortex. This creates oxymelanin and is seen as it reduces the natural colour through the different degrees of lift.

The colour control during lightening is not the same as with colouring though. Often when full-head lightening is done the result is quite yellow (although the control of warm pigments during lightening is better with high lift colour).

Choice of lightening method

High lift colour High lift colour provides a non-lightening solution for lightening hair. These types of colour are gentler than lightener and can be mixed with 6 per cent or 9 per cent volume hydrogen peroxide.

The colour control or colour targeting is generally better than lightening too, as high lift colour can deposit tones (e.g. ash, beige or warm tones) as the hair lightens. And because you are using a hair colour and not lightener, there is less moisture removed from the hair during the process, so a better hair condition can be guaranteed at the end.

BEST PRACTICE

The degree of lift required in emulsion lightener is controlled by the number of activators added into the mixing bowl with the oil. It is not boosted by stronger hydrogen peroxide levels. Always follow the manufacturer's instructions when using lightening products.

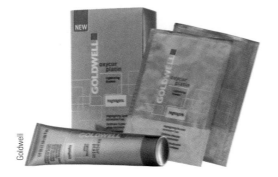

Goldwell

High lift colours are similar in composition to normal hair colours with one exception – they use an alkaline compound (e.g. resorcinol) which swells the hair shaft enabling a better penetration of the lightener into the polypeptide chains within the cortex.

Removing high lift colour You can remove high lift colour by emulsifying the colour, by adding a little warm water to the colour and gently massaging all over. This mixes the colour with the water and helps to release the products from the hair, enabling you to use a lighter action within the shampooing process. The hair can be conditioned as normal at the end, or an anti-oxidant can be applied to help close the cuticle and lock in the colour results.

HEALTH & SAFETY

Avoid inhalation of powder lightener. Be very careful when you dispense powder lightener into a bowl. The particles are very small and tend to 'dust' into the air very easily. This is a hazardous chemical compound which can cause respiratory conditions. You must avoid contact through inhalation. Wherever possible only use 'dust-free' powder lightener.

Emulsion lightener Emulsion lightener is a slower acting lightening process that is made up of two compounds that are added together and then mixed with hydrogen peroxide:

◆ oil (or gel) lightener.

◆ **activators**, (also known as **boosters** or controllers).

This type of lightener is specially formulated for use directly onto the roots of the hair and is suitable for contact with the scalp. It is kinder and gentler during the lightening process and is mixed with 20 per cent volume hydrogen peroxide for root, mid-length and ends application. The lift through the *undercoat* shades is aided and controlled by the addition of activators. These boost the power of the lightener while maintaining relatively low hydrogen peroxide strength.

Emulsion lighteners also contain additives which control the resultant colour as the lightener lightens the hair. As mentioned earlier, these tend to make hair yellow, so they have **matt emulsifiers** which neutralize unwanted yellow tones while the lifting process takes place. Heat may be used during the development of the process, but the process must be monitored closely (particularly if a colour accelerator or steamer is used to aid development) as these types of lighteners can often be more 'slippy' and mobile and might drip!

BEST PRACTICE

The degree of lift required in emulsion lightener is controlled by the number of activators added into the mixing bowl with the oil. It is not boosted by stronger hydrogen peroxide levels. Always follow the manufacturer's instructions when using lightening products.

Removing emulsion lightener Make sure that when the lightener is removed you rinse without massaging with only tepid or warm water. The client's scalp has been subjected to chemicals and could be sensitive, and the cooling action of the rinsing will stop the lightening process and make the client more comfortable. After the emulsion has been rinsed away, the hair can be shampooed with a mild colour shampoo and conditioned with an anti-oxidizing treatment.

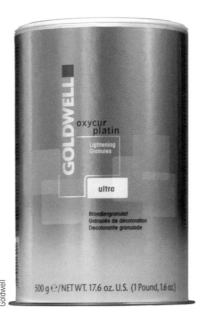

Goldwell

Powder lightener Powder lightener can be mixed with 6 per cent, 9 per cent or 12 per cent hydrogen peroxide, depending upon the level of lift required. Powder lighteners are fast acting and are used for a variety of highlighting techniques. When they are mixed in the bowl the consistency is that of a thick, 'porridge-type' paste. The stiffness of the consistency prevents spillages and enables the lightener to work like a poultice. As the process continues the lightener/peroxide mix will expand. This action is speeded up more if accelerated by heat, so a careful eye should be kept on the development timings.

Removing powder lightener The removal of powder lightener is similar to that of emulsion lightener, make sure that when the lightener is removed from the hair you rinse it without massaging, using only tepid or warm water. The removal of powder lightener can be far more problematic than that of emulsion lightener and this has more to do with the colouring technique that has been used. If different coloured highlights have been done with Easi-Meche™, foil, wraps, etc. these need to be removed carefully and individually as one colour may affect another. Although lightener has not been directly applied to the client's scalp, it still might be sensitive from the colouring technique. Therefore, the cooling action of the rinsing will stop the lightening process and make the client more comfortable. Afterwards the hair can be shampooed with a mild colour shampoo and conditioned with an anti-oxidizing treatment.

Lightening service required	Things you need to consider	Technique/application	Type
Whole head (on virgin hair)	**1. Test results:** (Skin/patch test, porosity elasticity etc.).	Follow manufacturer's instructions	
	2. Natural hair depth: Lighteners will lift five levels quite happily on hair with brown/ash pigments. However, strong red content will be difficult to remove. Hair beyond base 5 will not lift safely beyond base 9. Suggest other colouring options.	Lightener must be applied to mid lengths and ends first. A plastic cap should envelop the contents and can be developed with gentle heat until ready. When the hair has lightened two to three levels of lift, the root application can be applied.	Use only emulsion or cream based lightener. (Only certain products are suitable for application to the scalp.)
	3. Hair length: Lengths up to 10 cm lighten evenly, provided manufacturer's instructions are followed. Lengths over 15 cm are not recommended, as evenness of colour will be difficult to guarantee	Always follow manufacturer's instructions.	These are generally used with 6% hydrogen peroxide and sachet controllers to handle levels of lift.
	4. Hair texture: Finer hair needs extra care and lower hydrogen peroxide strengths i.e. 6%. Medium and coarser hair present fewer technical problems.		*High lift colour may be used instead of emulsion, check manufacturer's instructions for specific product suitability

(Continued)

(Continued)

Lightening service required	Things you need to consider	Technique/application	Type
	5. Hair condition: Only consider hair in good condition for lightening. (lightening removes moisture content during the process, hair that is porous or containing low moisture levels has insufficient durability for lightening).		
Full head (on previously coloured)	Specialist level 3 process – Therefore not recommended		
Root application (pre-lightened ends)	**1. Existing client:** Check previous records and current hair condition and carry out service. **2. New client:** Go through all the checks in the **full head application** table and find out the previous treatment history.	Roots only, without overlapping previous lightened ends.	Only emulsion or cream lighteners are suggested for application to the scalp.
Highlights (fine even meshes on virgin hair)	**1. Test results:** (Skin/patch test, porosity elasticity etc.).	Always follow manufacturer's instructions.	
Note – The success of highlights on coloured hair is very **poor** in comparison. This work is often undertaken in salons, but ends seldom lighten effectively, whilst the roots lighten very quickly. (*Specialist colour process - **synthetic colour** should be removed with a colour stripper)	**2. Natural hair depth:** Lighteners will lift five levels quite happily on hair with brown/ash pigments. However, strong red content will be difficult to remove and require stronger developer and/or additional heat. Hair beyond base 5 will not lift safely beyond base 9. Suggest other lightening technique. **3. Hair length:** Hair length will have an impact on evenness of colour. However a small tolerance is acceptable, and 'visually' indistinguishable on longer hair lengths	Plastic self-grip meshes (e.g. Easi-Meche™ L'Oréal). Foil meshes. Colour wraps.	High lift powder lightener with suitable hydrogen peroxide developer at 6%, 9% or for highest lift 12%. (Providing no product is allowed to make contact with the skin/scalp).

(Continued)

(Continued)

Lightening service required	Things you need to consider	Technique/application	Type
	4. Hair texture: Finer hair needs extra care and lower hydrogen peroxide strengths i.e. 6% Medium and coarser hair present fewer technical problems but generally take longer.		
	5. Hair condition: Only consider hair in good condition for lightening. (Lightening removes moisture content during the process, hair that is porous or containing low moisture levels has insufficient durability for lightening.)		

Cap highlights Highlight caps are a safe, simple and popular choice for cost-effective, single-colour or lightened highlights on short layered hair, as even a single colour application can achieve an attractive, multi-toned effect.

Woven highlights Woven highlights in foil, Easi-Meche™ or wraps are the preferred technique for multi-toning hair. The visual effects are unlimited and new exciting colour combinations and techniques are happening each year.

Toners and lightening toning

Permanent (and most quasi-permanent) colours are unsuitable for depositing tones on pre-lightened hair. If they were used, the effects could damage, if not destroy the hair. Permanent colours and some quasi-contain alkaline compounds and if you look back at the properties of pH upon hair, you will remember that alkalis swell the hair. If this were to happen after the hair has already been weakened from lightening, the hair is likely to break off!

Full head lightening seldom provides satisfactory results. There are usually some unwanted (golden or yellow) tones that need to be neutralized and this is achieved by using specially formulated lightener toners. Lightener toners are ranges of pastel shades that can be used to balance out and neutralize unwanted tones.

Toning is the process of adding colour to previously lightened hair. A variety of pastel shades, such as silver, beige and rose, are used to produce subtle effects. Different types of toners are available: read the instructions provided by their manufacturers to find out what is possible.

Toners and their effects

Level of depth	Tone required	Tonal effect	Pre-lighten to
10	Silver, platinum, mauve/violet	Cool	Very pale yellow
9	Ashen blondes, light beige blonde	Cool	Pale yellow
8	Beige blonde	Cool	Yellow
8	Sandy blonde	Warm	
7	Golden blonde	Warm	
7	Chestnut, copper gold	Warm	Orange
6	Red copper	Warm	
5	Mahogany	Cool	Red/orange
4	Burgundy, plum	Cool	

Safe methods of working for colouring and lightening services

Safety and preparation

Although the Health and Safety chapter covers many of the general aspects that you need to know, each technical procedure has specific things that relate to that area of hairdressing alone. Hair colouring is particularly problematic as it involves the application of a variety of potentially harmful chemicals. Therefore, the care that you take in handling products and preparing yourself and the client is absolutely critical to safe and successful colouring.

Records These should be found and put ready at the beginning of the day. The appointment book identifies all the expected clients, so all their treatment history – dates of visits, who provided the services, previous chemical services, records of any tests and any additional comments – can all be collated long before the clients arrive.

Similarly, when clients have been in, any results of tests or notes following treatments must be updated as soon as possible.

Tests Always refer to your test results before carrying out any colouring service. Check with the client that they have not had any positive reaction to the chemicals from the patch test and refer to your strand test for the agreed target shade. Finally, re-check the porosity and elasticity of the hair and update the client's record accordingly.

Materials After the records have been found it is advisable to get all tubes, cans or bottles of colour put aside and ready along with the client's record information. Doing this earlier has several benefits. It can save valuable time later when you need to mix them, particularly if you are running on a tight schedule.

HEALTH & SAFETY

Always gown your client properly so that they are protected from spillages of chemicals.

HEALTH & SAFETY

Always wear the PPE provided by the salon every time you apply colour.

BEST PRACTICE

Always carry out the necessary tests before you start, it could have a critical impact on the results.

Gowning Always make sure that the client and the client's clothes are adequately protected before any process is started. Most salons have special 'colour-proof' gowns for colouring and lightening processes. These gowns are resistant to staining and are made from finely woven synthetic fabrics that will stop colour spillages from getting through onto the client's skin or clothes. When you gown the client, make sure that the free edges are closed and fastened together. On top of this and around the shoulders you can place a colouring towel and over this a plastic cape. This needs to be fastened but loose enough for the client to be comfortable throughout the service.

HEALTH & SAFETY

After any treatment or tests have been carried out always update the client's records immediately. These tests are critical to the client's well-being and the salon's good name. You should record the:

- date
- the test carried out
- development times
- results
- recommended home-care or follow-up advice given.

Using barrier cream Barrier cream can be used as physical barrier to prevent staining around the client's face/hairline. It is also particularly useful if the client has any general sensitivity to chemical-based products. Remember it is not an excuse for poor slapdash application, allowing you to extend the colour application beyond the root area to the skin. However, it will help in areas where the colour seeps off the hair onto the skin.

Apply barrier cream to the skin with a finger or cotton wool close to the hairline, taking care not to get it onto the hair, as this could stop the colour from taking evenly.

It can be removed later after you have shampooed the colour from the hair and before any other services are conducted.

Seating position The chair back should be protected with a plastic cover. If this is not available, a colouring towel could be folded lengthwise and secured with sectioning clips at either end and the client should be sat comfortably, in an upright position, with their back flat against the cushioned chair pad.

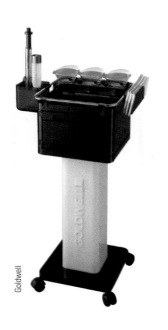

Goldwell

Trolley You should have your colouring trolley prepared and at hand with the materials you will need. Foils for highlighting should have been previously prepared to the right lengths and combs, brushes, sectioning clips, etc. should be all cleaned and sterilized and ready for use.

Protecting yourself Your personal hygiene and safety are also important. The care you take in preparing for work should be carried through in everything you do and this is made even more important when you are about to handle hazardous chemicals. Put on a clean colouring apron and fasten the ties in a bow. Then take a pair of disposable vinyl gloves and put them on ready for the application.

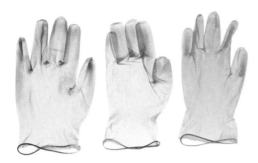

Use your time effectively – each salon allocates different times for different services. A re-touch may only take 20 minutes to apply on shorter hair whereas a long hair set of full-head woven highlights could be booked for an hour.

Preparation dos and don'ts

Dos	Don'ts
✓ When a client's hair is developing under a Climazone, Rollerball or any other colour accelerator, do check at intervals during the processing to see that they are comfortable and that the equipment is not too hot.	✗ Never handle electrical equipment with wet hands, always dry them first.
✓ Do check the equipment controls so that the timing and temperature settings are correct.	✗ Never leave colour spillages until later. Mop them up straight away while you still have your protective gloves on.
✓ Do check the manufacturer's instructions before you mix any products. They will give you the recommended amounts and quantities to mix together.	✗ Don't mix up too much product at one time, it is wasteful and expensive. If you need more you can always mix when you need it.
✓ Always do a skin test on the client before any colouring process.	✗ Never mix products up before they are needed. Colour products have a set development time and oxidization will start if they are exposed or mixed too soon.
✓ Do put screw tops and lids back on colouring products immediately. Their effectiveness will be impaired if they are exposed to the air for any longer than needed.	✗ Never attempt to do any colouring procedure without wearing the correct PPE.
✓ Do make a note of low levels of stock as product is removed from storage.	✗ Don't work in a cluttered environment. Always make sure that the work area is prepared properly and ready for use.
✓ Do make good use of your time. Always prepare your work area and the materials you will need before the client arrives; this saves valuable time later.	✗ Don't forget to complete the client details/records after doing the service. Make sure that all aspects – dates, times, changes in materials, etc. – are recorded accurately.

Colour consultation

It would be incorrect to say that one form of consultation is more important than another, but colouring is a complex area of work and if you do not make the right assessment before you start, the outcome could be disastrous.

BEST PRACTICE

Record the client's responses to your questions and the comments about how the results of any tests affected their hair and skin.

Colour consultation considerations

First of all	Things to consider
Does the client know of any reasons that would affect your choice of service?	Ask the client about their hair to find out if there are any known reasons why the service cannot continue – are there any contra-indications?
What colour would be best to suit their needs?	Should you be using temporary, semi-permanent or permanent colouring?
How can the desired effect be best achieved?	Does the colour need to be applied to the roots first, the mid-lengths and ends, or can it be applied all over? Would the effect benefit more from partial colouring such as highlights or lowlights?
How long will it last?	Will the colour fade off or does it have to grow out?
How much will it cost?	Is this affordable and something that can be kept up in the future?
How will it affect the hair?	Will the long-term effects be what the client expects?
Is the hair suitable for colouring?	Have you tested the hair and skin beforehand to see if there are any contra-indications or hair condition issues that will affect the result?

Now consider

What are the client's expectations?	How will the colour enhance the style and natural colour of the hair? What are the benefits for them?
What are the results of your tests?	Examine the hair. Does it present any limitations for what you intend to do?
What is the hair condition like?	Are there any factors that will change the way in which colouring will work on the hair? What previous information is available?
What do the client's records say?	Does this information influence the choice and colour process?
How will you show the effect to the client?	Have you got any illustrations of the finished effect? Does the colour chart give a clearer picture of the shade the hair will go?
How long will the process take?	Is there enough time to complete the effect? Has anything changed as a result of the consultation? Would this service now need to be re-booked or do you have the time to complete it still?

What contra-indications are you looking for?

Following on from your initial considerations, you should now be looking for any contra-indications.

Colour contra-indications

Contra-indications – Look for the following:	How could you find out more?	How else would you know?
Skin sensitivity	Ask the client if they have ever had a reaction to hair or skin products in the past.	Patch test/skin sensitivity test.
Allergic reaction	Ask the client if they have ever had a reaction to hair or skin products in the past	Patch test/skin sensitivity test.
Skin disorder	Ask the client if they know about any current skin disorders.	Examine the scalp to see if there are any physical signs of skin abrasions, **discolouration**, swellings, infestation or infections.

(Continued)

(Continued)

Colour contra-indications

Contra-indications – Look for the following:	How could you find out more?	How else would you know?
Incompatible products	If you see the results of any previous colour ask what type it was, how was it done?	Look for discolouration or unnatural colour effects on the hair. Test for incompatibles.
Medical reasons	Ask the client if there are any current medical reasons why colouring cannot be performed.	Examine the hair. Look for signs of healthy active growth. If there are signs of weakened, damaged, broken or missing hair, ask for more information. Test for elasticity and porosity.
Damaged hair	Ask the client if there are any current known reasons why the hair is in its current state/condition.	Examine the hair. Look for signs of healthy active growth. If there are signs of weakened, damaged, broken or missing hair, ask for more information. Test for elasticity and porosity.

What type of colour should I use?

Type, PPE and timings	Preparation	Suitability	Effects
Temporary colour PPE – wear gloves and apron. Whole head application done at workstation takes five minutes.	No mixing required, colour applied straight from the can, bottle, etc. as coloured mousses, setting lotions, hair mascara.	No skin test required. Most hair types (including coloured and permed), although it can be more difficult to remove from lightened hair. Colour control – poor, shade guide targeting can only be used as an approximation.	The colour only lasts until the next wash. Subtle toning on grey hair. Hair condition may be improved. Surface colour without chemical penetration. Does not lift natural colour, only deposits.
Semi-permanent colour PPE – wear gloves and apron. Whole head application done at workstation or at basin takes five minutes. Left on up to 15 minutes.	No mixing required, although transference to an applicator may be necessary.	Skin test may be required. Most hair types (including coloured and permed), often used as a colour refresher between permanent colour treatments. Can cover small amounts of greying hair. Colour control – poor, shade guide targeting can only be used as an approximation.	Lasts up to six shampoos. Colour fades/diffuses after each wash. Does not lift natural colour, only deposits. No regrowth, natural colour unaffected.
Quasi-permanent (longer-lasting) colour PPE – wear gloves and apron. Whole head brush application done at	Mixed with developer or activators. These can be in liquid or crystal form. Measurement and mixing must be accurate.	Skin test required. Most hair types (including coloured and permed), often used as a colour refresher between permanent colour treat-ments. Will cover up to 30 per cent	Lasts up to 12 shampoos. Colour fades a small amount after subsequent shampoos.

(Continued)

(Continued)

Type, PPE and timings	Preparation	Suitability	Effects
workstation, takes up to 25 minutes. Alternatively, using an applicator bottle can save time and takes up to 15 minutes. Left on up to 40 minutes.		grey hair. Colour control – good, will achieve shade guide targeting.	Does affect natural colour, bonds with natural pigments. Can produce a regrowth.
Permanent colour (para-dye) PPE – wear gloves and apron. Regrowth brush application done at workstation, takes up to 25 minutes. Left on up to 40 minutes. Whole head colouring will depend on length and order of application.	Mixed with hydrogen per-oxide at 10, 20, 30 or 40 volumes (3 per cent, 6 per cent, 9 per cent, or 12 per cent). Measurement and mixing must be accurate.	Skin test required. All natural hair types and most coloured and permed hair (providing hair not too porous or damaged). Will cover all grey. Can lift up to two shades – high lift colour will lift three or four shades.	Permanent colour or para-dyes are made in a wide variety of shades and tone. Long lasting and grows out. Will change natural hair pigments.

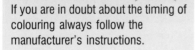

BEST PRACTICE

If you are in doubt about the timing of colouring always follow the manufacturer's instructions.

Note: All timings are approximated. Partial colouring techniques – highlights, slices, dip ends, etc. – may take longer depending on operator experience, the amount of colour applied and the technique used.

Measuring flasks and mixing bowls

Accurate measurement of hydrogen peroxide at any strength is essential. The amount used in relation to colour is a critical factor to a successful outcome and different types of colour are formulated to be used with particular developers. For example, a *L'Oréal DiaLight* should be mixed with *DiaActivator*™ developer. If you use a different developer, the consistency will be wrong and this will make the application difficult. All gel and cream colours, when mixed, will be stiff enough not to run or drip when either on the brush or on the hair. Using unmatched, alternative developers will do the opposite and could be a potential hazard for the client.

Measuring tools

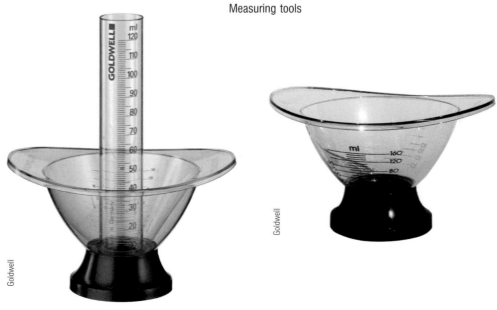

Goldwell

Goldwell

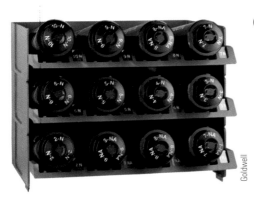

Colour rack

Goldwell

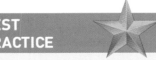

TOP TIP

When you measure developer into a measuring flask, you must make sure that your eyeline is at the same level as the liquid in the flask so that the measurement is accurate.

BEST PRACTICE

Always make sure that you remove all colouring products from the hair. This not only stops the action from developing further, but more importantly, it ensures that the client will not get any irritation or discomfort from chemicals deposited on the skin.

When you mix developer with colour from tubes, you will notice that all tubes have markings on the side showing the ¼, ½ and ¾ points. These enable you to squeeze from the bottom of the tube up to these points, knowing that your measurement will be accurate.

If you are mixing two or more shades of colour together, always mix these well in the bowl first before adding any developer. This allows the different pigments to be evenly distributed throughout the colour and also throughout the hair when it is applied!

Skin and hair tests

Skin or sensitivity test

The sensitivity test is used to assess the reaction of the skin to chemicals or chemical products. In the salon it is mainly used before colouring. Some people are allergic to external contact of chemicals such as PPD (found in permanent colour). This can cause dermatitis or, in even more severe cases, permanent scarring of skin tissue and hair loss. Some have an allergy to irritants to which they react internally.

To find out whether a client's skin reacts to chemicals in permanent colours, carry out the following test 24–48 hours prior to the chemical process, following the manufacturer's instructions.

Carrying out a skin test

Skin test procedure

1   Select and apply a small amount of a *dark colour*, within the range to be used, on a cotton bud. (Follow the manufacturer's explicit details.)

2   Clean an area of skin about 5mm square, behind the ear.

3   Apply a little of the colour directly to the skin.

4   Do not cover the area and ask your client to report any discomfort or irritation that occurs over the next 24 hours. Arrange to see your client at the end of this time so that you can check for signs of reaction.

5   Record the details on the client's record file (it may be useful for future reference).

6   Make an appointment for the future service.

7   If there is a positive response – a contra-indication, a skin reaction such as inflammation, soreness, swelling, irritation or discomfort – do not carry out the intended service.

8   If the result is negative, i.e. no reaction, the service may proceed as planned.

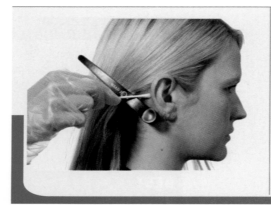

Patch test (Skin test)

A skin test should be done at least 48 hours before any permanent or quasi-permanent hair colouring service.

Apply a small amount of the natural base colour (i.e. if the target colour is 7.13 use base 7 or 7.0) behind the ear with a cotton wool bud.

Leave for 24–48 hours and ask the client to contact the salon if they experience any adverse reaction or discomfort.

Hair tests

BEST PRACTICE

You will be more likely to get a true test response by using natural base colours (especially darker shades) because these contain more PPD.

HEALTH & SAFETY

Never ignore the result of a skin test. If a skin test shows a reaction and you carry on anyway, there may be a more serious reaction that could affect the whole body!

Incompatibility test

	When is it done	How is it done
This will indicate if any *metallic salts* or other mineral compounds are present within the hair.	Prior to colouring, highlighting and perming treatments.	Place a small sample of hair in a mixture of 20 parts hydrogen peroxide (6 per cent) and one part ammonium-based compound from perm solution. If the mixture bubbles, heats up or discolours do not carry out the service.

Step		Process
1		As mentioned above, an incompatibility test will indicate whether there are any metallic salts present within the hair. It is very rare to find incompatibles present but hair restorers and compound henna are, typically, two types colour that would be incompatible with professional, quasi- and permanent colours.
2		Chemical incompatibility is tested for by mixing 20 parts of 6 per cent hydrogen peroxide with one part ammonium hydroxide. (If ammonium hydroxide is unavailable cold wave perm solution will do.)

(Continued)

(Continued)

Step		Process
3		Place a small amount of the hair to be tested in a bowl.
4		Add the mixed chemicals to the hair and leave for up to 30 minutes. ◆ A positive reaction will show signs of bubbling. ◆ heat will be generated. ◆ the hair will change colour (discolour).

Elasticity test		
	When is it done	**How is it done**
This determines the condition of the hair by seeing how much the hair will stretch and return to its original length. Overstretched hair will not return to the same length and indicates weakness and damage.	Before chemical treatment(s) and services. (Ideal for hair that has poor elasticity, e.g. from lightening or colouring.)	Take a dry strand of hair between your fingers, holding it at the roots and the ends. Gently pull the hair between the two points to see if the hair will stretch and return to its original length. (If the hair breaks easily it may indicate that the cortex is damaged and will be unable to sustain any further chemical treatment.) Do not conduct this test on *wet hair* as the hydrogen (and salt bonds) are already broken. This will give you a false result as the hair is bound to stretch. If the hair was lightened too, it will probably break off altogether.

BEST PRACTICE

Do not conduct an elasticity test on wet hair as this can give you a false result. For example, hair that has been lightened five or more levels will have no inner strength when wet and will always fail an elasticity test.

TOP TIP

When hair is wet it will be naturally weakened as most of the salt bonds and hydrogen bonds will be broken anyway.

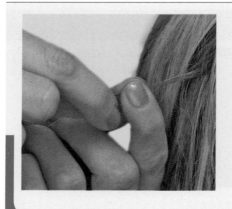

Elasticity test

An elasticity test is a good way of determining the internal condition of the cortex. Hair in good condition has sufficient inner strength and moisture levels to be able to stretch and return to its original length.

Take a single strand of dry hair and apply tension by pulling between the fingers to see how much the hair stretches.

Go to CHAPTER 6 Consultation p. 159, for more information on alpha and beta keratin.

Porosity test

	When is it done	How is it done
This test also indicates the hair's current condition by assessing the hair's ability to absorb or resist moisture from liquids. (Hair in good condition has a tightly packed cuticle layer which will resist the ingress of products.) Hair that is porous holds on to moisture: this is evident when you try to blow-dry it as the hair takes a long time to dry.	Before chemical services. If the cuticle is torn or damaged, the absorption of moisture and therefore hydrogen peroxide is quicker, so the processing time will be shorter. Over-porous hair will quickly take in colour but will not necessarily be able to hold colour as the cuticle is damaged and allows the newly introduced pigments to wash away.	Take a single strand of dry hair between your fingers and thumbs, holding out away from the head. Now run your finger and thumb, backwards, down the hair from points to roots. If it feels roughened, as opposed to coarse, it is likely that the hair is porous. As cuticle layers lie with their free edges towards the point ends, you are far more likely to be able to feel the tiny ridges of any lifted cuticles.

Strand test

	When is it done	How is it done
Most colouring products just require the full development time recommended by the manufacturer – check their instructions. (However, some hair conditions take on the colour faster than others do. A strand test will check the colour development and see if it needs to come off earlier.)	A strand test or hair strand colour test is used to assess the resultant colour on a strand or section of hair after colour has been processed and developed. A strand test is also useful prior to lightening natural pigments from hair or prior to removing synthetic pigments (i.e. decolour or colour reducer) to see how the hair will respond.	1 Rub a strand of hair lightly with the back of a comb to remove the surplus colour. 2 Check whether the colour remaining is evenly distributed throughout the hair's length. If it is even, remove the rest of the colour. If it is uneven, allow processing to continue, if necessary applying more colour. If any of the hair on the head is not being treated, you can compare the evenness of colour in the coloured hair with that in the uncoloured hair.

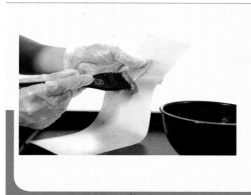

Test cutting

A way of finding out how hair will react and respond to a selected colour.

Cut a small amount of hair from an unnoticeable area on the client's head.

Mix up your target colour with the selected peroxide according to manufacturer's instructions and apply to the test cutting. Leave to develop for recommended time, then rinse and dry to check the result.

TOP TIP

This would be vitally important if there was a problem at some later stage, particularly if it involved any legal action taken against the salon.

Recording the results Make sure that you record the details of all tests that you conduct. Update the client's record card or computer file immediately after you have done the test. Don't leave it until later, you might forget! These records are essential information that will be needed again and help to show that a competent service has been provided at that time.

Colour selection

Colour selection, i.e. the process you go through in choosing the right target shade for your client's hair and the correct mixture of products to achieve that target shade, is based upon:

◆ Their personal choice (initially).

◆ The condition and quality of your client's hair (i.e. if it has already undergone processes such as highlights).

1 If the hair has been regularly coloured before and there is a clear regrowth, with ends that have faded, you may only need to do a straightforward regrowth application with the same colour. Then, later in the development process, the residual colour can be diluted and taken through to the rest to refresh the total effect. So in this instance a regrowth that takes 20 minutes to apply can be left for 30 minutes' development (depending on manufacturer/colour type). Then, in the last 15 minutes, it can be taken through to the ends, until it is ready to be removed.

   However, if your client's hair has been coloured before, you also need to remember that it will not be possible to make the hair lighter by colouring. Permanent colour does not reduce permanent (synthetic) pigments in the hair. (If this is required you will have to use a colour remover first.)

2 If you need or want to counteract and neutralize unwanted tones in the hair, you will need to apply the principles of the colour wheel. If the client wants to reduce or 'calm down' unwanted red tones then you will be choosing a colour slightly darker in depth but which has the matt tones capable of neutralizing that effect. Conversely, if your aim is to eliminate ashen 'GREEN' tones (e.g. the discolouration resulting from swimming in chlorinated swimming pools) then you will be introducing warmer tones to the hair. So in this situation a 'greeny'-looking base 6 blonde will be improved by a shade depth 6 but with a tone warmth .03 – for more information see the section on depth and tone earlier in this chapter.

If you had to reduce a tonal effect that was too yellow, say on a head that had been lightened, then (although the principle of toning lightened hair is slightly different) you would still be applying the principles of the colour wheel. Therefore, a violet-based ash colour should be used to neutralize the unwanted tones.

3 If your client has never had any colour on their hair before (virgin hair) then colour targeting is easy. Your client will be able to choose practically any shade on the permanent shade chart, providing it is at the same depth or darker. (It is possible to lighten a shade or two with colour in certain situations.)

4 If your client has grey or greying (i.e. white) hair then you will have to decide and agree on what reduction of grey is necessary. If the client wants to cover all the grey, then this is only achievable by using or adding base shades to the target colour, i.e. a natural shade or a natural shade plus the target shade.

The amount of base added to the target shade is directly proportional to the amount of grey. Grey hair is referred to as a percentage of the whole head. Therefore, a client who has about a quarter of their hair that is grey is referred to as 25 per cent grey. Similarly, a client one tenth of whose hair is grey is 10 per cent grey.

Existing hair condition

The hair's existing condition is a major contributing factor in the way in which it will respond when it is coloured. Porous hair will absorb the colour at a different rate. The porosity of hair is never even along the hair length, let alone across the hairs throughout the head. This is because the porosity of the hair relates to areas of damaged cuticle. Areas of high porosity occur at sites along the hair shaft where cuticle is torn or missing. At these points, moisture or chemicals can easily enter the inner hair without cuticle layer resistance.

This changes the rate of absorption, which ultimately affects the final evenness of the colour and the hair's ability to retain colour in subsequent washing etc. pH balancing conditioners help to even out the hair's porosity and return **chemically treated hair** back to a natural pH 5.5.

During processing the only other factors that affect the achievement of an even and expected final colour result (providing your selection is correct) are:

◆ timing

◆ temperature

Pre-softening resistant (white) hair

White hair can be very resistant to colouring, especially lighter shades ranging from bases 8 up to 10. Sometimes it is necessary to prepare the hair, prior to colouring, by lifting the cuticle slightly, so that the target shade can work better.

If your client is 100 per cent white/grey, you may have problems getting an even result. You can **pre-soften** the client's hair by using 20 volume 6 per cent hydrogen peroxide, by applying it directly to the resistant areas. The easiest way to apply would be at a backwash where you could apply the peroxide directly to the areas on dry hair with a colouring brush. (Alternatively, if your salon uses a *thinner* form of developer rather than crème, you may be able to apply it to the hair via a water spray.)

Leave the peroxide on the hair for five minutes then remove any excess with a towel.

Finally, move the client back to the workstation and dry the client's hair with a blow-dryer. You are now ready to apply the permanent/quasi-permanent colour as planned.

Timing the colour development

Colour saturation is proportional to the length of time that the colour is on and under-processed hair cannot achieve the same saturation as hair that has had full development. So, the longer that the colour is left on, the more density (saturation) it has.

This can be explained in another way. Imagine that you wanted to redecorate a plain, smooth, white wall. First of all, you choose the colour and shade of paint that you want it to be. Then, after some preparation, you take a brush and start by applying the first coat. When this is dry you look at the colour, only to find that the effect is uneven and patchy. You can see that the tone you wanted is there but it is often thin and almost transparent in places. So you repaint the wall. When this extra layer of paint dries, the saturation of colour is better and more even, but still a little patchy in places. Finally you apply a third coat to the areas that are still patchy and when it dries the colour has an even density throughout. This effect is called saturation; it is achieved by the even-ness of the density of the colour throughout the hair.

The effects of temperature during colouring

Temperature is also a contributing factor to colour development. The warmer the salon environment the quicker the colour processing will be. We know that when colour is introduced to heat, it takes even more quickly. This can be localized to the client or relate to the whole salon. For instance, the salon temperature may be cool but the colour can be speeded up, by putting the client under a Climazon™ or Rollerball™.

But, remember, the human body produces heat too. In fact up to 30 per cent of body heat is emitted through the top of your head! (This is why wearing a hat in winter keeps you warm.) This heating effect has a critical impact on the development of colour and even more precarious when lightening!

Therefore, with this extra heat around the scalp area, you can see there are potential problems in controlling the colour and aspects of the client's safety. To help control the process you must make sure that, when the colour is applied to the root area, the hair is lifted away from the scalp so that the air is able to circulate and ventilate the scalp evenly. This ensures that there are no 'hot spots' anywhere that might take more quickly or become a safety hazard to the client.

HEALTH & SAFETY

When the scalp becomes warm during the processing the skin attempts to regulate the overheating by producing sweat. At this point when the skin is moistened by sweat the colouring products become more mobile and will spread more easily onto and even into the skin! This is extremely dangerous and will cause scalp burns as chemicals enter the skin through the hair follicles!

Initially, the client will not be able to distinguish between the heat from the processing and the burning sensation from the chemicals. By the time that they do, the longer-term damage is done. Chemical burns continue to act upon the skin long after the colour has been removed. You must avoid this happening.

If this does occur, the client must have medical attention immediately.

TOP TIP

Remember once you have finished with the towels to immediately put them into a basin of water or the washing machine.

TOP TIP

White hair is very resistant to colouring but some colours are guaranteed to work. Find out from your colour ranges, which ones will give 100 per cent coverage on white hair.

BEST PRACTICE

Under-processed colours will not last as long, so follow your manufacturer's instructions for development times.

BEST PRACTICE

Only work on manageable amounts of hair at any one time. Always secure the hair that you aren't working on out of the way with sectioning clips.

Colour selection checklist

◆ What is the client's target shade?

◆ What is the percentage of white/grey hair, does it need to be pre-softened?

◆ What is the difference in depth between the natural hair and the target colour?

◆ If the target shade is lighter than the natural shade, is it achievable by colouring alone?

◆ What colouring products would be needed to achieve the effect?

◆ What developer will be needed to achieve the effect?

◆ If the hair appears porous or porous in areas, do you need to do a test cutting first?

◆ If the hair has a small percentage of white/grey, what amount of base shade will you need to add to the target shade to stabilize the effect?

BEST PRACTICE

You don't have to re-colour hair as a full head every time. You can refresh the colour when you do a re-touch service.

BEST PRACTICE

Always prepare your client, work area and equipment before you start any colour service.

Refreshing the colour of the lengths and ends

When you are re-colouring the roots on longer hair you will often find that the ends of the colour need refreshing too. This does not mean that a full head colour is necessary: the refreshing can be done during the application.

Appearance	1st step	2nd step	3rd step	4th step
When the colour looks the same at the ends as the target shade.	Apply to regrowth	Allow to develop and then 15 minutes before full development time.	Add 15–20cc of tepid water to the mixture in the bowl then apply this to the lengths and ends.	Leave for a further 5–10 minutes, to complete the development process.
When the tonal quality has faded but the colour is still the same depth.	Apply to regrowth	Allow to develop then 25 minutes before full development time.	Add 15–20cc of tepid water to the mixture in the bowl then apply this to the lengths and ends.	Leave for a further 15–20 minutes, to complete the development process.
When both the tonal quality and depth has faded on the ends.	Apply to regrowth	Add 15–20cc of tepid water to the mixture in the bowl then apply this to the lengths and ends immediately.	Leave all the colour on for full development for 35–40 minutes.	

Regrowth application: quick checklist

Regrowth checklist	
Consultation	◆ Find out what needs to be done. ◆ Are there any modifications needed to do the regrowth?
Prepare the client	◆ Make the usual protective preparations. ◆ Brush the hair through to remove the tangles. ◆ Apply a barrier cream to the hairlines (if necessary).
Prepare the materials	◆ Make sure that you have everything you need at hand. ◆ Put on your disposable gloves and apron. ◆ Mix the products correctly.
Method/technique	◆ Divide the hair into four equal quadrants. ◆ Start the application with a brush to the roots at the top of the head, working down and along each quadrant. ◆ Pick up a horizontal section of hair within a back quadrant and with the tail of the brush. ◆ Apply the colour/bleach to the regrowth evenly. ◆ Repeat down the back of the head and through the sides.
Development	◆ Monitor the colour development throughout the processing. ◆ Apply heat if needed to speed up the development process. ◆ Check with the client throughout to ensure their comfort.
Removal	◆ When processing is complete, take the client to the basin and rinse the hair with tepid/warm water, gently massage to **emulsify** the colour. ◆ Rinse thoroughly until the colour is removed. ◆ Shampoo and condition with an anti-oxidizing agent.

STEP-BY-STEP-REGROWTH APPLICATION

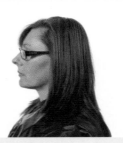

1 Before
Prepare the client by protecting them with a clean gown, towel and cape.

Put on your apron and gloves.

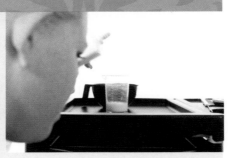

2 Prepare your trolley with the materials you need.

Mix the colour according to manufacturer's instructions.

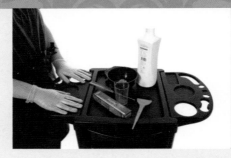

3 When measuring hydrogen peroxide you should always get down to eye level as this ensures accurate measurement.

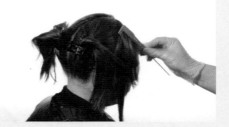

4 Prepare the client's hair by brushing through to remove any tangles.

Then divide the hair into four quadrants ('hot cross bun') and section each one out of the way.

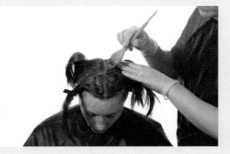

5 Start applying the colour directly to the regrowth without overlapping onto the previously coloured hair.

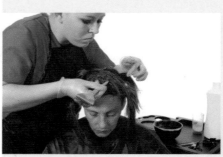

6 After applying the colour to the 'hot cross bun' area you can start to take sections within the quarters, horizontally.

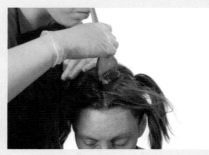

7 Work down through each section and move the hair that has been coloured over, and out of the way.

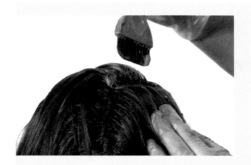

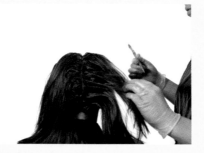

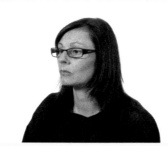

8 Work down through each section and move the hair that has been coloured over, and out of the way.

9 With all of the sections completed, just quickly check where you have applied and the hairlines to make sure that everywhere has been covered.

Then allow to develop for the recommended time.

10 Final effect.

Full head application: quick checklist

Full head colour checklist	
Consultation	◆ Find out what needs to be done. Are any changes needed for the application, colour(s) or lightener?
Prepare the client	◆ Make the usual protective preparations.
	◆ Brush the hair through to remove the tangles.
	◆ Apply a barrier cream to the hairlines.
Prepare the materials	◆ Make sure that you have everything you need to hand.
	◆ Put on your disposable gloves and apron.
	◆ Mix the products correctly.
Method/technique	◆ Divide the hair into four equal sections.
	◆ Start the application with a brush to the mid-lengths and ends at the top of the head, working down and along each quadrant.
	◆ Pick up a thin 5mm horizontal section of hair within a back quadrant and with the tail of the brush.
	◆ Apply the colour/lightener to the mid-length and ends evenly.
	◆ Repeat down the back of the head and through the sides.
1st part of development	◆ Allow the mid-length and ends to develop sufficiently first.
	◆ Monitor the colour development throughout the processing.
	◆ Apply heat if needed to speed up the development process.
	◆ Check with the client throughout to ensure their comfort.
2nd part of development	◆ Pick up each of the horizontal sections of hair with the tail of the brush.
	◆ Apply the colour/lightener to the root area evenly.
	◆ Repeat down the back of the head and through the sides.
	◆ Monitor the colour development throughout the processing.

(Continued)

(Continued)

Full head colour checklist	
	◆ Apply heat if needed to speed up the development process.
	◆ Check with the client throughout to ensure their comfort.
Removal	◆ When processing is complete, take the client to the basin and rinse the hair with tepid/warm water, then apply gentle massage to emulsify the colour.
	◆ Rinse thoroughly until the colour is removed.
	◆ Shampoo and condition with an anti-oxidizing agent.

STEP BY STEP: FULL HEAD APPLICATION

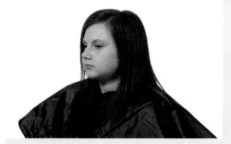

1 Before.

Prepare the client by protecting them with a clean gown, towel and cape.

Put on your apron and gloves.

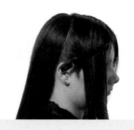

2 Prepare the client's hair by brushing through to remove any tangles.

Then divide the hair into four quadrants ('hot cross bun') and section each one out of the way.

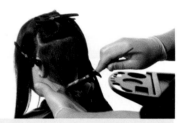

3 A full head colour on longer hair must be applied to the mid-lengths and ends first because these areas will need longer time to develop.

Mix your colour according to the manufacturer's instructions, then, starting with one of the lower, back sections, apply your colour to the mid-lengths and draw down to the ends.

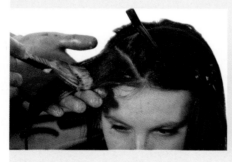

4 The sections for **full head application** to mid-lengths and ends are three or four times the thickness of that applied to the roots.

With all the back sections done, you can start to work on the sides in a similar way.

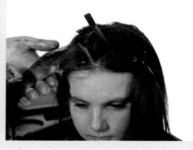

5 Again, draw the colour through the lengths, to cover all the ends.

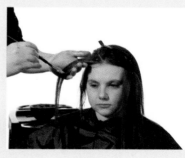

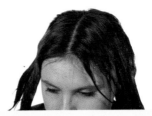

6 When the mid-lengths and ends are complete, you can leave the colour to develop for the recommended timings.

You can use an accelerator to speed up the process.

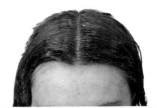

7 After the mid-lengths and ends have developed, you can apply the root application.

See re-touch colour steps for more details.

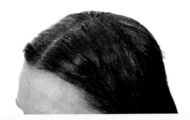

8 Develop all of the colour until processing is complete.

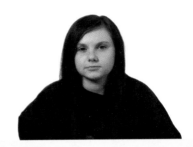

9 Final effect.

Cap highlights: quick checklist

Cap highlights checklist	
Consultation	◆ Find out what effect your client is trying to achieve.
	◆ How much lightened or coloured hair in relation to natural colour is expected – 5 per cent, 10 per cent, 25 per cent?
	◆ How will you explain the effect to the client?
	◆ Do you have any visual aids to help?
	◆ Explain everything that you are going to do.
Prepare the client	◆ Make the usual protective preparations.
	◆ Brush the hair to examine the growth patterns and to remove any tangles. Look for areas where highlights would be conspicuous or unsightly.
	◆ Look for natural part/parting areas. Confirm how the hair is to be worn.
	◆ If the hair has slightly longer layers or tends to tangle, apply some talcum powder to the hair and work through with your hands. This will help the hair to come through the holes, reducing any discomfort from tugging and picking the sections.
Prepare the materials	◆ Check the quality of the highlight cap. When a cap has previously been used for colouring it starts to wear.
	◆ Look for enlarged holes or splits where colour/lightener can seep through on to the hair.
	◆ Make sure that you have everything you need at hand.
	◆ Put on your disposable gloves and apron.

(Continued)

(Continued)

Cap highlights checklist	
	◆ Mix the products correctly.
	◆ Ask the client to take hold of the front of the cap, ensuring it is centrally positioned at the forehead.
	◆ Pull the cap down smoothly, ensuring that the fit hugs the contour of the head correctly.
Pull the highlights through	◆ Start at the nape area.
	◆ Pull the highlights through by taking enough hair to complete each one in a single movement. Always pull through at an acute (narrow angle) to the cap.
	◆ Complete the pattern of repeated highlights, i.e. the percentage required, all over the head.
Apply the lightener or colour	◆ Carefully apply the mixture to all of the highlights evenly.
	◆ Lift the pasted hair slightly with the tail of a comb for even ventilation, so that no hair is trapped and can overheat or overdevelop.
Development	◆ Carefully place a clear, polyethylene cap on and around the highlights, to stop any spillages and to aid an even development.
	◆ Monitor the colour development throughout the processing.
	◆ Apply heat if needed to speed up the development process.
	◆ Check with the client throughout to ensure their comfort.
Removal	◆ When processing is complete, rinse thoroughly until all the product is removed (a slight shampoo may be needed).
	◆ Lift the flanges of the cap into the basin area and remove in one smooth and even pull.
	◆ Shampoo and condition with an anti-oxidizing agent.

STEP-BY-STEP: CAP HIGHLIGHTS

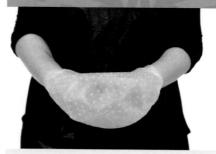

1 Wash, dry and then talc the cap – then check the highlight cap for splits, holes and tears.

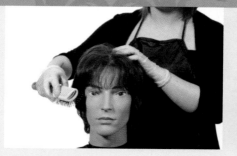

2 Brush/comb through the hair to remove any tangles before placing the cap on the modelling head.

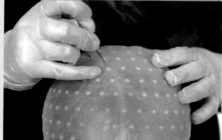

3 Make sure that the cap fits closely down to the scalp area.

Start at the top and lift through a small section of hair.

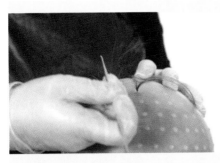

4 The section – if you have removed the tangles properly – should be even and slip through the holes easily.

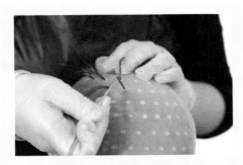

5 Carry on taking sections through in an evenly balanced pattern all over the cap.

That is, every hole, every other hole or every third hole.

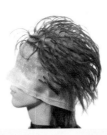

6 With most of the hair pulled through you can carefully brush it through to keep it out of the way from areas yet to be worked on.

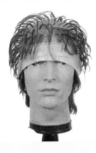

7 When you have finished, check that you have an evenly balanced highlighting pattern.

Fold back the rim so that the fold will collect any runny product or drips.

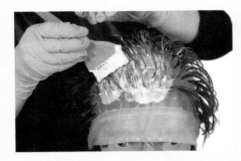

8 After mixing the required products, i.e. colour or lightener, start to apply evenly from the brush without 'blobbing' or dripping.

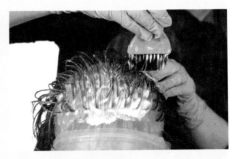

9 Continue all over the cap's surface.

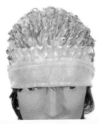

10 Allow the product to develop according to manufacturer's instructions.

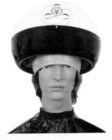

11 Apply heat with an accelerator or steamer as required.

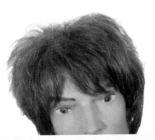

12 Rinse the product off at the basin, remove the cap and shampoo/condition in the normal way.

Final effect.

STEP-BY-STEP: CAP HIGHLIGHTS

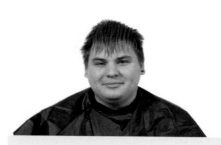

1 Before.

Prepare the client by protecting them with a clean gown, towel and cape.

Put on your apron and gloves.

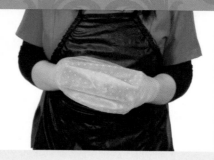

2 Wash, dry and then talc the cap – then check the highlight cap for splits, holes and tears.

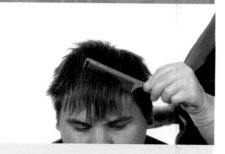

3 Brush/comb through the hair to remove any tangles before placing the cap on the client's head.

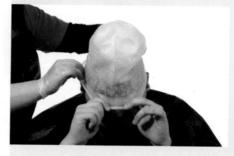

4 Check where the front of the cap is and ask the client to take hold of the cap at the centre of the forehead. Pull down at the back and carefully around the ears.

Make sure that the cap fits closely down to the scalp area.

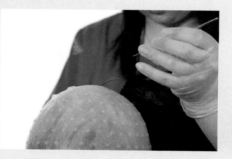

5 Start at the top and lift through a small section of hair with the crochet hook.

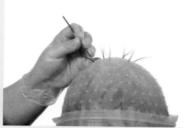

6 Carry on taking sections through in an evenly balanced pattern all over the cap.

That is, every hole, every other hole or every third hole.

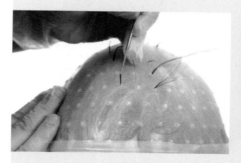

7 Be careful not to pull as this can be extremely painful for the client.

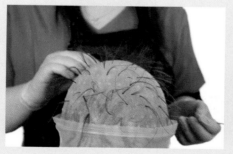

8 When you have finished, check that you have an evenly balanced highlighting pattern.

Fold back the rim so that the fold will collect any runny product or drips.

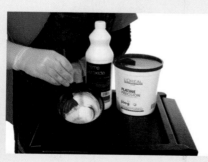

9 Never mix up your product until you are ready to use it.

Always follow the manufacturer's instructions when mixing.

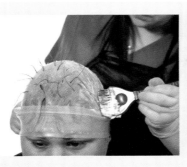

10 After mixing the required products, i.e. colour or lightener, start to apply evenly from the brush without 'blobbing' or dripping.

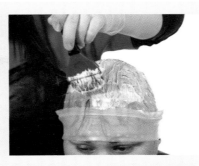

11 Continue all over the cap's surface.

Allow the colour/lightener to develop under an accelerator or steamer for the correct length of time.

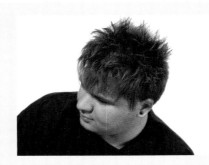

12 Final effect.

Woven highlights: quick checklist

Woven highlights checklist	
Consultation	◆ Find out what effect your client is trying to achieve.
	◆ How much lightened and/or coloured hair in relation to natural colour is expected? What percentage of each is needed – 5 per cent, 10 per cent, 25 per cent?
	◆ How will you explain the effect to the client?
	◆ Do you have any visual aids to help?
	◆ Explain everything that you are going to do.
Prepare the client	◆ Make the usual protective preparations.
	◆ Brush the hair to examine the growth patterns and to remove any tangles, look for areas where highlights would be conspicuous or unsightly.
	◆ Look for natural part/parting areas and confirm how the hair is to be worn.
Prepare the materials	◆ Make sure that you have everything you need at hand including foils cut to the required length.
	◆ Put on your disposable gloves and apron.
	◆ Mix the products correctly.
Method/technique	◆ Divide the hair into four equal sections.
	◆ Start at the back of the head at the nape.
	◆ Divide the remaining hair and section and secure it out of the way.
	◆ Pick up a horizontal section of hair and, with your pin-tail comb, weave out of the section a mesh of fine amounts of hair.
	◆ Underneath the mesh, place a foil long enough to protrude beyond the hair length.
	◆ Apply the colour/lightener to the mesh evenly.
	◆ Fold in half and half again – fold the edges too, if required.
	◆ Continue on to next section with the alternating colour(s) or lightener.
	◆ Repeat up the back of the head and through the sides.

(Continued)

(Continued)

Woven highlights checklist	
Development	◆ Monitor the colour development throughout the processing.
	◆ Apply heat if needed to speed up the development process.
	◆ Check with the client throughout to ensure their comfort.
Removal	◆ When processing is complete each foil must be removed individually by rinsing thoroughly until all the product is removed – this ensures that the colours do not run and bleed together.
	◆ Shampoo and condition with an anti-oxidizing agent.

BEST PRACTICE

If you used dry heat to accelerate the development of permanent colours, don't let the heat dry out the products as this will stop the colour from developing further.

STEP-BY-STEP: WOVEN HIGHLIGHTS

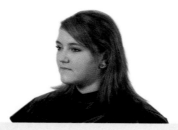

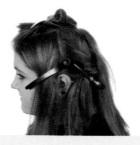

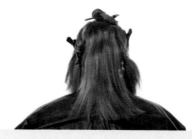

1 A full head of highlights provides tonal colour effects to all of the hair. Sometimes done with colour to form lowlights but more often done with lightener or lightener and colour to create multi-tonal effects.

Prepare a trolley with foils, colouring bowl, brush, sectioning clips and tail comb.

Brush through the hair to remove any tangles.

2 Section off the hair first to gauge the width of your foils and the effect over the head.

3 Section off any hair that you are not working with and create a section no wider than the foil you are putting in.

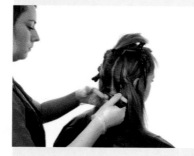

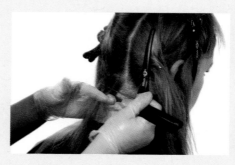

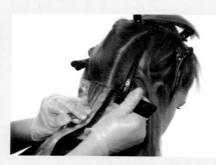

4 Then, holding your first section, weave off a uniform amount of hair that will become highlights.

5 Lift them off the held section, and hold them with your finger and thumb.

Neatly place a foil beneath the highlights and pull the highlights onto the foil to trap it in place.

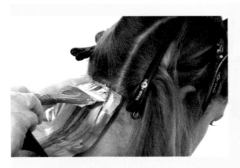

6 With your other hand, apply colour/lightener to the section starting near the root.

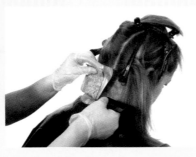

7 You can fold the foil in half and then the sides of the foils, to make parcels that stop the colour product seeping out.

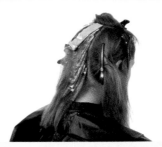

8(a) Carry on working upwards, repeating the process in a uniform way.

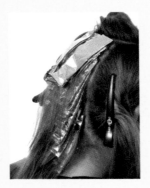

8(b) As Before.

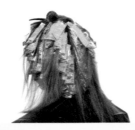

9 Full head of woven highlights.

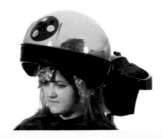

10 Use a steamer (or accelerator) for the recommended development time.

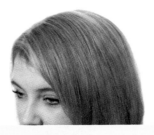

11 Final effect.

STEP-BY-STEP: T-SECTION HIGHLIGHTS

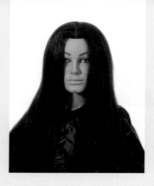

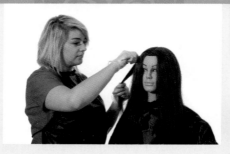

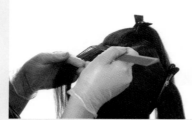

1 A set of **T-Section highlights** follows the parting through the top and extends down the sides to colour the front hairline.

Prepare a trolley with foils, colouring bowl, brush, sectioning clips and tail comb.

Brush through the hair to remove any tangles.

2 Check where the width of your foils will impact on the width and proportions of the head.

3 Section off any hair that you are not working with and create a section no wider than the foil you are putting in.

Then, holding your first section, weave off a uniform amount of hair that will become highlights.

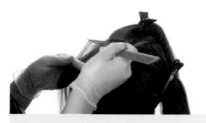

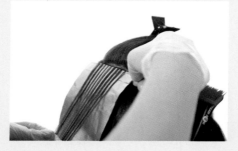

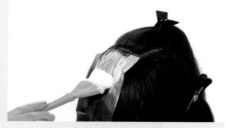

4 Lift them off the held section and hold them with your finger and thumb.

5 Neatly place a foil beneath the highlights and pull the highlights onto the foil, to trap it in place.

6 With your other hand, apply colour/lightener to the section starting near the root.

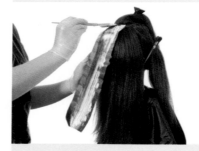

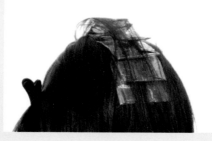

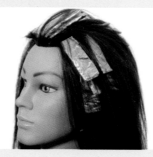

7 Extend the colour/lightener down to colour all of the hair.

Fold the foil up in half, making sure that no product seeps out at the sides.

8 You can fold the sides of the foils up to make parcels that encapsulate all of the product.

Carry on working upwards, and through the top to the front hairline.

9 Start at the bottom of the sides and repeat the process as you work up to the parting area.

BEST PRACTICE

Colouring faults can often be avoided if you are careful how you work in sectioning and moving the hair.

STEP-BY-STEP–SHOESHINE

1 Before.

Prepare your work area and materials.

Wash and cut the hair so that it is lifted away from the head.

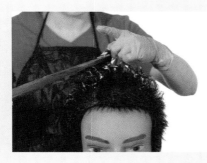

2 Apply spray to help it stand up.

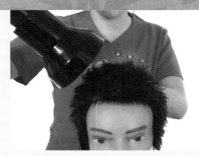

3 Make sure that the hair is totally dry and standing in 'peaks'.

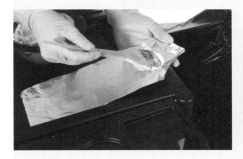

4 Depending on whether you are 'shoe shining' with colour or lightener, prepare a section of foil by applying the pre-mixed product to the central part.

Make sure that the product is 'stiff' enough to work with.

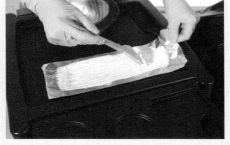

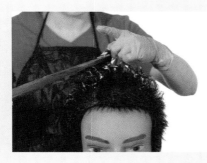

5 Now turn the foil upside down and sweep it across the points of the hair very lightly so that only the last centimetre or so gets coloured.

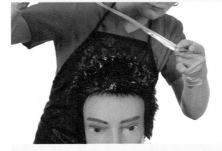

6 'Polish' the surface of the hair in the areas requiring colour.

Develop for the recommended time.

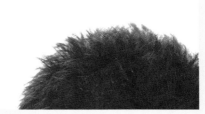

7 Finished effect.

STEP-BY-STEP: COLOUR SLICING

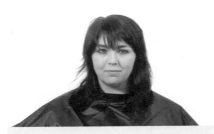

1 Colour **slicing** is a way of introducing colour to emphasize the hairstyle in some way.

Before.

Prepare the client by protecting them with a clean gown, towel and cape.

Put on your apron and gloves and prepare your trolley with the mixed colour, your foils, bowl, brush, etc.

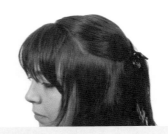

2 Section off the area and secure any hair not being coloured out of the way.

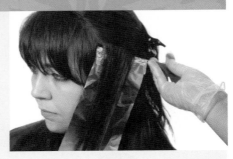

3 Hold the area for intended colouring to see where it appears in the mirror.

Then take a slice of hair and place it in a long enough foil.

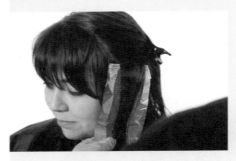

4 Apply the colour to the hair.

Note: unless the slice is to be worn on the surface hair, you don't need to go right to the root, it will never be seen.

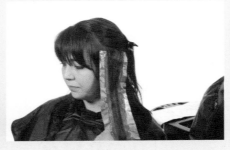

5 Don't allow the colour to seep near the edges.

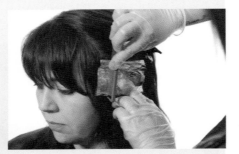

6 Fold your foil to encapsulate the hair and the colour.

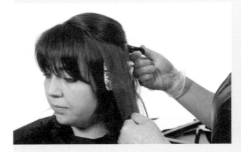

7 Repeat the slices wherever they are required.

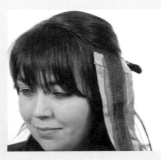

8 Apply the foil.

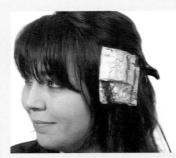

9 Secure the foil.

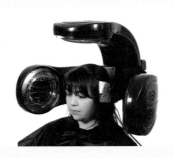

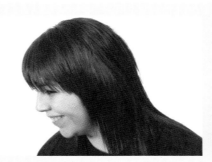

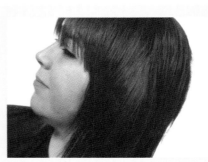

10 Allow to develop for recommended time. If you use an accelerator it will help to speed up the process.

11 Final effect.

What went wrong?

Sometimes things do go wrong, and you need to think quickly about how you will resolve the issues. There are all sorts of colouring problems, so the table below addresses some of the more common faults.

Problem or fault	Possible reasons why	Corrective actions
Colour patchy or uneven	◆ Insufficient coverage by colour. ◆ Poor application. ◆ Poor mixing of chemicals. ◆ Sectioning too large. ◆ Overlapping, causing colour build-up. ◆ Under-processing – colour was not given full development.	◆ Spot colour the patchy areas.
Colour too light	◆ Incorrect colour selection. ◆ Peroxide strength too high causing lightening. ◆ Under-processed. ◆ Hair in poor condition.	◆ Choose a darker shade. ◆ Check strengths and re-colour. ◆ Check strengths. ◆ Re-colour. ◆ Apply restructurants.
Colour fades quickly	◆ Effects of sun or swimming. ◆ Harsh treatment: over-drying, ceramic straighteners, etc. ◆ Hair in poor condition. ◆ Under-processing.	◆ Recondition before next application.

(Continued)

(Continued)

Problem or fault	Possible reasons why	Corrective actions
Colour too dark	◆ Incorrect colour selection. ◆ Over-processing. ◆ Hair in poor condition. ◆ Metallic salts present.	◆ Process correctly. ◆ Senior assistance required.
Colour too red, or Root glare	◆ Peroxide strength too high revealing undertone colour. ◆ Hair not lightened enough. ◆ Under-processing.	◆ Apply matt/green tones.
Discolouration	◆ Hair in poor condition. ◆ Undiluted colour repeatedly combed through. Incompatibles present.	◆ Use colour wheel to correct unwanted tones. ◆ Senior assistance required.
White hair not covered	◆ Resistance to peroxide/colour. ◆ Lack of base shade within the mixed colours.	◆ Pre-soften. ◆ Re-colour with correct amount of base and tones.
Hair resistant to colouring	◆ Cuticle too tightly packed. ◆ Under-processed. ◆ Incorrect colour selection. ◆ Poor mixing/application.	◆ Pre-soften. ◆ Re-colour. ◆ Senior assistance required. ◆ Senior assistance required.
Scalp irritation or skin reaction	◆ Chemicals not removed from hair properly after processing. ◆ Peroxide strength too high.	◆ Wash hair again and condition with anti-oxidants.
Breakage	◆ Lightening/highlighting hair that has previously had lightener on it before.	◆ Use restructurant on remaining hair to strengthen the weakened hair.

Provide aftercare advice

You have had a great success, the client really thinks that your work is fab, and is even going to recommend you to their friends. Therefore, it is time to finish off the job properly. Colour work is difficult at any time and there are so many factors that can affect the result.

You need to make sure that you have provided the best possible advice, so that your client can maintain their look and stop that colour from washing down the drain. It is so easy to ruin a great look, but you can prevent that by telling them about the products that will work with your colour(s) to enhance and keep it looking fresh.

It is not just about the shampoos and treatments either, styling products are going to affect the hair as well. So create a plan for your clients and give them your *prescribed* regime. That way they can keep the information and have the list of the right things that they *need* and *should* buy.

Clients need your help to look after their hair at home. You need to give them the right advice so that they can make the most of their new colour and style between visits.

SUMMARY

As a final reflection on what you have covered in this chapter, you should now have a clearer picture of all the essential aspects relating to colouring and lightening hair. In particular, you should now have a basic understanding of the key principles of:

1   Why preparation is essential to the service.

2   The contra-indications that are specific to colouring and lightening hair and the tests that must be performed before the service is provided.

3   The range of different colour effects that can be created by full head or partial techniques.

4   The techniques involved for creating the different effects.

5   How to use and maintain the tools and equipment associated with colouring and lightening hair.

6   Providing advice to the clients about how to maintain their hair colour and hair condition.

And collectively, how these principles will enable you to provide a variety of colouring and lightening services and effects to your clients.

ASSESSMENT OF KNOWLEDGE AND UNDERSTANDING

Project 1

For this project you will need to collect and test a range of hair samples. You will need to create three sets of sample batches of:

1   grey/white hair

2   coloured hair (with high lift colour)

3   lightened hair

4   coloured hair (base 6)

5   natural virgin hair (base 6).

Each of the different types listed above will be coloured with:

◆   a base shade 8

◆   a copper shade 8

◆   an ash/beige shade.

Mark each hair sample so that you know which one is which. Now mix up your three selected shades with 6 per cent (20 volume) hydrogen peroxide, then apply a little of each colour to each of the three collected sample batches. Allow time for the full development, then rinse each one and dry it off.

Record the changes for each sample:

◆   Which ones reached target shade?

◆   Which ones had no effect?

◆   Which ones have little or no coverage?

◆   Which ones have discoloured?

Write up the findings of your project in your portfolio. If you have enough of each sample repeat the exercise again but now with 3 per cent (10 volume) hydrogen peroxide for a differing set of results.

Case study

Your salon is recommended to a client who has moved to the area. She walks into the salon with lightened hair and requests a root re-touch. The hair is coarse, dry and below the shoulders.

She says that her work had tended to move her around and previous attempts by other salons have resulted in inconsistent colouring.

How would you deal with this?

List the process of events that should take place in your portfolio. Include in your responses:

- Consultation aspects, questions, examination and tests.
- Selection of suitable products and equipment.
- The precautions you would take.
- The advice and conclusion you would provide.

Project 2

For this project you will need to collect and test a range of hair samples.

You will need to create sample batches of:

- grey/white hair
- coloured hair (base 6)
- natural virgin hair (base 7)
- natural virgin hair (base 6)
- natural virgin hair (base 5).

Each of the different types listed above will be lightened to test the effects upon each prior to highlighting.

Mark each hair sample so that you know which one is which. Now mix up your lightener with 9 per cent (30 volume) hydrogen peroxide and then apply a little lightener to each of the sample batches.

Allow time for the full development, then rinse each one and dry it off.

Record the changes for each sample:

- Which ones reached a suitable shade for highlights?
- Which ones were unsuitable for highlights?
- Which ones had no effect?

Write up the findings of your project in your portfolio.

Case study

Your client recently had her hair highlighted at another salon while on holiday. The client did not think that the result was at all satisfactory. The resultant highlight effect was uneven and also patchy in places that were too gold.

How would you deal with this situation?

Make notes of what you would say and do. List the questions you would ask and the order in which you would ask them. Retain notes for your portfolio.

Here are some things you should consider:

- Find out why the hair was not successfully treated at the other salon.
- Find out whether the client returned there to complain and what the outcome was.
- Record what you think might have caused the unsatisfactory results.
- Record what you think would have been a successful course of action.
- Find out whether the hair is in a fit state for further treatment.
- Record the results of your discussion with your client, and what you have agreed.

Revision questions

A selection of different types of questions to check your colouring knowledge.

Q1	A _____ test will identify a client's sensitivity to colour products.	Fill in the blank
Q2	A quasi-permanent colour lasts longer than semi-permanent colour.	True or false
Q3	Which of the following products are likely to be an incompatible?	Multi selection
	Permanent colour containing PPD ☐ 1	
	Retail permanent colour containing PPD ☐ 2	

Vegetable henna   ☐ 3

Compound henna   ☐ 4

Single step applications for covering grey, i.e. *Just for men*   ☐ 5

Single step toners for application to lightened hair   ☐ 6

Q4   Lighteners and high lift colours are the same.   True or false

Q5   Which of the following tests do not apply to colouring services?   Multi choice

Skin test   ○ a

Incompatibility test   ○ b

Porosity test   ○ c

Development test curl   ○ d

Q6   Permanent colours alter the pigmentation of hair within the cuticle.   True or false

Q7   Which of the following colour products do not require the addition of hydrogen peroxide as a developer?   Multi selection

Powder lightener   ☐ 1

Semi-permanent colour   ☐ 2

Quasi-permanent colour   ☐ 3

Temporary colour   ☐ 4

Vegetable henna   ☐ 5

High lift colour   ☐ 6

Q8   Green tones within hair are neutralized by adding _____ tones.   Fill in the blank

Q9   Hair lightened from natural base 7 should be capable of maximum lift to: Multi choice

Red   ○ a

Pale yellow   ○ b

Yellow   ○ c

Yellow/orange   ○ d

Q10   Lightened hair that appears too yellow can be neutralized by adding mauve.   True or false

13 Perming

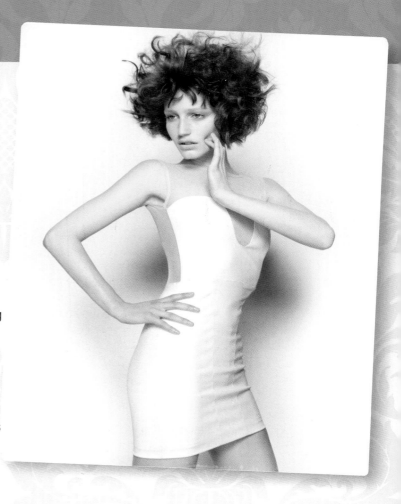

LEARNING OBJECTIVES

◆ Be able to maintain effective and safe methods of working

◆ Be able to prepare for perming and neutralizing

◆ Be able to perm and neutralize hair

◆ Understand how to work safely when perming and neutralizing hair

◆ Know about the tests for perming and neutralizing

◆ Understand the basic science for perming and neutralizing

◆ Know the products, equipment and their uses

◆ Understand perming and neutralizing techniques and problems

◆ Know how to provide aftercare advice to clients

KEY TERMS

acid wave
ammonium thioglycolate
brick wind
cold wave lotions
directional wind
disulphide bonds
end papers
exothermic perms

fish-hooked
hair (and skin) tests
incompatible
neutralizer
nine-section wind
perm solution
post-damping
post-perm treatment

polypeptide chain
pre-damping
pre-perming treatment
reducing agent
skin tests
spiral wind

Unit topic

Perm and neutralize hair.

INTRODUCTION

Ask one hundred clients with finer hair types what they really want and 90 per cent will say 'lasting volume'. There is only one service in hairdressing or barbering that can deliver this and that is the permanent wave.

Perming is a complex technical operation that many people get wrong – it involves the accurate and careful:

◆ Evaluation of the client's needs in relation to lift, volume or curl.

◆ Matching perming products to the client's hair.

◆ Sectioning of hair and positioning and winding the perming rods.

◆ Application of potentially damaging acid and alkali chemicals.

◆ Neutralizing and rebalancing the hair at the end of the process.

◆ Explanation and advice for clients on how they can manage their *new* hair.

If you can get all of the above right, then no-one will ever know that the hair has been permed. But people seldom do, they tend to cut corners by using the wrong size curlers or the wrong lotions, they leave the development too long, or they haven't explained to the client, what they need to do. The simplest mistake of all is down to poor advice, because in order for the client to achieve a new look, they need to be able to change the ways and routines that they normally use to maintain their hair. It is because of this single factor that perming has *fallen by the wayside*. People don't like change and they find it hard to change the ways that they do things and with perming – like hair extensions – they have to.

Successful perming relies *heavily* upon having good knowledge and the experience in knowing how different hair textures, types and densities will react when the perm is applied. Without this knowledge, the only thing that can be guaranteed is failure, but like many things in life, it is easy when you know how.

Perm and neutralize hair

PRACTICAL SKILLS

Learn how to carry out a consultation before the service

Preparing yourself and your client correctly

Recognizing contra-indications during consultation

Providing advice to clients about their hair

Maintaining accurate client records

Carrying out a variety of perming and neutralizing methods and techniques

Providing advice to your client about how to maintain their hair between salon visits

Learn how to monitor the perming process

UNDERPINNING KNOWLEDGE

Learn about the salon's perming products

Learn how to recognize hair and skin conditions, defects and disorders

Learn how to recognize contra-indications and other things that can affect intended services

Learn about the tools and equipment that you can use for perming

Learn about hair tests and how they affect perming services

Learn about the effects of perming products upon different types of hair

Learn about the pH scale and how different pH levels affect hair and skin

How does perming work?

Go to **CHAPTER 8** Style and finish hair for more information on temporary and permanent bonds.

In the styling chapter we looked at the different bonds within the **polypeptide chains** of the hair and their properties. If you look back again at the chapter, you will see that there are *temporary bonds*, i.e. those that are broken during shampooing, and *permanent bonds*, i.e. those that are not affected. The permanent linkages, i.e. **disulphide bonds** are only changed during perming or relaxing. The chemicals used in these services, will change the natural, physical tendency of the hair.

Polypeptide chains and disulphide cross links

The polypeptide chains have three different cross-linkages or bonds that join them to other polypeptide chains.

Two of them: The Salt bonds and Hydrogen bonds are temporary and are broken down when the hair is wet.

One other: The Disulphide bond is permanent and is only changed during chemical services such as perming and relaxing.

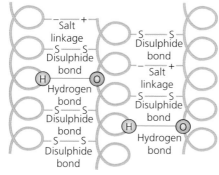

Polypeptide chain   Polypeptide chain   Polypeptide chain

Each disulphide bond is a chemical bond linking two sulphur atoms, between two poly-peptide chains lying alongside each other. During perming, some of these links or bridges are chemically broken, making the hair softer and more pliable, allowing it to be moved into a new position of wave or curl. Only 10 per cent to 25 per cent (depending on lotion strength) of the disulphide bridges are broken during the action of perming. If too many are broken, the hair is damaged permanently.

The principle of perming

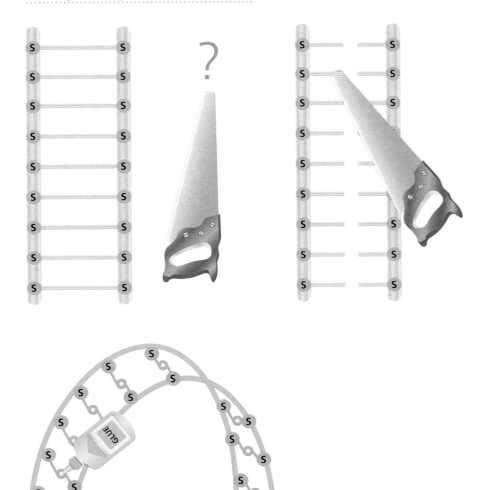

The illustration above tries to explain it in another way:

1   The ladder represents the hair and disulphide bonds as rungs holding the ladder together.

2   When perm lotion is applied, the rungs/disulphide bonds are broken.

3   During perming, the hair is bent around a curler. The disulphide bonds are then re-formed in the neutralizing process, into their new locations; permanently waving the hair.

The science version

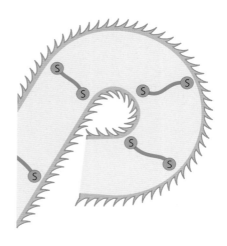

Disulphide bridges

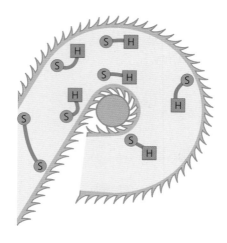

Reduction: breaking disulphide bridges

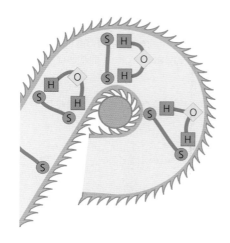

Oxidation: Forming new disulphide bridges

Knowledge Check

Science of the permanent wave

1   The hair is first wound with tension on to a curler or rod. This is the moulding stage. Then you apply perm lotion to the hair, which makes it swell. The lotion flows under the cuticle and into the cortex. Here it reacts with the keratin, breaking some of the disulphide bonds between the polypeptide chains. This softening stage allows the tensioned hair to take up the shape of the curler: you then rinse away the perm lotion and neutralize the hair. This fixing stage permanently rearranges the disulphide bonds into the new shape.

2   This process can also be described in chemical terms. The softening part that breaks some of the cross-links is a process of reduction. The disulphide bridges are split by the addition of hydrogen from the perm lotion – The chemical in the perm lotion that supplies the hydrogen is a **reducing agent**. The keratin is now stretched in its waved/curled state.

3   The final part of the process, the fixing stage, re-creates the bonds, *but now at different positions* between polypeptide chains. This occurs when oxygen is introduced during the neutralizing process as it readily links with the hydrogen atoms within the hair – the chemical in the **neutralizer** that supplies the oxygen is called an oxidizing agent or oxidizer.

Safe effective methods of working

Protect the client

Gowning   **Perm solution** is normally applied by post-damping – where the lotion is applied and absorbed into previously wound sections of hair – the solutions tend to be very watery and mobile. This, potentially, could be a hazard to the client unless you take adequate precautions. The majority of perm lotions are alkaline. If they drip or soak into clothing, they will be held against the skin. This is potentially very dangerous as it could cause irritation, swelling and even chemical burns!

Make sure that you protect your client well so that this never happens. Put on a chemical-proof gown and secure into place, a clean, fresh towel around their shoulders. On top of this, you should fix a plastic cape, ensuring that it is comfortable around the neck.

Barrier cream After gowning, you can now apply the barrier cream to the hairline.

Protect yourself Your salon must provide all the personal protective equipment (PPE) that you may need in routine daily practices. Perming involves the handling and application of chemicals, so this is one of those occasions where you have a duty to protect yourself from their hazardous effects. Always read the manufacturer's instructions and follow the methods of practice that they specify.

Minimize waste Get into the habit of not being wasteful, all the resources that you use cost money and the only way that you can be more effective is to make the most of your time. Think about what goes down the sink; water is the first thing that comes to mind.

All business premises have metered water so, in principle, every shampoo and conditioning rinse can be a calculated cost. But sometimes people rinse far longer than they need to or leave taps running between shampoos and that's where the additional cost mounts up. This is even worse if the water is hot – we've now got the additional cost of heating it too!

Different types of perm

A perm is a major change for a client – they will have to live and cope with the result and its effects for months. Choosing the right sort of lotion to match the client's needs is very important as there are several different types of perming lotions and each type comes in a variety of different applications for resistant, normal coloured and lightened hair. There are even perms that are suitable for highlighted hair, i.e. a perm that is able to differentiate between lightened, coloured and normal hair on the same head!

As you can see, the chemistry can be very complex and can do a job where the hair isn't over-processed or damaged during the service.

- **Cold wave lotions** contain an alkaline compound called **ammonium thioglycolate**. These types of perm are most widely available and simplest to use with applications for all hair types and tendencies and most conditions. These solutions tend to have a pH at around 9.0 so they are a fairly strong alkali that will swell the hair and affect around 20 per cent of the disulphide bridges. They reduce the natural moisture levels within the hair and are therefore better on normal to greasy hair types. They are particularly good for achieving strong, pronounced movement and curl and therefore create lasting effects that can withstand the high maintenance of regular blow-drying, setting etc.

- **Acid wave** lotions provide alternatives for perming when the hair is particularly delicate and needs to retain higher moisture levels or requires softer, gentler movement. They have lower pH values at around 6–7 and are therefore much gentler in the way that they work. They are suited to drier, more porous hair types too. Acid perms are two-part solutions and require the components to be mixed together just before application so that the perm is self-activated.

TOP TIP

Barrier cream applied around the hairline will also help prevent the action of chemicals harming the client during processing.

HEALTH & SAFETY

You are obliged to wear and use the PPE provided for you, these being disposable non-latex gloves, a waterproof apron and barrier cream.

HEALTH & SAFETY

Remove and dispose of waste items as soon as possible. Don't leave cotton neck wool, plastic caps, etc. around at the basins. Put them into a covered bin. Wash, dry and replace perm curlers back into the trays as soon as possible.

HEALTH & SAFETY

Your salon will provide disposable vinyl gloves for your personal safety when you are handling any chemicals in the workplace.

HEALTH & SAFETY

Dermatitis is an occupational hazard for hairdressers. You reduce the risk by wearing vinyl gloves when using chemicals. The gloves provide you with a guaranteed barrier against the action of harsh chemicals upon the skin.

Go to CHAPTER 6 Consultation p. 144, for more information on consultation techniques.

◆ **Exothermic perms** tend to be similar to acid waves in their chemical composition and therefore can have similar benefits. The only difference is that these perms need heat in order to work and this is self-generated when the perm is mixed together before applying to the hair/curlers.

Preparing for perming and neutralizing

Consultation

The consultation for perming would follow the same procedures as that for other services.

Knowledge Check

The Control of Substances Hazardous to Health Regulations 2003

1   The Control of Substances Hazardous to Health Regulations (COSHH) 2003 lay out the potential risks that hairdressing chemicals can have. You need to make yourself aware of the information provided by the manufacturers about their handling, storage and safe disposal. Generally, perm solutions should be stored in an upright position, in a cool, dry place away from strong sunlight. When they are used, they should be applied in a well ventilated area and if there is any waste – materials that cannot be saved and used another time – it should be disposed of by flushing down the basin with copious amounts of cold water.

You will need to consider:

◆ The hair and style requirements – does it warrant or need permanent support?

◆ Any signs or contra-indications to perming – is there any hair damage or condition issues, hair or scalp disorders, diseases, lifestyle requirements?

◆ **Hair tests** – have you conducted the necessary hair tests and looked at the client's treatment history?

◆ **Skin tests** – have you conducted the necessary skin tests and looked at the client's treatment history?

◆ Suitable perms – what are the client's expectations and which type of perm would be appropriate?

◆ Costs – have you explained the costs and benefits to the client?

◆ Home care and maintenance – have you explained how the client's hair should be handled and maintained between salon visits?

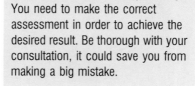

BEST PRACTICE

You need to make the correct assessment in order to achieve the desired result. Be thorough with your consultation, it could save you from making a big mistake.

Things to look for

Contra-indications for perming	
The following list indicates situations when perming should **not** be undertaken	
Hair condition	◆ Particularly porous – possibly coloured, or lightened. ◆ Hair is weakened, broken or damaged. ◆ Hair fails an elasticity test or has low elastic properties. ◆ Incompatible chemicals are present on the hair – *Just for Men*, *Grecian 2000*, compound henna, etc. ◆ Varied levels of porosity throughout the lengths – poorly co-loured or lightened.
Scalp condition	◆ Clear indications of abrasions or sensitive areas. ◆ Evidence of physical or chemical changes on the hair or scalp. ◆ Evidence of scalp disease or disorder.
Lifestyle	◆ Client has neither the time nor the ability to style their hair carefully. ◆ Client is not prepared to maintain their perm with the correct recommended products. ◆ Client swims a lot in public (chlorinated) pools.
General	◆ Client is considering other chemical processes before or after a perm – other chemical services can have a severe detrimental effect on the quality of the hair and the durability of the perm. ◆ Client has existing medical conditions that may affect the out-come.

Analysis/examination

During your consultation, look for the following and consider your options for perming:

◆ **Hair texture** – For medium textured hair, use perm lotion of normal strength. Fine hair curls more easily and requires weaker lotion. Coarser hair can often be more difficult to wave and may require a stronger lotion for resistant hair, although this is not true with Oriental hair.

◆ **Hair porosity** – The porosity of the hair determines how quickly the perm lotion is absorbed. Porous hair in poor condition is likely to process more quickly than would hair with a resistant, smooth cuticle.

◆ **Previous treatment history** – 'Virgin' hair – hair that has not previously been treated with chemicals – is likely to be more resistant to perming than hair that has been treated. It will require a stronger lotion and possibly a longer processing time.

◆ **Length and density of hair** – Longer, heavier hair generally requires a firmer or tighter curl than shorter hair because the hair's weight will cause it to stretch. Short, fine hair can become too tightly curled if given the normal processing time.

HEALTH & SAFETY

Some medical conditions affect the way that hair responds. For example, clients with thyroid problems may find that perms don't seem to take properly or are not long-lasting.

Go to p. 414 Pre-perming treatments, later in this chapter for more information on hair porosity.

Go to p. 413 Hair tests, for more information on making a test curl.

HEALTH & SAFETY

Clients that have been taking health supplements such as cod liver oil over long periods of time will notice an effect on the way that the perm takes in the hair. When cod liver oil supplements are taken, increased levels of moisture are deposited.

◆ **Style** – Does the style require firm curls or soft, loose waves or just body and bounce?

◆ **Size of rod, curler** – Larger rods produce larger curls or waves, whereas smaller rods produce tighter curls. Longer hair generally requires larger rods. If you use very small rods in fine, easy-to-perm hair, the hair may frizz. If you use rods that are too large you may not add enough curl.

◆ **Incompatibility** – Perm lotions and other chemicals used on the hair may react with chemicals that have already been used – for example, in home-use products. Hair that looks dull may have been treated with such chemicals. Ask your client what products are used at home and test for incompatibility.

Other things to find out

Things that the client needs or will want to know

◆ How long will it last?

◆ Is perming suitable for their hair type, condition and texture?

◆ Is perming a cost effective solution for them?

◆ How much will it cost?

◆ How will it affect the hair?

◆ What are the long-term effects and handling issues for the client?

Things that you need to know

◆ What are the client's expectations?

◆ How will the perm enhance or support the style and the hair?

◆ What are the benefits for them?

◆ What are the results of your tests?

◆ Examine the hair – does it present any limitations for what you intend to do?

◆ What is the hair condition like?

◆ Are there any factors that will change the way in which perming will work on the hair?

◆ What previous information is available?

◆ What do the client's records say?

◆ Does this information influence/affect the choice and perm process?

◆ How will you show the effect to the client?

◆ Have you got any images/pictures of the finished effect?

◆ How long will the process take?

◆ Is there enough time to complete the effect?

◆ Has anything changed as a result of the consultation?

◆ Would this service now need to be re-booked or do you still have the time to complete it?

TOP TIP

Always record the details of the consultation/service for future reference.

Perm related tests

Test	What happens?	How is it done?
Elasticity test	◆ This tests the tensile strength of the hair. Hair in good condition has the ability to stretch and return to its original length, whereas hair in poor or damaged condition will stretch and will not return to original length. This lack of elasticity will make the hair difficult to manage and maintain. A clear indication for this would be to ask the client how long their set or blow-dry lasts after it has been done. When the styling drops or can't be sustained in the hair, it is a clear indication that the hair has lost this vital attribute of elasticity.	◆ Take a single hair strand and hold firmly at either end then stretch between your fingers. If it breaks easily, the cortex may be damaged and perming could be harmful.
Porosity test	◆ The purpose of this test is to find out how well protected the inner cortex is by the cuticle layers. Porous hair has a damaged cuticle layer and readily absorbs moisture. This presents a problem when drying, as this hair takes longer to dry and often lacks the ability to hold a style well.	◆ Do this by taking a small section of dry hair and sliding from the points, through to the roots, between your fingertips; you can then feel how rough or smooth it is. Rougher hair – as opposed to coarse hair – is likely to be more porous, and will therefore process more quickly.
Incompatibility test	◆ Hairdressing products are formulated from *organic chemistry*. These are incompatible with inorganic chemistry compositions and will cause damage to the client's hair. This test will identify whether metallic salts are present within the hair, a clear contra-indication that the perm may be carried out.	◆ Protect your hands by wearing disposable gloves. ◆ Place a small cutting of hair in a mixture of one part 6 per cent hydrogen peroxide and 20 parts ammonium thyioglycolate. Watch for signs of bubbling; heating or discolouration: these indicate that the hair already contains incompatible chemicals. ◆ The hair should not be permed, nor should it be coloured or lightened. Perming treatment might discolour or break the hair, and might burn the skin.
Pre-perm test curl	◆ If you are unsure about how your client's hair will react under processing you could conduct a pre-perm test curl – Sometimes this can be done on the head and in other situations where there isn't sufficient time etc. you will need to cut a sample for testing.	◆ Wind, process and neutralize one or more small sections of hair. The results will be a guide to the optimum rod size, the processing time and the lotion strength. Remember, hair needn't have the same porosity along its entire length.
Development test curl	◆ This test is always carried out after the hair has been damped with perm solution and during the processing time. ◆ This test determines the curl development so that the processing can be stopped when the hair reaches its optimal stage this is at the point where the desired curl has been achieved and before there is any damage to the hair.	◆ Unwind – and then rewind – rods during processing, to see how the curl is developing. If the salon is very hot or cold, this will affect the progress of the perm – heat will accelerate it, cold will slow it down. When you have achieved the 'S' shape you want, stop the perm by rinsing and then neutralizing the hair.

Recording the results Make sure that you record the details of any test that you conduct. Update the client's record card immediately after you have done the test. Don't leave it until later, you might forget! These records are essential information and may be needed again for future use.

Pre-perm and post-perm treatments

Matching the correct perm lotion to hair type is an essential part of the hair analysis. However, many perming solutions come in only a coloured, normal, or resistant formula and this alone will not be sufficient for all hair conditions. Dry, porous hair will absorb perming solutions more readily, therefore, special attention needs to be given. **Pre-perming treatments** are a way to prepare the hair, as slightly porous hair may have an uneven porosity throughout the lengths. Hair that is nearer the root will have a different porosity level to that at mid-length hair, or that of the ends. Therefore, the hair's porosity levels will need to be balanced before the perm lotion is applied. This enables the hair to absorb perm lotion at the same rate, evening out the development process and ensuring that the perm doesn't over-process in certain areas.

TOP TIP

A pre-perming treatment is applied before winding on damp hair and combed through to the ends.

TOP TIP

Temperature has a major impact on perming. This could be general salon temperature or by added heat from a hood dryer. In either case remember that processing times will be reduced considerably.

After perming and neutralizing, it is also necessary to rebalance the hair's pH value back to that of 5.6. **Post-perm treatments** do this by removing any traces of residual oxygen from the neutralizing process.

Preparing to perm

1 Prepare your trolley.

2 Protect your client with a gown and towels.

3 Shampoo the hair to remove grease or dirt with a pre-perming, soapless shampoo – failure to remove build-up of styling products could block the action of the perm lotion.

4 Towel-dry the hair – excess water/moisture will dilute the lotion, but if the hair is too dry the perm lotion won't spread evenly through the hair.

5 Apply a pre-perm lotion to help even out porosity – if the hair needs it. Make sure you have read the instructions carefully. Too much pre-perm lotion may block the action of the perm itself.

6 Check that your client's skin and clothing are adequately protected.

Tools and equipment

◆ **Rods or curlers** Choose the correct sizes

◆ **End papers,** For use while winding

◆ **A tail comb and clips** For sectioning and dividing

◆ **Cotton (neck) wool strips** To protect your client

◆ **Disposable vinyl gloves** To protect your hands

◆ **Perm lotion and a suitable neutralizer/normalizer** For perming and neutralizing the hair. Make sure that you read the instructions carefully

◆ **A water spray** To keep the hair damp

◆ **A plastic cap and a timer** For the processing stage

◆ **Barrier cream** For the hairline

◆ **Tensioning strips** To bridge between curlers keeping the rubbers away from damaging the hair

Winding techniques

In order to produce an even curl result the hair must be permed in a tidy, logical order. When sectioning is done properly, it makes the rest of the process simple and quick, but when not, you would have to re-section the hair during the perm, and this may spoil the overall result.

Step-by-step – nine-section perm wind

◆ Following shampooing and towel-drying, comb the hair to remove any tangles.

◆ Make sure you have the tools you will need, including a curler to check the width of the section size.

◆ Now divide the hair into nine sections, as follows (use clips to secure the hair as you work):

◆ divide the hair from ear to ear to give front hair and back hair.

◆ divide the back hair into lower, nape hair and upper top back hair.

◆ divide the front hair, approximately above the mid-eyebrow, to give a middle and two sides.

◆ divide the top section along the same lines, to give a middle and two sides.

◆ divide the nape section likewise, to give a middle and two sides.

Once the hair has been divided into the **nine-section wind** and firmly secured with clips you can start to wind in the perm rods. The diagram on sectioning shows these sections, the numbering refers to the order in which the sections are wound. You start winding at the occipital area down the back of the head in an organized and controlled way. The sectioning techniques for perming can be adapted and used for many other techniques.

Six-section wind In the figure above – the six-section winding technique amalgamates the zones 5 and 2, 4 and 1 and 6 and 3, to form only three rear panels at the back of the head. This means that the wind is started centrally, at the top rather than halfway down the back. This is easier to manage than the nine-section wind, although it will take a little more care in sectioning accurately.

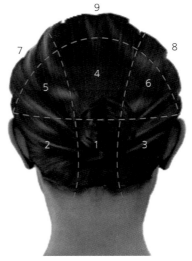

Sectioning nine-section wind

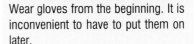

BEST PRACTICE

Wear gloves from the beginning. It is inconvenient to have to put them on later.

Go to p. 418 on winding techniques below for more information on directional and brick-type winding.

TOP TIP

Note that the tension of the held section is even throughout. There should be no slack or pulling from one side to the other.

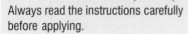

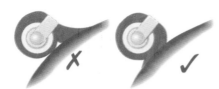

BEST PRACTICE

Always read the instructions carefully before applying.

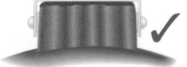

Step-by-step – winding

1 Divide off a section of hair, of a length and thickness to match the curler being used – see the diagram above.

2 Comb the hair firmly, directly away from the head. Keep the hair together, so that it doesn't slip.

3 Place the hair points at the centre of the curler. Make sure the hair isn't bunched at one side and loose at the other.

4 Hold the hair directly away from the head. If you let the hair slope downwards, the curler won't sit centrally on the base section: hair will overlap, and the curler will rest on the skin.

5 Before winding, make sure the curler is at an angle suited to the part of the head against which it will rest when wound.

Knowledge Check

The **National Occupational Standards (NOS)** for hairdressing at Diploma Level 2 require demonstration of a *nine-section*, directional and brick winding technique. The latter is a quicker version and is more commonly used in salons.

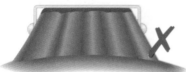

6 Hold the hair points with the finger and thumb of one hand. The thumb should be uppermost.

7 Direct the hair points round and under the curler. Turn your wrist to achieve this. The aim is to lock the points under the curler and against the main body of hair – if they don't lock, they may become 'buckled' or '**fish-hooked**'. Don't turn the thumb too far round or the hair will be pushed away from the curler and won't lock the points.

8 After making the first turn of the curler pass it to the other hand to make the next turn. The hands need to be in complete control: uncontrolled movement, or rocking from side to side, may cause the ends to slip, the hair to bunch or the firmness to slacken.

9 After two or three turns the points will be securely locked. Wind the curler down to the head. Keep the curler level – if it wobbles from side to side, the hair may slip off or the result may look uneven.

10 At the end, the curler should be in the centre of the section. If it isn't, unwind it and start again.

11 Secure the curler. Don't let the rubber fastener press into the hair – it might damage it.

STEP-BY-STEP: WINDING

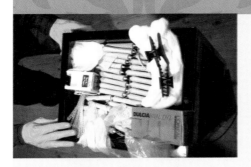

1 Prepare a trolley with all the correct perming equipment:

Clips, cotton wool, perm curlers, perm solution, plastic cap, pin-tail comb, water spray and end papers.

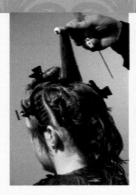

2 For a standard, 6 section wind, divide off the hair into areas of equal proportions. Each area needs to be no wider than the size of the curler.

Start the perm wind with a horizontally positioned curler, just under the crown.

Take a section no wider or deeper than the curler

Comb the hair with an even tension and place an end paper around the ends and extending beyond the points of the hair

Wind the curler down with an even tension and secure the hair by fixing the band across.

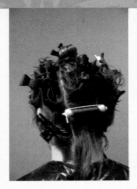

3 Continue to wind the complete back section down to the nape.

Keep the hair moistened (but not saturated) as you work.

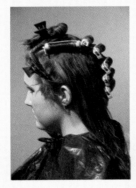

4 Moving around to the side, start again at the top and fix your first curler.

Continue down to the nape and then complete both sides in the same way.

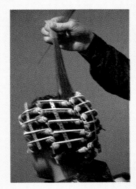

5 The last section on a standard layered hairstyle would normally be the top (particularly if body and curl was needed on top).

Continue through to the front.

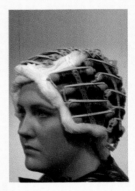

6 When the perm wind is finished, you can place cotton neck-wool around the hairline to protect the client from any drips.

Perm bridges can then be used to lift the rubber bands away from the hair, as this removes any 'crimping'.

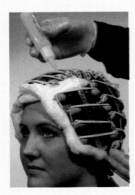

7 Prepare the correct lotion and apply directly to the curlers, ensuring that only a 'thin ribbon' of solution dampens the hair.

Go all over the curlers at least twice.

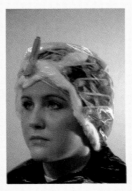

8 Carefully place a plastic cap on, and around the curlers and twist and fix with another curler.

Check that the client is comfortable and leave to develop (with or without heat and for the manufacturer's recommended timings).

Check the development and when ready, start the neutralizing process.

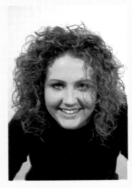

9 Finished effect.

Other winding techniques There are various winding techniques, used to produce varied effects. The following are the most commonly used.

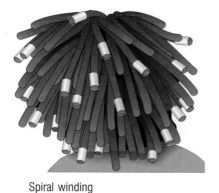

Spiral winding

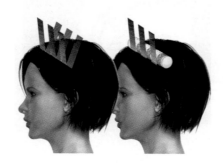

Weaving winding

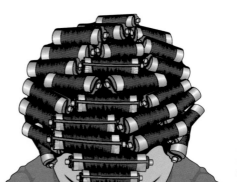

Staggered or brick winding

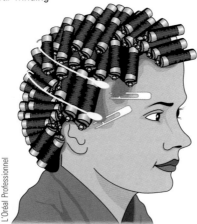

Directional winding

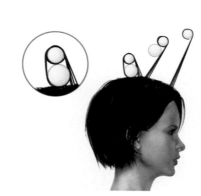

Double winding

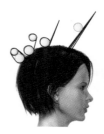
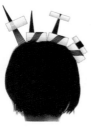

Piggyback winding

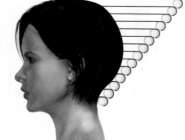

Stack winding

Directional winding – Like directional winding in setting, the perm is wound in the direction in which it is to be finally styled. This technique is suitable for shorter hairstyles, as the root movement created is able to support the weight of the hair.

Brick winding – Again like 'brick winding' in setting, the perm curlers are placed in a pattern resembling brickwork. The benefit of using this method relates to the staggering of the partings, as by doing this you avoid creating gaps in the hair. This technique is suitable for short hairstyles.

Spiral winding – This is a technique for long hair, to produce cascading curls. The technique can be done with conventional curlers, but is best suited to spiral curlers or sponge 'bendy' rollers. These curlers are placed in the hair in a *vertical plane*, which allows the hair to fall in spiralled shapes.

Perming tools and equipment

Tools and equipment

- ◆ **Pin-tail comb** The parallel, metal pin-tail comb is better for sectioning than a plastic tail comb as you can achieve cleaner, neater sections.

- ◆ **End papers** Fibre end papers are standard throughout the industry and have replaced the 'old-fashioned' tissue type. Fibre papers absorb lotion/neutralizer better than tissue and this will give a better end curl. Make sure before you start that you have enough to complete the work.

- ◆ **Plastic rod curlers** These are the most commonly used and can be either solid in their construction or hollow, which allows a better flow of lotion, water or neutralizer through them.

  Sizes are graded in order of colour and will range from minute, **green** curlers to extra-large **black** curlers.

- ◆ **Spiral winders** These are longer in length than the standard curler and this allows for them to be used on longer length hair. They can be solid in construction, forming a uniform shape throughout their length, or foam-covered bendable rollers for a comfortable and easy application.

- ◆ **Bowl and sponge** Whereas perms are normally applied directly from a bottle to the wound hair, neutralizer is often applied with a sponge. The benefits for this allow the sponge to foam up the lotion, creating stiffer foam that stays where it is applied, rather than using a watery solution.

- ◆ **Neck wool** Essential PPE for the client. It is applied all around the hairline before the lotions are applied so that any drips of perm lotion or neutralizer don't make contact with the client's skin or clothes.

Processing and development

Perm lotion may be applied before winding (pre-damping) or when winding is complete (post-damping).

Pre-damping can be used on long hair to ensure the solution penetrates evenly through the hair length. When pre-damping, you have to work quickly to avoid over-processing the hair. Your work should be complete within 35 minutes. Follow the manufacturer's instructions on the type of application to use.

Post-damping is the normal and accepted and more convenient way to work, as you can wind the hair **without wearing gloves** and the time taken in winding doesn't affect the overall processing time.

TOP TIP

Dry cotton neck wool is not as absorbent as slightly moistened cotton wool.

TOP TIP

Never try to damp down without cotton neck wool.

Applying the perm lotion All contemporary perming systems are individually packed, ready for direct application to the hair. Historically, the bulk bought lotions were dispensed from large bottles into a bowl and applied using cotton wool, a sponge, or a brush.

- ◆ Underlying hair is often more resistant to perming – e.g. at the nape of the neck – so you could apply lotion to those areas first.

- ◆ Keep lotion away from the scalp. Apply it to the hair section, about 12mm from the roots.

- ◆ If post-damping, apply a small amount of the perm lotion to each rod – do not over-saturate as the lotion will flood onto the scalp and will drip on to the client. This could cause either irritation or burning on the scalp or skin.

- ◆ It is better to apply the lotion again once the first application has started to absorb into the hair.

Go to **p. 413** for more information on the development of a test curl.

HEALTH & SAFETY

Take care not to splash your client's face while rinsing. Even dilute perm lotion can irritate the skin. If perm lotion enters the client's eye, flush out immediately with cold running water. Ensure the water drains downwards away from the face. Seek help.

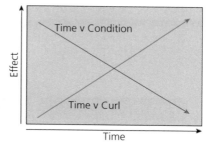

HEALTH & SAFETY

Time is proportional to damage, you must check the perm and stop the development at the correct point.

Go to **p. 423** for more information on timing the perm and developing the test curl.

◆ Don't overload the applicator and apply the lotion gently. You will be less likely then to splash your client.

◆ If you do splash the skin, quickly rinse the lotion away with water.

Processing – factors and timings Processing begins as soon as the perm lotion is in contact with the hair and this timing is critical. Processing time is affected by the hair texture and condition, the salon temperature and whether heat is applied, the size and number of curlers used and the type of winding used.

The perm needs to be checked during the development so that over-processing is avoided. The optimum processing ensures that the curl is maximized while there is no detrimental effect to the hair condition.

The figure below shows two intersecting lines; both have a time element, but each one has a different resultant effect. The green line has an increase in curl development over time, where the red line has a decrease in hair condition/damage over time. Ideally, where the two lines cross, it will denote the optimum perm processing. At this point a curl development check will show a good 'S' movement without loss of essential hair moisture/and subsequent impaired condition.

Hair texture and condition Fine hair processes more quickly than coarse hair and dry hair more than greasy hair. Hair that has been processed previously will perm faster than virgin hair.

Temperature A warm salon cuts down processing time – in a cold salon it will take longer. Even a draught from an open window will affect the time required. Usually the heat from the head itself is enough to activate perming systems. Wrap your client's head with plastic cap to keep in the heat. Don't wrap the hair in towels as these will absorb the lotion and slow down the processing.

Some perm lotions require additional heat from computerized accelerators, Rollerball™ or dryers. Don't apply heat unless the manufacturer's instructions tell you to – you might damage both the hair and the scalp. And don't apply heat unless the hair is wrapped, as the heat could evaporate the lotion or speed up the processing too much.

Curlers Processing will be quicker with a lot of small sections on small curlers than with large sections on large curlers – the large sections will also give looser results.

Winding The type of winding used, and the tension applied, can also affect processing time. Hair wound firmly processes faster than hair wound slackly – in fact, if the winding is too slack it will not process at all. Hair wound too tightly may break close to the scalp. The optimum is a firm winding without tension.

Neutralizing

Introduction

The successful outcome of a perm is dependent on the correct processing and the way the hair is re-balanced during the action of neutralizing.

In this section we will look at:

1 The principles of neutralizing perms.

2 How neutralizing works.

3   Choosing a neutralizer.

4   Neutralizing techniques.

5   What to do after perming.

Re-balancing the hair

Neutralizing is the process of fixing the curl or movement into the hair, while returning the hair back to a balanced chemical state. An industry term, 'neutralizing' is a little misleading. In chemistry, a 'neutral' chemical condition is neither acidic nor alkaline (pH 7.0). During neutralizing, the (previously) processed hair is returned to the skin's healthy, slightly acidic natural state of pH 5.6. Re-balancing the pH value of the hair is essential for maintaining hair in good condition. If the hair is not re-balanced the hair will be dry, porous and the perm will be very difficult to manage afterwards.

How neutralizing works   As described earlier, perm lotion acts on the keratin in the hair. The strongest bonds between the polypeptides are the disulphide bonds. Perm lotion breaks some of these, allowing the keratin to take up a new shape. This is how new curls can form.

Neutralizing re-builds new disulphide bonds on new sites along the polypeptide chains. If you didn't neutralize the hair it would be weak and likely to break, and the new curls would soon fall out.

Choosing a neutralizer   Perming lotions are produced with matching neutralizers – they are designed to work together so that the chemical pH values can be re-balanced accurately. Always use the neutralizer that matches the perm lotion you've used.

A neutralizer may be supplied as an emulsion cream, a foam, or a liquid. Always follow the manufacturer's instructions. Some can be applied directly from the container, others are applied with a sponge or a brush.

Neutralizing technique   Neutralizing follows directly on from perming. Imagine that you have shampooed, dried and wound the hair. The hair is now perming, and you are timing the perm carefully and making tests to check whether it is complete. You will also be reassuring the client that they have not been forgotten! As soon as the perm is finished, you need to be ready to stop the process immediately.

Preparation

◆   Collect all the materials you will need beforehand.

◆   Make sure there is a basin available for the period needed.

First rinsing

◆   When the perm is ready, move your client to the back wash basin and make sure they are comfortable.

◆   Carefully remove the cap. The hair is in a soft and delicate stage, so don't put unnecessary tension on it. Leave the curlers in place.

◆   Run the water. You need an even supply of warm water. The water must be neither hot, nor cold as this will be uncomfortable for the client. Hot water will also irritate the scalp and could burn.

BEST PRACTICE

Read labels and check contents of boxes – before use.

BEST PRACTICE

Remember to re-balance the pH values of the hair by using an anti-oxidant conditioner.

◆ Check the pressure and temperature against the back of your hand. Remember that your client's head may be sensitive after the perming process.

◆ Rinse the hair thoroughly with the warm water. This may take about five minutes or longer if the hair is long. *The rinsing stops the perm process* – until you rinse away the lotion, the hair will still be processing. Direct the water away from the eyes and the face. Make sure you rinse all the hair, including the nape curlers. If a curler slips out, gently wind the hair back onto it immediately.

Applying neutralizer

◆ Make sure your client is in a comfortable sitting position.

◆ Blot the hair thoroughly using a towel – you may need more than one. It may help if you pack the curlers with cotton wool.

◆ When no surplus water remains, apply the neutralizer. Follow the manufacturer's instructions. These may tell you to pour the neutralizer through the hair, or apply it with a brush or sponge, or use the spiked applicator bottle. Some foam neutralizers need to be pushed into the hair. Make sure that neutralizer comes into contact with all of the hair on the curlers.

◆ When all the neutralizer has been applied, start timing the process according to the manufacturer's instructions.

◆ After, gently and carefully remove the curlers. Don't pull or stretch the hair. It may still be soft, especially towards the ends, and you don't want to disturb the curl formation.

◆ Apply the neutralizer to the hair again, covering all the hair. Arrange the hair so that the neutralizer does not run over the face. Leave for the recommended time.

Second rinsing

◆ Run the water, again checking temperature and pressure.

◆ Rinse the hair thoroughly to remove the neutralizer.

◆ You can now treat the hair with an after-perm (anti-oxidant) or conditioner. Use the one recommended by the manufacturer of the perm and neutralizer, to be sure that the chemicals are compatible.

Anti-oxidant conditioning An anti-oxidant conditioner should now be applied to remove any last traces of chemicals within the hair, they neutralize the effect of the chemical process by helping to restore the pH balance of the hair to pH 4.4–5.5 and smooth down the hair cuticle, improving the hair's look, feel, comb-ability and handling.

After neutralizing At the end of the neutralizing process, you will have returned the hair to a normal, stable state.

◆ The reduction and oxidation processes will have been completed.

◆ The hair will now be slightly weaker – fewer bonds will have formed than were broken by the perm.

◆ Record any hair or perm faults on the client's record card. Correct faults as appropriate.

◆ Under-neutralizing – not leaving neutralizer on for long enough – results in slack curls or waves.

◆ Over-oxidizing – leaving the neutralizer on too long or using oxidants that are too strong – results in weak hair and poor curl.

The hair should be ready for shaping, blow-drying or setting.

Perming faults and remedies

Fault	Action now	Possible cause	In future
The perm is slow to process	◆ Increase warmth but do not dry out. Check the winding tension and the number of curlers.	◆ Winding was too loose. ◆ The curlers were large, or too few were used. ◆ The wrong lotion was used. ◆ The sections were too large. ◆ The salon is too cold. ◆ Lotion was absorbed from the hair. ◆ Too little lotion was used.	◆ Wind more firmly or use smaller curlers. ◆ Use smaller curlers and more of them. ◆ Double-check labels on bottles. ◆ Take smaller sections. ◆ The temperature should be comfortable. ◆ Don't leave cotton wool on the hair. ◆ Don't skimp on the lotion or miss sections.
The scalp is tender, sore or broken	◆ Seek advice from a qualified first-aider.	◆ The curlers were too tight. ◆ The wound curlers rested on the skin. ◆ Lotion was spilt on the scalp. ◆ There was cotton wool padding soaked with perm lotion between the curlers. ◆ The hair was pulled tightly. ◆ The perm was over-processed.	◆ Don't apply too much tension when winding. ◆ Curlers should rest on the hair. ◆ Keep lotion away from the scalp. ◆ Renew the cotton wool as necessary or don't use it. ◆ Don't overstretch it. ◆ Time perms accurately.
There are straight points or roots	◆ Re-perm, if the hair condition permits.*	◆ The curlers or sections were too large. ◆ Sections were overlooked. ◆ Too few curlers were used. ◆ The winding was too loose. ◆ Lotion was applied unevenly.	◆ Take sections no longer or wider than the curler used. ◆ Check that all hair has been wound. ◆ Put curlers closer together. ◆ Be a little firmer next time. ◆ Take care to apply it evenly.
There are 'fish-hooks'	◆ Remove by trimming the ends.	◆ The hair points were not cleanly wound. ◆ The hair points were bent or buckled. ◆ The hair was wrapped unevenly in the end papers. ◆ Winding aids were used incorrectly.	◆ Comb the hair cleanly. ◆ Place hair sections evenly on to the curlers. ◆ Curl from the hair points. ◆ Take more care – practise winding.

(Continued)

(Continued)

Fault	Action now	Possible cause	In future
Hair is broken	◆ Nothing can be done about the broken hair. ◆ After discussion with your senior or trainer, condition the remaining hair.	◆ The hair was wound too tightly. ◆ The curlers were secured too tightly. ◆ The curler band cut into the hair base. ◆ The hair was over-processed. ◆ Chemicals in the hair reacted with the lotion.	◆ Wind more loosely next time. ◆ Secure them more loosely next time. ◆ Keep it away from the hair base. ◆ Follow the instructions more carefully. ◆ Test for incompatibility beforehand.
The hair is straight	◆ Re-perm, if the hair condition permits.*	◆ The wrong lotion was used for hair of this texture. ◆ The hair was under-processed. ◆ The curlers were too large for the hair length. ◆ The neutralizing was incorrectly done. ◆ Rinsing was inadequate. ◆ Conditioners used before perming were still on the hair. ◆ The hair was coated and resistant to the lotion.	◆ Choose the lotion more carefully. ◆ Time perms accurately. ◆ Measure the curlers beforehand. ◆ Follow the instructions more carefully. ◆ Rinse more thoroughly. ◆ Prepare the hair more carefully. ◆ Check for substances that block the action of perm lotion, shampoo if necessary.
The hair is frizzy	◆ Cut the ends to reduce the frizziness.	◆ The lotion was too strong for hair of this texture. ◆ The winding was too tight. ◆ The curlers were too small. ◆ The hair was over-processed. ◆ The neutralizing was incorrectly done. ◆ There are fish-hooks.	◆ Assess texture correctly – select suitable lotions – read manufacturer's instructions. ◆ Practise and experiment to avoid this. ◆ Choose more suitable curlers. ◆ Time perms accurately. ◆ Follow the instructions more carefully. ◆ Avoid bending hair points when winding.
The perm is weak and drops out**	◆ Re-perm, if the hair condition permits.*	◆ Lotion was applied unevenly. ◆ The neutralizer was dilute. ◆ Neutralizing was poorly done. ◆ The hair was stretched while soft. ◆ The curlers or sections were too large.	◆ Apply lotion more evenly. ◆ Follow the instructions more carefully. ◆ Be more careful. ◆ Handle the hair gently. ◆ Use more curlers.

(Continued)

Fault	Action now	Possible cause	In future
Some hair sections are straight	◆ Re-perm if the hair condition permits.*	◆ The curler angle was wrong. ◆ The curlers were placed incorrectly. ◆ The curlers were too large. ◆ Sectioning or winding was done carelessly. ◆ Perm lotion or neutralizer was not applied correctly.	◆ Wind correctly. ◆ Use smaller curlers. ◆ Practise before perming again. ◆ Make sure that all curlers get the correct application of chemicals.
The hair is discoloured		◆ Metallic elements or compounds present.	◆ Test for incompatibility.
Unknown/ unexpected result	◆ Seek assistance from a senior operator/follow their instructions.		◆ Learn from this experience and modify your process accordingly.

*Don't re-perm the hair unless its condition is suitable. For example, you should not re-perm if the hair is over-processed.
Conditioning treatments and/or cutting may help. Discuss the problem with a senior member of staff.

**Before attempting to correct this fault – make sure that the hair is not over-processed. Dampen the hair to see how much perm there is.

Provide aftercare advice

As we have already said at the beginning of this chapter, perming is complex and can only be successful if the clients know what to expect and how they can manage their hair. Clients need your help to look after their hair at home. You need to give them the right advice so that they can make the most of their new perm and style between visits.

Remember to tell them how a new perm needs particular care in the way that it is handled and that stretching during styling will weaken the result and could even cause the perm to fail prematurely.

You should tell them what sorts of products they could use that would benefit the condition and manageability of their hair. You should also make a point of telling them what they should avoid, as some products will work against the new perm.

Explain the benefits of maintaining their hair in good condition, as hair in good condition is easier to manage, it lasts longer, looks better and is noticeable to everyone else as well.

SUMMARY

As a final reflection on what you have covered in this chapter, you should now have a clearer picture of all the essential aspects for perming hair. In particular, you should now have a basic understanding of the key principles of:

1 Why preparation is essential to the service.

2 The contra-indications that are specific to perming hair and the tests that must be performed before the service is provided.

3 The techniques involved for creating different permed effects.

4 How to use and maintain the tools and equipment associated with perming.

5 Providing advice to the clients about how to maintain their perm and their hair's condition.

And collectively, how these principles will enable you to provide a variety of permed effects to your clients.

ASSESSMENT OF KNOWLEDGE AND UNDERSTANDING

Project 1

For this project you will need to collect and test a range of hair samples.

Over a period of time, collect and fix together a variety of different hair samples.

You will need to create three batches of:

◆ grey/white hair

◆ coloured hair

◆ double processed hair

◆ lightened hair

◆ previously permed hair

◆ natural virgin hair.

For each type, record the differences in tendency, texture and condition.

Use a little perm lotion in each scenario.

1 Perm your first batch of samples with the correct/ matched lotion for the correct length of development time with a medium size curler.

2 After you have rinsed and neutralized each one, note any changes in tendency, texture and condition in your portfolio.

3 Repeat the process again with a second batch of samples using:

◆ Tinted lotion on the grey/white hair.

◆ Normal lotion on the tinted, lightened and double processed hair.

◆ Resistant lotion on the previously permed and virgin hair.

Now record your findings again after over-processing the samples and see the differences.

Note: Keep your third batch for a later project with neutralizing.

Project 2

Use the remainder of your hair samples from Project 1. Perm them and prepare them, ready for neutralizing.

Try out different ways of neutralizing. Note the different effects produced and record them for your portfolio. Carry out this project in the following ways:

◆ Without rinsing the hair sample, apply the neutralizer and time as directed by the instructions. What are the effects produced when the hair is still wet and the effects when it has been dried?

◆ Using another permed hair sample, rinse the hair but do not apply any neutralizer. What are the effects produced when the hair is still wet and the effects when it has been dried?

◆ On the third sample, leave out both rinsing and neutralizing phases. What are the effects produced when the hair is still wet and the effects when it has been dried?

◆ Rinse and neutralize the fourth sample as directed by the perm manufacturer. What are the effects produced when the hair is still wet and the effects when it has been dried?

◆ Retain these samples and compare the results when the hair has dried out. Then check again after 12, 24 and 48 hours.

◆ List and try out different types of neutralizer, with varying times of application. Compare the results.

◆ Repeat these experiments using hair of different textures. Make sure that you have a correctly permed and neutralized sample with which to compare your results.

Revision questions

A selection of different types of questions to check your knowledge.

Q1 A development test _____ will identify when optimum movement is achieved.
Fill in the blank

Q2 Cold wave perms are usually post-damped.
True or false

Q3 Which of the following factors are likely to be affected by perming?
Multi selection

Elasticity	☐ 1
Natural colour	☐ 2
Thickness	☐ 3
Texture	☐ 4
Porosity	☐ 5
Abundance	☐ 6

Q4 Neutralizers contain hydrogen peroxide.
True or false

Q5 Which of the following chemical bonds are permanently rearranged during perming?
Multi choice

Salt bonds	○ a
Hydrogen bonds	○ b
Disulphide bonds	○ c
Oxygen bonds	○ d

Q6 Time and temperature have a direct impact upon perm development.
True or false

Q7 Which of the following tests are *not* applicable to perming?
Multi selection

Strand test	☐ 1
Incompatibility test	☐ 2
Peroxide test	☐ 3
Porosity test	☐ 4
Elasticity test	☐ 5
Skin test	☐ 6

Q8 The rearrangement of chemical bonds takes place within the _____ .
Fill in the blank

Q9 The chemical compound responsible for modifying the hair's structure during perming is?
Multi choice

Hydrogen peroxide	○ a
Ammonium hydroxide	○ b
Ammonium thioglycolate	○ c
Sodium perborate	○ d

Q10 Smaller perming rods produce tighter curl effects.
True or false

14 Develop creativity

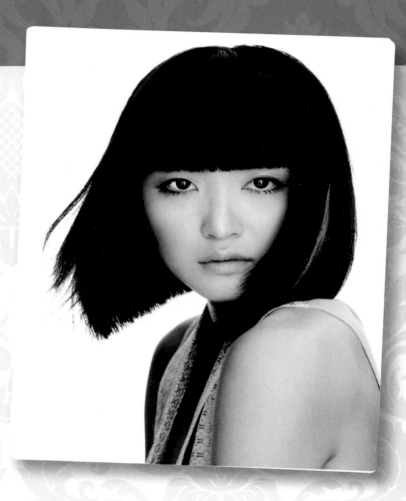

LEARNING OBJECTIVES

◆ Be able to research ideas in relation to themes

◆ Be able to plan and create a mood board

◆ Present your ideas and themes to others

◆ Be able to re-create your ideas as finished hair effects

KEY TERMS

asymmetrical
avant-garde
balance
contrast
emphasis

harmony
mood board
movement
ornamentation
project

proportion
symmetrical
total look

Unit topic

Create and agree original design with hair.

INTRODUCTION

Hair creativity is an everyday, commonly used term that relates to a number of complex things that our clients associate with, such as *artistic interpretation, geometric lines and angles, and the basic concepts of design.* When put into words like that, it sounds like something that we will never grasp. But like many things in life, what things sound like, and what they really are, can be two very different things.

As hairstylists for men or women, we have to develop a number of different skills, but all focused on the same thing.

We need to have:

◆ An appreciation of shape, dimension, image, colour and textures.

◆ An understanding of things that have balance, or imbalance.

◆ The skills to express our creativity by moulding, shaping and forming our client's hair.

◆ The ability to explain our ideas and interpretations to our clients and peers through *mood boards* and other visual media.

Hairstyling involves things that are considered aesthetic, artistic, often scientific, but always practical. The hairstylist who can bring these skills together and can manage to make themselves understood by their clients will always be in demand.

This chapter sets out to capture some of these essential components and will help you to develop your own creativity that you could use with your clients, in competitions, photo shoots and public demonstration.

Developing your creativity

PRACTICAL SKILLS

Designing images based on themes

Creating a mood board to convey ideas in a visual form

Learn how to create images based on themes

Learn how to present ideas to others

UNDERPINNING KNOWLEDGE

Learn the basic principles of design

Learn how colour is used in design

Learn how to resource information and research ideas

Where do I get my creative ideas from?

Inspiration can come from almost anywhere, at any time. Movies, TV, magazines, videos, the Internet, even from someone you see on the street – anything, anywhere can trigger the creative processes. One of the biggest sources for inspiration from popular culture is music and that is because it touches everyone, but in different ways.

Admittedly, you can't *see* music but if you think how it makes you *feel* happy, excited or sad, you can see that something you listen to and hear is able to spark-off other senses such as feelings, memories, hopes and dreams. Many others find inspiration in nature. For example, the perpetual rhythm and movement of ocean waves have inspired painters, poets, composers and hairstylists. The shapes, colours, patterns and textures of plants, animals and minerals are also a great source of visual ideas. At times, you may find yourself looking to the past for inspiration. A hairstyle from an earlier era might inspire you to re-invent it in a way that works for today.

Modern inspiration in fashion often starts on the streets and in the clubs. Hair design usually follows the fashion trends and helps to finish off the **total look**.

Once inspired, you will need to decide which tools such as scissors, razors, clippers, straighteners and tongs you will need. Then you will have to think about which techniques you will use to create the effects too.

It is always a good idea when working out a design to first practise on your modelling block. As you develop or practise a technique, there is always the chance that your original concept will turn into something entirely different. There are no failures if the experience is a lesson learned. If you are open to change, the creative process will be exciting and satisfying.

As a creative stylist, you will need to develop a visual understanding of which hairstyles work best on different face shapes and body types. It takes time and experience to train your eye to recognize the best design elements.

You cannot achieve a trained eye simply through reading this, or any other book and it won't necessarily come from looking at pictures either. It may help you to review these pages repeatedly, but do not lose your patience if it takes a while to understand these concepts.

TOP TIP

The things that you want to do for your clients can be tried out and perfected on your modelling block first.

How is an image created?

Different people understand *image* in different ways. If we look the word up in a reference book, its meaning is given as 'representation, likeness, semblance, form, appearance, configuration and structure'. Collectively, these words form the basic elements of design.

If you don't give yourself the opportunity to experiment and *play* with creative effects, how will you ever improve? Quite simply you can't. You have to learn by experience and that means that sometimes, you will get things wrong. In the beginning, you might find that, in working on your modelling block you have more disasters than successes, but does that matter, your block isn't going to complain or be upset?

Over time, your practise will pay off and you will develop your own set of rules for things that you can and cannot do, or put another way, things that work and things that don't. When you do find success, it is rather like following a recipe. You mix, add and blend various ingredients, which together, combine to take on a new form that is completely different from what we started with. If you follow the recipe, the result is almost guaranteed, but if you do not, then a disaster may occur.

The only difference between you and an experienced stylist is that the experienced stylist can visualize the final effect of what they are trying to create and then work out the process and the things they need to do in a sequential order to achieve that final effect.

All that you need to do at this stage is understand the basic elements of design and how they impact an overall effect.

> **TOP TIP**
>
> Don't expect new things to work immediately, you must be patient as they will take some time to perfect.

The basics of good hair design

To begin to understand the creative process involved in hairstyling, it is critical to learn the five basic elements of three-dimensional design.

These elements are:

- Line
- Form
- Space
- Texture
- Colour

Line

Line defines *form* and *space*. The presence of one, nearly always means that the other two are involved. Lines create the shape, design and movement of a hairstyle. The eye *naturally* follows the lines in a design. They can be straight or curved. There are four basic types of lines:

> **TOP TIP**
>
> The basics of good hair design can be applied to your block. That way you will see how these rules apply to hair.

Horizontal lines Horizontal lines create width in hair design as shown in Figures 15.1 and 15.2. They extend in the same direction and create different levels, or elevations, as well as baselines for frames.

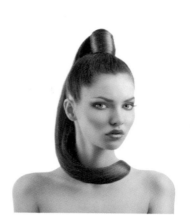

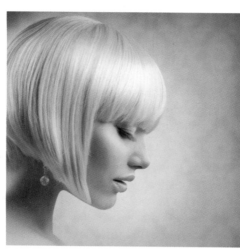

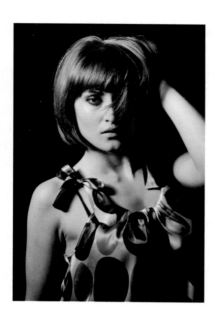

Vertical lines Vertical lines create length, height or depth in hair design. They make a hairstyle appear longer and narrower as the eye follows the lines up and down.

Diagonal lines Diagonal lines are positioned between horizontal and vertical lines. They are used to emphasize and accentuate, or minimize and diminish facial features. They do this by diverting attention from one area or detail and moving the eye line to another. Therefore, diagonal lines can also be used to create interest in hair design.

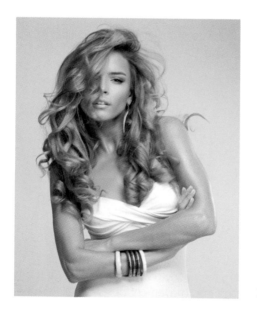

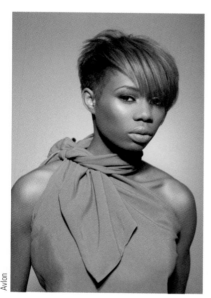

Avlon

Curved lines Curved lines are lines moving in a circular or semi-circular direction, and soften a design. They can be large or small, a full circle or just part of a circle. Curved lines may move in a clockwise or counter-clockwise direction. They can be placed horizontally, vertically or diagonally. Curved lines repeating in opposite directions create a wave.

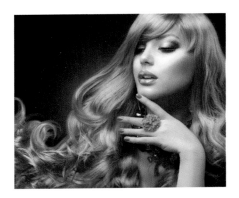 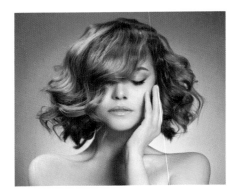

Designing with lines The type of line, direction or combination you choose defines a hairstyle:

◆ *Single lines* An example of this is the one-length hairstyle. These hairstyles produce classic effects and are best for clients requiring the lowest maintenance when styling their hair.

◆ *Parallel lines* are repeating lines in a hairstyle. They can be straight or curved. The repetition of lines creates more interest in the design. A finger wave is an example of a style using a series of curved, parallel lines.

◆ *Contrasting lines* are horizontal and vertical lines that meet at a 90-degree angle. These lines create a dramatic hard edge. Contrasting lines in a design are usually for confident clients who are able to carry off a strong look.

◆ *Transitional lines* are usually curved lines that are used to blend and soften horizontal or vertical lines.

◆ *Convergent or divergent lines* are lines with a definite momentum, with forward or backward movement.

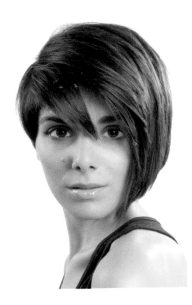 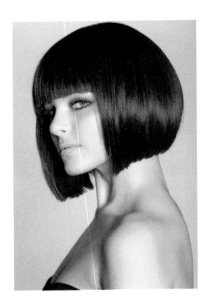 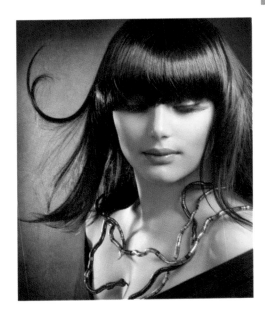

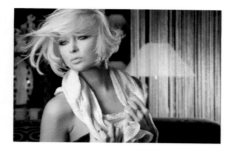

Shape and form

Form is the mass or general outline of a hairstyle. It is three-dimensional and has length, width and depth. Form or shape creates mass, which can also be called volume. The two-dimensional silhouette is usually the part of the overall design that a client will respond to first. These can be in the *negative,* where the outline produces a dark silhouette against a light background, or the reverse, a *positive* as shown in Figure 15.14. Generally, simple forms are best to use and are more pleasing to the eye. The hair form should be in proportion to the shape of the head and face, the length and width of the neck, and the shoulder line.

Space *Space* is the area surrounding the form or the area the hairstyle occupies. We are more aware of the (positive) form than the (negative) spaces. In hair design, with every movement the relationship of the form and space change. A hairstylist must keep every angle in mind; not only of the shapes being created, but of the spaces surrounding the shapes as well. The space may contain curls, curves, waves, straight hair or any combination.

Textural content

Textural content refers to wave patterns that must be taken into consideration when designing a style for your client. All hair has a natural wave pattern: straight, wavy, curly or extremely curly. For example, straight hair reflects light better than other wave patterns, and we see that as shine. It is also worth mentioning that straight hair produces the most shine when it falls as a *single sheet* and is cut to a single length, as shown in Figure 15.16. Wavy hair can be combed into waves that create horizontal lines, as shown in Figure 15.15. Curly hair and extremely curly hair are not able to reflect much light and can sometimes be coarse to the touch. Curly hair creates a larger form than straight or wavy hair does.

> **TOP TIP**
>
> A design line in hair can be created by a cut base line, layer patterning, hair colour or directional movements. Sometimes you need to stand back in order to see the overall effect that these lines have upon your hairstyle.

> **TOP TIP**
>
> Texture in design concepts has a different meaning to texture in reference to the thickness of individual hairs.

Go to **CHAPTER 8** Styling and finishing hair for more information about styling techniques.

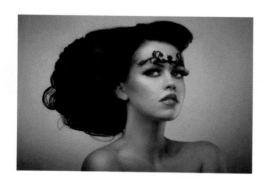

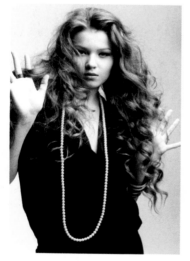

Creating texture with styling tools Texture can be created temporarily with the use of heat and/or wet styling techniques. Hair straighteners, or hot rollers can be used to create a wave or curl. Curly hair can be straightened with a blow-dryer or straightening irons.

Crimpers can be used to create interesting and unusual wave patterns like zigzags. Hair can also be wet-set with rollers or pin curls to create curls and waves. Finger waves, braids and plaits are another way of creating temporary textured pattern changes.

Creating texture with chemicals Wave pattern changes can be permanent through the chemical services of perming and relaxing. They last until the new growth of hair is long enough to alter the design. Curly hair can be made straighter with relaxers and straight hair can be curled with permanent waves.

Tips for designing with wave patterns:

◆ When using many wave pattern combinations together, you create a look that is very busy. This is fine for the client who wants to achieve a multi-textured look, but may be less appropriate for more classic, professional effects.

◆ Smooth wave patterns accent the face and are particularly useful when you want to narrow a rounder head shape.

◆ Curly wave patterns take attention away from the face and can be used to soften square or rectangular features.

Hair colour

Hair colour plays an important role in hair design, both visually and psychologically. It can be used to make all or part of the design appear larger or smaller. Hair colour can help define texture and line, and it can tie design elements together.

Warm and cool tones	
Warm colours/tones	**Cool colours/tones**
Reds – if orange based or tomato red	Reds – if blue or violet based
Oranges	Blues
Yellows – if golden based	Pinks or Beige
Browns	Greys – ashen based colours
	Greens

BEST PRACTICE

The aspects of warm and cool tones have a dramatic effect on the appearance of hair, and if you choose the wrong colour tones for your client, it could be a disaster.

Dimension with colour Light colours and warm colours are *advancing* and demand to be noticed, or create the illusion of volume. Dark and cool colours recede or move *backwards*, toward the head, creating the illusion of less volume. The illusion of dimension, or depth, is created when colours that are lighter alternate with those that are darker.

You should avoid mixing warm and cool colours within the same hair effect, as they are discordant with what the eye *expects to see* and accepts as normal. But if you want to create strong contrasts and you have the model/client with the confidence to wear it, you can produce some very striking effects!

TOP TIP

Colour has an immense effect on the overall aspects of a hairstyle. *Sometimes less is more.*

Lines and linear effects with colours Because the eye is always drawn *naturally* to the lightest colour, you can use a light colour to draw a line in a hairstyle in the direction you want the eye to travel. A single line of colour, or a series of repeated lines of colour, can create a bold, dramatic accent.

To give another explanation of the linear effects of light lines within a hairstyle, the most popular form of colouring over the past 40 years is highlighting. So if you now think of which colour options for highlighting have been the most popular, then lightened highlights always comes out on top.

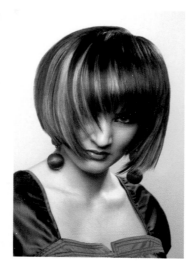

Colour selection The choice of colour for clients is another important aspect to consider. There are two ways of providing colour.

- Harmonizing colour
- Contrasting colour

Most clients want a hair colour that suits them and, therefore, you should choose harmonizing tones as these are colours that are compatible and complementary with the skin tone of the client. For example, if a client has a gold tone to their skin, warm hair colours are more flattering than cool hair colours. Similarly, if a client has an olive skin tone, then cooler colours will be more suitable. For a more conservative or natural look when using two or more colours, choose colours with similar tones within two levels of each other.

Some clients will always want to follow fashion, regardless of whether it suits them or not. And often in these situations, clients are drawn to things that are totally inappropriate. Contrasting effects occur when one colour is placed against another and the result doesn't complement the client, or the colours create stark effects. It doesn't mean that they should never be used, but it does require a bit more thoroughness during consultation, so that these effects can be explained and you can find out if the client has the confidence to wear them.

When using high **contrast** colours in most salon situations, you should use one colour sparingly. A strong contrast can create an attention-grabbing look and should only be used on clients who can carry off a *bold* look and have the confidence to wear it.

Style design

In day to day salon work, hairstylists seldom have the opportunity to let their creativity have a 'free rein' with their clients' hair, contrary to what many hairstylists believe. Day to day 'commercial work' is very routine, even mundane! So having the opportunities to do something really creative are few and far between.

The opportunities tend to come around in certain situations:

1 Your client wants a total re-style and a new colour effect.

2 Through hair demonstrations or promotional activities.

3 When you take part in hair competitions.

What aspects of a hairstyle create a great image?

- Have you ever studied great hair images closely?
- What is it about those images that gives them impact or appeal?

Now, what is it about 'everyday' commercial work that makes it seem routine? You could say that it is make-up or clothes – we could say it is the lighting, or say that it's something to do with the client? All these factors contribute to the final effect, but yet we haven't been looking at the hair.

The hair design elements There are five elements of hair design:

- **Proportion**
- **Balance**

- ◆ Movement
- ◆ Emphasis/accent
- ◆ Harmony

The more you understand about these design elements, the more confident you will feel about creating styles that please your clients and the people that comment about those styles, to your clients.

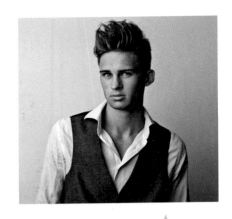

Proportion Proportion is the comparative relationship of one thing to another. For example, a 60-inch television set might be considered out of proportion or scale in a very small bedroom.

Therefore, a person with a very small chin and a very wide forehead might be said to have a head shape that is not in proportion. A well-chosen hairstyle could create the illusion of better proportion for such a client.

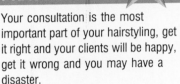

Body proportion Considering your client's body proportions are an essential part of consultation. So the design of a hairstyle must take into account the client's body shape and size. Challenges in body proportion become more obvious if the hair form is too small or too large. When choosing a style for a woman with large hips or broad shoulders, for instance, you would normally create a style with more volume.

But the same large hairstyle would appear out of proportion on a petite woman. A general guide for classic proportion is that the hair should not be wider than the centre of the shoulders, regardless of the body structure.

Balance You can establish balance when equal or appropriate proportions create symmetry. In hairstyling, it can be the proportion of height to width. But balance can be **symmetrical** or **asymmetrical**.

To measure symmetry, divide the face into four equal parts. The lines cross at the central axis, the reference point for judging the balance of the hair design. You can then decide if the hairstyle looks pleasing to the eye and is in correct balance.

Symmetrical balance occurs when an imaginary line is drawn through the centre of the face and the two resulting halves form a mirror image of one another. Both sides of the hairstyle are the same distance from the centre, the same length and have the same volume when viewed from the front.

Balance or imbalance in art The term symmetry or symmetrical refers to things being even, and asymmetry or asymmetrical refers to things being uneven. Therefore consider the following:

- ◆ Does balance relate to symmetry?
- ◆ Does imbalance relate to asymmetry?
- ◆ If balance and symmetry convey harmony, does imbalance and asymmetry portray discord?

The vast majority of commercial work undertaken in salons today leads us, as hairdressers, to ensure that both sides of the haircut are of an even length, that weight is proportionally distributed, and that degrees of curl or straightness are maintained throughout the hairstyle.

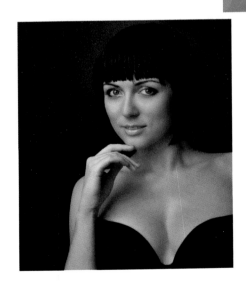

What we are required to do by the majority of clients is to produce a finished effect that may have originated from a picture, which is then modified to suit the client and becomes the perfect example of symmetry. This may be a nice style, but does it still have the same impact as the original picture? Why not? Well, we had to take the fringe shorter, so the client could see out, or we needed to calm down the volume so that it would be suitable for work, etc.

What is often happening with the best fashion images is that we automatically convert a high impact, dynamic, *asymmetrical* image into a recessive, passive *symmetrical* style.

If you have never thought about this before, start looking very closely at your favourite style images, you are going to *learn the secret of good design*.

Going back to the questions:

◆ Does balance relate to symmetry?

◆ Does imbalance relate to asymmetry?

The truth is that the best images, which are often asymmetrical in appearance, contain the visual excellence in artistic or aesthetic balance.

The following illustrations try to explain this key principle or concept in art.

In Figure 15.20, we have a 'see-saw' with equal masses on each of the opposing ends. As these masses are of equal weight, we arrive at equilibrium, an apparent balance which is symmetrical and harmonized.

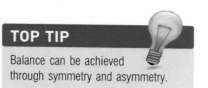

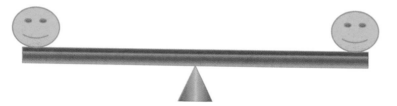

Figure 15.20   Balance-Symmetry

In Figure 15.21, we have a 'see-saw' which has a weight on one end and another heavier weight counterbalanced across the pivotal point. We now arrive at another form of equilibrium or artistic balance that is asymmetrical. But this image has far more impact on the eye because the image is *advancing* and like all good images – *it jumps off the page*.

Figure 15.21   Imbalance-Asymmetry

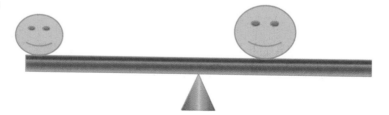

If you don't believe what you are seeing here, why not try this as an experiment. Try creating a simple see-saw and place two similar objects on either end. Now try to move one of those objects inwards, towards the central pivot and see if it will still balance.

Now use another object of a larger mass and counterbalance this on the see-saw. *Hey presto, you have created artistic balance.*

This key principle can be used in many ways in your hairdressing too. Not just in the ways of apportioning balance or volume but in colours as well. When you put slices of colour into hair, never put the same amount on either side of the parting, use different amounts on either side. Second, if you do use slices as a colour effect, *always* use odd numbers either side instead of even ones.

✓ 1 and 3s

✓ 3s and 5s

✗ 2s and 4s

✗ 4s and 6s

TOP TIP

Odd numbers work well for colour slices.

Movement The direction that the hairs take, individually and collectively, affects the overall style. The position and line of the hair gives direction to the style. The variation of this line produces direction within the style. The more varied the line direction, the more movement will be seen, showing as texture, wave or curl.

A fluid or flowing line gives a softer effect, whereas broken lines of movement create a harder visual impact. The more breaks within the style continuity, the greater the contrasts produced.

As far as movement is concerned within hair design, texture also plays a part in the visual effect of the hair. Texture is the term given to the way an object feels:

◆ rough or smooth;

◆ fine or coarse.

In hairdressing, we can *see* the textural effects and we can also *feel* the textural aspects.

TOP TIP

Emphasis can also be referred to as accent or accentuation.

Emphasis/accent Emphasis creates focus and in a design it is emphasis that draws the eye first, before it travels to the rest of the design. A hairstyle may be well balanced, with movement and harmony, and yet still be boring.

Emphasis or accent within a hairstyle can be created by the following:

◆ Wave patterns

◆ Colour

◆ Change in form/shape

◆ Ornamentation.

Choose an area of the head or face that you want to emphasize. Keep the design simple so that it is easy for the eye to follow from the point of emphasis through to the rest of the style. You can have multiple points of emphasis as long as you do not use too many and as long as they are decreasing in size and importance. Remember, *less is often more*.

Harmony Harmony is the creation of unity in a design and is the most important of the art principles. Harmony holds all the elements of the design together. When a hairstyle is harmonious it has the following elements:

◆ An overall form of interesting shapes.

◆ Coordinated colours and textures.

◆ Balance and movement that together strengthen the design.

A harmonious design is never too busy and it is in proportion to the client's facial and body structure. A successful harmonious design includes an area of emphasis from which the eyes move to the rest of the style.

The principles of design may be used in modern hairstyling and make-up to guide you as you decide how best to achieve a beautiful appearance for your client. Your job is to accentuate a client's best features and to *play down* features that do not add to the person's appearance. Every hairstyle you create for every client should be properly proportioned to body type and correctly balanced to the person's head and facial features. The hairstyle should attractively frame the client's face.

An artistic and suitable hairstyle will take into account physical characteristics such as the following:

◆ Shape of the head, including the front view (face shape), profile and back view.

◆ Features (perfect as well as imperfect features).

◆ Body posture.

> **TOP TIP**
>
> Harmony in a hairstyle refers to a form of balance.

Demonstrations, competitions and photo shoots

When you understand the aspects and elements of good design, you will want to apply them and show-off your skills in the best possible ways. Public demonstration, hair competitions and photo shoots are the *normal avenues* for this creative outlet.

Public demonstrations

Hairdressing demonstrations form a very important part in training and salon promotion. Public demonstration provides the opportunity to generate new sales, through increasing the numbers of clients within the salon and helping to promote the products sold and used within the salon.

Go to **CHAPTER 4** Promotion and display pp. 102–104, for more information about internal promotions.

All external events need thoughtful planning and as you progress onwards to the next level, you will find that you will be required to help in this area of promotion.

Photography and photo sessions

The power of a good photograph is undeniable. It instantly says more about your work and the image you want to project than any *advertorial* will. However, while fun, photo-sessions are not easy. They can be time-consuming, expensive – and sometimes disappointing if not properly coordinated.

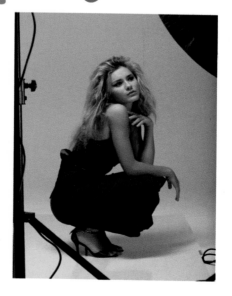

Think about themes Define your look. Questions to consider:

◆ Will the look be classic, fashionable, avant-garde or themed?

◆ Will the finished effect be the result of a service, say a colouring or cutting, or created by specific products?

◆ Will the look have more impact in black and white or colour?

◆ What clothes and accessories are best suited to the look?

- What image or effect are you trying to create – natural, classic, dramatic or romantic?

- Have you created a **mood board** to provide a visual representation of your intended effects?

Putting a photo shoot together Once you've decided on the look you're going to go for, start to create your photographic team.

Your model Picking a suitable model can be a tricky task. A common mistake is to choose a pretty girl with unsuitable hair, or vice-versa. Ideally she should have a combination of both. And remember, a conventionally pretty face isn't always *photogenic*, so study each prospective model carefully.

- Look for regular features and bright, clear eyes.

Avoid prominent chins and noses, over-full lips or dark circles under the eyes. The skin should be clear – even the most skilful of make-up artists won't be able to disguise completely obvious blemishes – and she should have a long, slim, unlined neck and a good profile to give the photographer maximum scope.

- Make sure that the hair suits the type of work you plan to do.

All models have limitations on what they will let you do in relation to cut, colour or perm. So your choice needs to be the right length, shade, texture and style. The model must also have the right features to fit your look – a sweet face is no good if you want an 'aggressive', moody or 'edgy' image.

The photographer If you can, get the help of a professional, *or someone who is learning to be a professional*. Choose someone who specializes in hair, beauty or fashion photography. All photographers, even if they are students, will have a portfolio, so have a look at the effects that they like to create to check their ideas are in tune with yours.

Make-up Good make-up is vital for a successful shoot, whereas bad make-up will ruin your work. If you know someone in this area of work, or who is a keen amateur, use them, but don't expect the impossible – a make-up artist, however good, can't completely change a model's face.

Clothes and accessories Time to *beg, borrow or steal*. The things that you dress your model in are going to have a dramatic impact on the overall success of the final images. Don't forget, if you choose current fashions, they will be out of date very quickly. If you choose historical themes or fantasy ideas, they can take away the impact of what you are trying to focus upon, or miss your target audience completely.

What type of clothes work best? Obviously this depends on the image you want to achieve and whether you are working with a professional stylist. If you don't want your shots to date too quickly then go for neutral fashions that don't scream out a particular season. Necklines should be simple and jewellery effective. But don't overload – if in doubt, leave out.

Have a plan Think about the designs and put together a mood board by cutting out images you like from magazines. Once you've decided on the styles, work out how you are going to achieve them. By creating a mood board you will be able convey a visual representation to everyone else involved.

TOP TIP

A pretty face is not enough to carry a great hairstyle off. They will need the hair/hairstyle too.

Go to **Creating a mood board**, p. 444 for more information on mood boards.

Draw up a list of the equipment and products you'll need and check them off when packing your session tool kit. The general rule is to take everything – and then add anything else that might come in handy!

On the day Have a clear idea of the looks you want to create but have in mind several alternatives as back-up. Pay attention to detail and make sure you see the digital stills, perhaps as output to a laptop's screen before changing and moving on to the next look. Picking up on faults isn't always easy. Those to look out for include gaps in the style, stray hairs on clothes/face, rumpled clothes, pins showing or too much product/make-up and the larger the image is shown on the screen, the more obvious the defects will be.

Be decisive and don't settle for second best. If you're not completely happy with an image, say so nicely and make the necessary changes. Keep the backgrounds or backdrops simple so as not to distract from the hair. White backdrops are good for any hairstyles and are a *classic* look for fashion effects. If you do want to use colour, keep to lighter colours or pastel shades so that they don't detract from the purpose of the shot.

Hairdressing competitions

Entering hairdressing competitions can be great fun and a great way of showing your creativity too. It is however, very challenging and requires a lot of personal discipline, dedication and thorough practise in order to achieve the right look that will catch the eye of the judges.

Competitions vary enormously between internal college events, to regional and national heats, and these vary greatly in the way that entrants take part.

For example:

The *L'Oréal Colour Trophy* is a national competition. It is initially short-listed at a regional level by photographic entry. Entries are sent out to participating salons or colleges early in the new year and the closing date for final entries is in March. Then after a preliminary judging, selected entrants are invited to take part at the regional finals, where they have to demonstrate their work '*live*' in front of a large audience, and against the clock. Winners from each of the regions are then invited to take part in the grand final in a 'top' London hotel in late spring.

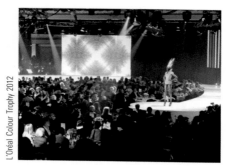

L'Oréal Colour Trophy 2012

The National Hairdressers Federation (NHF) holds competitions at regional levels and is very popular in supporting students as well as the experienced professionals. Their competitions allow allcomers to participate and finalists from individual regions are then invited to take part at national level.

At the top of British hairdressing: The *British Hairdressing Awards* attract the very best stylists from the top salons. These again are shortlisted by photographic entry. In this competition entrants enter a variety of categories ranging from Regional, **Avant-garde**, Artistic Team, London and British Hairdresser.

If you visit *Salon International* each year in Autumn at *ExCel* (London Exhibition Centre), you can see the nominees' work as they take a prominent gallery position within the main hall.

Many hairdressing organizations, colleges and major manufacturers run or sponsor competitions. If it's something that you would like to do, find out who is organizing competitions in your area and send off for a competition brief detailing the entry requirements.

Good practice – tips for taking part in competitions

◆ Watch the trade press for news about when and where competitions are taking place.

◆ Go along to competitions and watch what happens. See what type of work is successful in competitions and keep an eye on emerging trends and fashions.

◆ Ask trainers and tutors for advice. Also take advice from people who have entered or know about competitions.

◆ Read the rules carefully and know exactly what is required.

◆ Take time to find exactly the right model, one with the right type of hair, the right age and with looks that fit into the competition rules. A beautiful girl with good deportment helps considerably, but if her hairline is not up to scratch she may put you out of the competition.

◆ Understand that competition work is very different from salon work. Colouring in particular can often be a lot stronger on a competition floor than the salon floor.

Regular competitors stress the importance of preparation:

◆ Check and prepare your equipment.

◆ Take time to find the right model, particularly if you are trying to express a specific image or theme.

◆ Product knowledge and application is imperative, never attempt to style a model's hair without testing the product's effects on her hair beforehand.

◆ Practise, practise and prastice.

Regular entry to competitions keeps you up to date, you get a feel for the emerging under currents, fashions and trends which is vitally important. The motivation gained by attending competitions is infectious, and it is then passed on to younger members of staff. Competitions give you the opportunity to see what your competitors are doing. There is always something to be learnt by watching other salon teams and stylists work.

Competition day! You have prepared your model and you have practised the look for hours. Now the day of the competition has arrived. Stage fright has struck, but keep calm, there is nothing to worry about, everyone including the 'great names' suffer from nerves at this time. It is not just the stylists but the models too!

Stick to the rules:

◆ The style you do must conform to the competition rules. For example, if a day style is required, don't go over the top with elaborate 'hair up' or hair ornaments. If it's free style, a wider choice is allowed.

◆ Once you and your fellow competitors have finished your models, you'll be asked to leave the floor so the judges can take over. These people who are normally qualified hairdressers, hair and beauty journalists and occasionally, previous winners, choose the most competently designed and dressed head of hair. Depending on the type of competition and the marking criteria, the judges will award points covering all aspects of style ranging from technical detail, shape, movement, use of colour and artistic adaptation.

ACTIVITY

Competitions always have a brief for what is required and acceptable. Spend some time interpreting what is wanted, it may prevent a disappointment later on.

Creating a mood board for competitions or photo shoots

In order to take part in any of these events you will need to create a visual plan of what you are trying to produce. This way you will be able to get ideas on how you can develop your plans further and have a visual representation that you can share with others.

Purpose of a mood board A mood board is an alternative way of communicating ideas or methods of work to a target audience. It provides a way of *setting the scene* and prepares a storyline, or narrative to share concepts and express moods or feelings behind the image.

What is a mood board? A mood board is a visual representation of your ideas and thought processes and gives people a glimpse of the *story* behind your image. The simplest form of a mood board would be a large poster, probably A2 in format/size and could be made up as a collage. That is a *pastiche* of different media including:

- images;
- text;
- objects;
- textiles; and
- accessories.

Other mood boards could take on the form of a *mini-installation*. For example, a designed set or stage, on which you could add objects and other media to create a three-dimensional representation of your ideas.

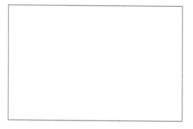
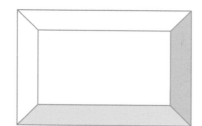

Developing a theme The hardest part of the planning process for a creating a mood board is developing the theme. This is the part where you need to make decisions about your **project** and its purpose.

You will need to consider the following from the outset:

Developing your theme	
Factors influencing your decisions	**Aspects to consider**
Where can you find sources of information?	◆ Internet – Searches, YouTube, Flickr ◆ Library ◆ Magazines ◆ Films ◆ TV ◆ Shows and demonstrations ◆ Other leading stylists' work ◆ Photographs

(Continued)

2D and 3D Mood Boards

(Continued)

Developing your theme

Factors influencing your decisions	Aspects to consider
What genre of hairdressing will your theme address?	◆ Avant-garde
	◆ Current fashion
	◆ Theatrical
	◆ Historical
	◆ Fantasy
	◆ Film or famous people
	◆ Futuristic
What is the purpose of the hairstyle?	◆ School prom
	◆ Public demonstration
	◆ Competition
	◆ Photo shoot

After collecting the variety of objects and elements that you will use to create your mood board, you can then start building the image. At this stage, you might find that your original ideas have changed quite considerably. Don't worry, as this always happens and the more time that you build-in to the creation stage, the more likely you are to change your ideas.

Finally, when you have pieced together all the textures, colours, information and feelings, you should try out your ideas by doing a small evaluation to a small audience of people. If you have stimulated the right feelings, you will find that your work will create lots of conversation and 'prompt' several questions. If all this happens, you know that you are on the right track.

SUMMARY

As a final reflection on what you have covered in this chapter, you should now have a clearer picture of all the essential aspects for developing your own creativity. In particular, you should now have a basic understanding of the key principles of:

1 How an image can be created.

2 The basics of good hair design and the aesthetic design components involved in creating an image.

3 How you can take part in external demonstrations, hairdressing competitions and photo shoots.

4 Developing a mood/story board for communicating your image and theme to other people.

And collectively, how these principles will enable you to become a better hairdresser or barber.

ASSESSMENT OF KNOWLEDGE AND UNDERSTANDING

Project

Choose one of the seasons listed below as your theme for a simple, A2 mood board.

1 Spring

2 Summer

3 Autumn

4 Winter

Research your chosen season by thinking about the colours, textures and pictures that convey these feelings and express this type of image. After your initial planning, find suitable elements that will project this theme on your mood board.

Finally, create your A2 mood board by putting your ideas together and fixing your colours, textures and other media to it.

Now answer the following questions:

Q1   Which is the most useful source of information for researching any form of theme?

Internet ☐
Twitter ☐
Dictionary ☐
Journals ☐

Q2   A visual representation of a collection of ideas is called a _____?

Q3   A picture is a 3D image

True or False

Q4   Which of the following are features of design?

Colour ☐
Magazines ☐
Shape ☐
Balance ☐
Books ☐
Camera ☐

Q5   Which of the following is not a form of visual media?

Books ☐
Magazines ☐
Television ☐
Radio ☐

Q6   Imbalance is the opposite to balance

True or False

Q7   Which of the following creates a softer effect?

Diagonal lines ☐
Straight lines ☐
Sharp angles ☐
Curved lines ☐

Q8   What H describes things that work well together H _____?

Q9   A stark contrast describes things that do not go together?

True or False

Glossary

Abrasion Broken, damaged skin (grazed).

Absorption The act of taking up or taking in water, e.g. a sponge absorbs water.

Accelerator A machine that produces radiant heat (infrared radiation) which can speed up chemical hair processes such as colouring or conditioning.

Accessories (hair) See ornamentation.

Accident book A record of accidents within the workplace required by health and safety law. Incidents in the accident book should be reviewed to see where improvements to safe working practices could be made.

Acid A substance that gives hydrogen ions in water and produces a solution with a pH below 7.

Acid conditioner A conditioner which has an acidic pH and helps to restore the hair's natural pH.

Acid mantle The layer of acidity maintained on the skin's surface which gives the skin slightly antiseptic properties.

Acid wave These lotions provide alternatives for perming when the hair is particularly delicate and needs to retain higher moisture levels or requires softer, gentler movement. They have lower pH values at around 6–7 and are therefore much gentler in the way that they work.

Acne A condition causing spots to appear, normally seen around the face, cheeks and mouth due to the overproduction of sebum from the sebaceous glands.

Activator A chemical used in bleaches or some perm lotions to start or boost its action.

Acute Sharp, severe or having pronounced symptoms.

Added hair A general term that covers the addition of hairpieces, wefts and extensions.

African type hair Any hair type which is tightly or loosely coiled, resembling black African hair.

Aftercare advice Recommendations given to the client following a service to maintain the finished result and enable the benefits to be continued at home.

Albinism A condition of the hair and skin where there is an absence of pigment.

Alkaline A substance or compound having the qualities of an alkali.

Allergy A sensitivity and possible intolerance to certain products, chemicals or compounds. See also patch test.

Aloe vera (shampoo ingredient) A popular, mild natural base ideal for healthy hair and scalps that can be used on a frequent basis.

Alopecia A general term covering a wide range of thinning or bald hair.

Alopecia areata Small circular patches of baldness, which eventually grow back, or move to other areas.

Alopecia totalis A term referring to the total lack of hair on the body.

Alpha keratin Hair in its natural state, prior to styling, i.e. the state the hair is in before stretching and setting it into a new shape.

Ammonia A strong smelling gas that is very soluble in water. An alkaline component of many high lift colours and ammonium-based compounds found in bleach lighteners.

Ammonium thioglycolate An active, alkaline substance in perm lotions that reacts with the disulphide bonds.

Anagen The stage of hair growth during which the hair is actively growing.

Anatomy The science of the structure of organic bodies.

Anchor A beard shape that resembles an anchor from the centre of the bottom lip and around and up the chin.

Anti-dandruff treatment A shampoo or conditioning treatment that is used to combat dandruff.

Anti-oxidant (conditioner) A conditioner that stops the oxidation process of chemical services.

Antiseptics Substances that reduce the growth of micro-organisms that cause disease.

Apocrine gland A type of sweat gland attached to the hair follicles in the armpits, pubic regions and nipples.

Appointment An arrangement made for a client to receive a service on a particular date and at a particular time.

Appointment system A system of organizing the volume of work (client services or treatments) undertaken by a salon. This may be completed manually or by a computerized system.

Appraisal A process of reviewing work performance over a period of time and planning future work objectives.

Arrector pili (muscle) The muscles that are attached to the walls of the follicle and, when contracted, raise the hair upright forming 'goose bumps'.

Artificial colour Any form of colour that is not a naturally occurring pigment. This is also called synthetic colour.

Ash/ashen tones Hair colour shades that contain blue, violet tones producing 'cooler' effects.

Astringent A substance which causes contraction and is applied after shaving to close the pores.

Asymmetrical Unevenly balanced, without an equal distribution of hair on either side.

Autoclave A device for sterilizing items in high temperature steam.

Avant-garde A genre of fashion that is considered progressive or exaggerated.

Awarding organization An approved examining body such as City and Guilds, VTCT, Edexcel, OCR, who define the examinations and assessment processes and conduct the certification administration.

Back-combing/back-brushing Pushing hair back to bind or lift the hair using a comb or brush.

Backwashes Washbasins where the client reclines backwards so that the neck rests in the basin.

Bacteria A tiny organism that can only be seen under a microscope.

Balance When equal or appropriate proportions create symmetry.

Baldness The loss of hair.

Barber's itch An infection of the hair follicles in the beard area of the face. Shaving makes it worse. Common Name **Folliculitis**.

Barrel curls A long hair dressing where wefts of hair are moulded into cylindrical shapes with an open centre. These are gripped into position and produce a chic, classic effect, popular for bridal work.

Barrier cream A cream that protects the skin against harmful moisture or infection.

Baseline A cut section of hair which is used as a cutting guide for following sections of hair. The baselines will determine the perimeter of the hairstyle, or part of the style, and may take different shapes according to the effects required.

BD Appointment abbreviation for blow-dry.

Beard and moustache shaping For a beard: shaping the facial hair shape around the mandible (jaw-line). For a moustache: shaping any facial hair worn above the upper lip.

Benefits Aspects that influence potential purchasers about the ways in which the functions of products or services may provide advantages for them.

Beta keratin The state the hair is in after it has been stretched and set into a new shape. See also alpha keratin.

Bleach A hairdressing product that dissolves/removes natural colour pigments from hair. It is available in powder, cream and oil forms.

Blending A technique for mixing different colours of hair extension fibres to create more naturally occurring effects, multi-toned effects and highlighted effects.

Blunt cutting Cutting sections of hair straight across (parallel) while holding the hair between the index and middle finger.

Body language Non-verbal communication provided by gestures, expressions and mannerisms that reveal the way a person is thinking or feeling.

Body odour (BO) The result of poor personal hygiene and lack of regular washing.

Booster An activator or colour development accelerator.

Braid Another name for a plait or plaiting.

Brick wind A technique of winding rods into the hair so that there aren't any uniform divisions or 'roller marks' after the perm is finished. When the hair has been wound in this formation it looks like a brick wall.

C/BW Appointment abbreviation for cut and blow-drying.

Camomile (shampoo ingredient) The best ingredient for use on oily scalps as it has a natural lightening effect.

Cane rows An effect created by multiple rows of scalp plaits that follow the contour of the head. Also known as corn rows.

Capillary A small 'hair-like' filament or tube, e.g. blood capillaries. These are the narrowest parts of the blood circulatory system that provide nourishment to the dermal papilla.

Catagen The stage of hair growth during which the hair stops growing, but the hair papilla is still active.

Caustic A very irritant substance, capable of burning or destroying tissue.

CBD Appointment abbreviation for cut and blow-dry.

Charge cards A form of payment where the complete amount of credit spent must be repaid by the cardholder each month to the card company.

Chemical reaction A process of two or more chemicals combining to create a different substance.

Chemically treated hair Hair that has been permed, coloured, bleached or relaxed.

Cheques An alternative form of payment to that of using cash.

Chignon A long 'hair-up' style forming a 'classic' knotted effect.

Chipping A cutting technique where the points of the scissors are used to 'chip' in to sections of hair, removing small chunks to create texture.

Cicatricial alopecia Baldness due to scarring of the skin arising from chemical or physical injury. The hair follicle is damaged and permanent baldness results.

Clarifying shampoo Strong, deep acting shampoo often used prior to chemical services to remove the build-up of styling products and dirt.

Cleanser Removes dead skin cells, sebum and debris from the skin.

Client consultation A service usually provided before the client has anything done to their hair to find out what the client wants, identify any styling limitations, provide advice and maintenance information and formulate a plan of action.

Clip-on hair extensions Pre-coloured wefts of hair that have clips or combs attached to them so that they can be affixed to the hair.

Clipper over comb A technique of cutting hair with electric clippers, using the back of the comb as a guide. This technique is often used on very short hair and hairline profiles.

Clippers Hair clippers are a mechanical cutting device operated by mains electricity or battery power. The cutting parts are created by two parallel blades with serrated teeth. The hand holds the direction of the clippers and subsequently, the cut. Hair is trapped within the teeth and the upper, moving blade oscillates back and forth to cut away all the hair that is exposed.

Club cutting or clubbing hair The most basic and most popular way of cutting sections of hair straight across (parallel) while holding the hair between the index and middle finger.

Coarse hair A texture of hair where the individual thickness of the hair is greater than that of fine or medium types. Coarser hair has more layers of cuticle than those on finer types.

Coconut (shampoo ingredient) Coconut contains an emollient which helps dry hair to regain its smoothness and elasticity.

Cohesive setting The wetting, moulding and drying of hair into a stretched position. See also alpha keratin.

Col (Rt or Fh) Appointment abbreviation for colouring, either root application or full head. Cold and hot bonded hair extensions.

Cold wave lotions These are alkaline perms and are the most widely available and simplest to use with applications for all hair types and tendencies and most conditions. These solutions tend to have a pH at around 9.0 so they are a fairly strong alkali that will swell the hair and affect around 20 per cent of the disulphide bridges.

Colour correction An overarching term that encompasses a variety of colouring problems and processes, such as removing artificial colour, removing or correcting banded colour and re-colouring hair that has been lightened back to a depth and tone similar to the hair's natural pigmentation.

Colour stripper A colouring product that is specially formulated to reduce the size of synthetic or artificial pigments within a client's hair and therefore removing depth and tone from previously coloured hair.

Colour test A diagnostic test to find out if a colour is suitable and/or achievable. It can be done by taking a test cutting or by applying colour on a small section of hair on the head.

Colour wheel (used during colour consultation) A diagram made up of colours that provides an at-a-glance, visual aid for showing complementary colours and opposite, neutralizing tones.

Communication Good communication is essential for establishing good customer service. We demonstrate this by listening to the client's requests, hearing and acting on what they are saying and always responding to clients in a polite but positive way.

Compatible Able to mix without an unwanted reaction.

Compound henna A mixture of vegetable henna and mineral elements that produce an incompatible hair dye. A contra-indication to all oxidation processes.

Concave When referring to this in cutting terms, a concave shape has a perimeter that creates a curved shape which is higher at the centre rather than lower (i.e. convex).

Conditioner A product that can be used to treat the hair or scalp, such as surface conditioners, penetrating conditioners, scalp treatments and leave-in conditioners.

Confidentiality Client confidentiality is a discreet and professional way of handling client information without disclosing private matters to other staff or personnel.

Consumer Protection Act (1987) Legislation protecting customers from unlawful sales practices and mishandling of personal information. The Act safeguards the consumer from products that do not reach reasonable levels of safety.

Contact dermatitis A skin disorder caused by intolerance of the skin to the direct contact with a particular substance or a group of substances. On exposure to the substance the skin quickly becomes irritated and an allergic reaction occurs.

Contagious Communicable or transmissible (infectious).

Contaminate To infect with germs.

Continuing Professional Development (CPD) A title given to a process of updating knowledge and experience on a continuous basis within a particular vocational sector.

Contra-indication   A limiting factor that affects the original/proposed plan of action, possibly allowing a treatment or service to continue, if and only when specific conditions are met. In some cases a contra-indication will stop a proposed service altogether.

Contrasts   A marked difference, e.g. between colours, say black and white.

Convex   When referring to this in cutting terms, a convex shape has a perimeter that creates a curved shape which is lower (dips) at the centre. See also concave.

Cornrows/cornrowing   A styling effect created by plaiting hair into small three stem plaits close to the scalp. Several cornrows produce linear or curved designs across the head.

Corrosive   A substance that destroys organic tissue by chemical means.

Cortex   The inner part of the hair where hairdressing chemical processes change or modify the natural hair, i.e. where permanent colour is deposited and where perms make physical changes to the hair.

COSHH   An abbreviation for Control of Substances Hazardous to Health. COSHH safety regulations affect the way in which chemicals are handled at work. These health and safety regulations are created for your safety and must be adhered to.

Cowlick   A hair growth pattern that appears at the front hairline where strong movement makes part of the hair stand away from the rest. This limits styling options and can be made worse by removing weight and length.

Credit card   An alternative form of payment to using cash. These cards are held by those who have a credit account where there is a pre-arranged borrowing limit.

Cross checking   A final checking technique for assessing the continuity and accuracy of the haircut. Where you find an imbalance in weight, or extra length that still needs to be removed, it provides you with the opportunity to remove it in order to create the perfect finish.

Curtain rail   A narrow band of hair that is left around the jaw-line.

Customer care/Client care   A way of providing a service to customers that promotes goodwill, comfort, satisfaction and interest. Maintaining goodwill ultimately results in regular repeated business.

Cuticle   The outer protective layers of the hair that produce an overlapped effect (like tiles on a roof).

Cutting angle   The angle at which the scissors, razor etc. cuts the hair.

Cutting comb   A type of comb that is between 12–20cm long. It is used for general cutting and is rigid and parallel throughout its length, or it is used for barbering and is tapered and more flexible. Most cutting combs have two different teeth patterns; one end finer with closer teeth for precision work or finer hair and the other end coarser with wider apart teeth for coarser hair and de-tangling.

D/C   Appointment abbreviation for dry cutting.

Dandruff   A commonly occurring skin dysfunction where there is an over-production of epidermal cells. White scaling flakes are shed from the scalp and can be seen on the shoulder area of darker apparel. Dandruff is not contagious.

Data Protection Act   Legislation designed to protect the client's right to privacy and confidentiality. See also confidentiality.

Database   An archive or repository of information held on a computer, relating to business records including client and staff names, sales, products, etc.

Debit card   A method of payment where the card authorizes immediate debit of the cash amount from the client's account.

Debris   A polite term referring to loose material that needs to be cleared away after different forms of styling, e.g. hair fragments, bands, glue, etc.

Defining crème   A finishing product which gives control to unruly hair.

Defining wax   A finishing product that provides textural effects to short or long hair when used throughout the ends of the hair.

Demonstrate   Display and explain a physical instruction.

Denman brush   A parallel, flat brush with removable cushioned bristles. It is used for general brushing, de-tangling hair before shampooing and drying straight hair of any length.

Density   The amount of hair follicles that populate a particular area of the skin or scalp.

Deodorant   A substance that removes or conceals offensive odours.

Depth   The term used to describe the lightness or darkness of hair.

Dermatitis   A form of eczema which results in a red, sore, hot and itchy rash, usually between the fingers. This is known to be caused by contact with hairdressing chemicals and solutions. The condition is avoided by the wearing of PPE (such as disposable vinyl gloves).

Dermatologist   A (qualified) medical specialist for skin conditions.

Dermis   The lower layers of newer skin below the outer epidermis.

Detergent   A cleansing agent found in many washing materials and virtually all shampoos. It has a 'polar' molecule structure, where one end is attracted to dirt and grease and the other to water. When it comes into contact with dirt, it surrounds it and lifts it away from a surface, forming an emulsion.

Dexterity   The skill and ease of using the hands.

Diffuser   An attachment for a blow-dryer which suppresses and disperses the blast of hot air and turns it into a multidirectional diffused heat.

Directional wind   A technique of winding rods in the direction in which it is to be finally styled so that, when finished, the hair will move in a particular direction.

Discolouration   An incongruent colour effect which can result from poor colour application, incorrect colour choice or can even indicate the presence of incompatibles.

Disconnection   An area within a haircut where a continued style line is broken or disjointed. A deliberate and distinct difference exists creating two levels within the layering patterns or perimeter baselines.

Disease   An abnormal condition affecting the body of an organism.

Disentangling   The process of removing tangles and knots from hair. It is usually carried out with a wide tooth brush or de-tangling comb.

Disinfectant   A chemical agent that will kill most germs and bacteria (unlike sterilization which kills 100 per cent of germs and bacteria). A typical example would be Barbicide®.

Disulphide bonds   The chemical bonds within the hair that are permanently rearranged during perming, relaxing and neutralizing.

Double booking   An error in the appointment system where clients' bookings overlap.

Double crown   A common hair growth pattern which appears as two whorls of hair at, or around, the crown area. This feature limits styling options and will dictate how short and the direction of how the hair can be worn.

Dressing   The process of achieving finish to previously set hair.

Dry hair   A condition in which the hair loses natural moisture levels affecting the handling, maintenance and style durability. It is often as a result of chemical treatments or heat styling.

Dry wax   A non-greasy finishing product that provides textural effects to short or long hair when used throughout the ends of the hair.

Eczema   A skin condition which appears as a reddening of the skin accompanied with itching and sometimes inflammation. It is thought to be associated with stress although one of its forms, dermatitis, can be triggered by contact with chemicals. See also dermatitis.

Effective communication   Professional communication that is not ambiguous and provides clear instruction or information.

Effectiveness   The quality of output achieved in a work setting.

Effleurage   A light stroking massage movement applied with either the fingers or the palms of the hands and used during shampooing and conditioning.

Elasticity test A test to check the hair's ability to stretch and return to its normal length. This is a good indicator of the hair condition and strength of the internal structure of the hair.

Electricity at Work Regulations (1989) These regulations state that electrical equipment in the workplace should be tested every 12 months by a qualified electrician. The employer must keep records of the equipment tested and the date it was checked.

Emphasis The creation of focus in a hair design that draws the eye first before it travels to the rest of the design.

Emulsify In colouring terms, the process of adding a little water to the processed hair in order to loosen the colour from the hair, without adding detergent, before shampooing.

End papers Protective paper wrapping, used around the points of the wound sections during perming to reduce/eliminate the risk of 'fish hooks', i.e. buckled ends.

Enquiry A question presented by clients or business contacts to find out more information.

Epidermis The older, upper, protective layers of skin that constantly migrate towards the surface.

Epilation The extraction of hair.

Ethmoid bone The bone that lies between the eye sockets.

Eumelanin Naturally occurring dark brownish or black pigments within the cortex of the hair.

Evacuation procedures The arrangements made by the salon for emergency purposes, e.g. exit routes, assembly points, etc.

Exfoliation The removal or shedding of a thin outer layer of skin from the epidermis. This is done by using a gentle abrasive substance to remove the surface skin.

Exothermic perms These perming lotions tend to be similar to acid waves in their chemical composition and therefore can have similar benefits. However, they need heat in order to work and this is self-generated when the perm is mixed together before applying to the hair/curlers.

Face or facial shapes The size and shape of the facial bone structure. Face shapes include oval, round, square, heart, diamond, oblong and pear.

Fading (colour reference) The loss of intensity of coloured hair due to harsh treatment, heat styling, wrong shampoos or environmental damage.

Fading (cutting reference) A method of blending one graduated, layered area 'seamlessly' to another, within a haircut. Or graduating very short layers out and on to the skin, e.g. classic men's barbering where short hair is faded out on to the neck.

Feathering A cutting term relating to a tapered or tapering effect.

Features The aspects of a product or service that state its functions, i.e. what it does.

Finger waves The process of moulding or styling hair in a pattern of alternating waves, using the fingers and a comb.

Fish hooks A term used to describe the buckling at the points of the hair, due to incorrect winding during perming or styling.

Fish tail plait (herringbone plait) A four-strand plait which is achieved by crossing four pieces of hair over each other to create a 'herringbone' look.

Flat brush A type of brush that has a handle that extends to the brush head with a flat and not curved profile. Flat brushes and paddle brushes are used for general brushing.

Flat twists Where the hair is twisted and rolled by hand, flat to the scalp.

Follicle A 'tube-like' indentation within the skin from which the hair grows.

Folliculitis Inflammation of the hair follicles which may be caused by bacterial infection.

Fragilitas crinium The technical term which is commonly known as split ends.

Franchise A business which is licensed to operate under the branding and reputation of another.

Freehand Refers to a cutting technique where the hair is cut without holding and is cut with natural fall, e.g. fringes.

Freehand cutting A cutting technique carried out without holding the hair. This is usually to compensate for the natural fall of hair, e.g. cutting a fringe.

French plait A three-strand plait that starts, centrally, near the front hairline and continues closely to the scalp to the nape and continues as a freely hanging plait beyond. This is also known as Congo plait or Guinea plait.

French pleat A method of styling longer hair into a vertical roll positioned at the back of the head.

Friction (massage technique) A firm, vigorous rubbing massage technique made by the fingertips and used during shampooing.

Frontal bone The bone that forms the forehead.

Full head application (of colour or bleach) A colouring technique that requires a sequence of applications to the mid-lengths, ends and regrowth area.

Furunculosis Raised, inflamed, pus-filled spots giving irritation, swelling and pain.

Germinal matrix The living part of the hair root where nutrients, carried in the blood supply, are converted into keratin (making hair and skin).

Goatee A narrow beard which circles the mouth and chin.

Grade Attachment combs for clippers that provide a range of different, pre-defined cutting lengths.

Graduation A cutting technique that is created by a sloping variation which joins longer hair that over-falls shorter hair in one continuous, blended, cutting angle.

Greasy hair A condition caused by the over-production of natural oils, i.e. sebum, which exudes from glands within the scalp onto the surface and eventually the hair.

Grievance A cause for concern or complaint.

Grips and hairpins A variety of metal or plastic items for securing the hair into position.

Guideline The first or starting section of hair that is held and cut to the required length and then used as a template for the following sections.

H/L FH or HL ½H Appointment abbreviation for full head or half head highlights.

Hair bulb The lower club-shaped part of the hair that is attached to the germinal matrix.

Hair colour The resultant effect from two colour aspects within the hair. These are depth (the lightness or darkness of a colour) and tone (the degree of red, gold, ash, etc.).

Hair extensions Pieces of artificial or natural hair that are added, either temporarily or for a longer period, to a client's natural hair to provide instant length, volume or movement.

Hair growth patterns These are double crown, widows peak, cowlick, nape whorl, natural parting and regrowth.

Hair shaft The portion of hair that projects above the epidermis.

Hair tendency Refers to a hair's straightness, wave, body or curl.

Hair tests There are a number of tests that can be carried out prior to a service to help evaluate the effects of processing upon the hair. These tests could reveal contra-indications to services or provide information on how the hair can be processed under certain conditions, e.g. porosity test, elasticity test, pull test, etc.

Hair texture Refers to the thickness or thinness of individual hairs, either coarse, medium or fine.

Hairdressing and Beauty Industry Authority (HABIA) HABIA is part of the Consumer Services Industry Authority (CSIA) and is the standards setting body responsible for National Occupational Standards in hairdressing and beauty therapy.

Hairspray A fixative originally derived from shellac, now made from water soluble compounds and is also known as lacquer.

Halitosis Bad breath.

Hard water Water containing minerals which do not easily lather. Hard water contains magnesium and calcium salts.

Harmony The creation of unity in a design. It is the most important of the art principles and holds all the elements of the design together.

HASAWA The abbreviated term referring to the Health and Safety at Work Act (1974).

Hazard Something with a potential to cause harm.

Head lice An infestation of animal parasites. A very contagious contra-indication. The trichological term for head lice is pediculosis capitis.

Health and Safety (First Aid) Regulations (1981) Legislation that states that workplaces must have appropriate and adequate first-aid provision.

Health and Safety at Work Act (1974) Legislation that lays down the minimum standards of health, safety and welfare requirements in all workplaces.

Heat protection spray Used in conjunction with electrically heated styling tools. The product laminates the outer layer of the hair so that it is protected from the damaging effects of heat.

Heated rollers Used for dry setting techniques. These are electrically heated rollers that are used as an alternative to wet setting. Heated rollers produce softer results than wet setting.

Heated tongs An item of heat styling equipment that provides movement, lift, volume, waves or spiralled curls on dry hair.

Henna A natural colorant derived from the Lawsonia plant. Its leaves are mixed with water to create a red hair dye.

Herpes simplex The scientific name for cold sores.

Highlight cap A technique for highlighting hair where small sections or wefts of hair are drawn through a close fitting 'rubberized' cap and coloured or lightened. A convenient option for people who have a sensitivity to colouring and cannot have colour applied by other means.

Highlights/Hi-lites A term for a very popular partial colouring technique, where small sections of natural hair are isolated (with foil, wraps, meche, etc.) and coloured or lightened to give a multi-toned effect.

HL or H/L Appointment abbreviation for highlighting.

HL T sect Appointment abbreviation for highlight, top and sides only.

Holding angle The angle at which the hair is held out from the head when completing a haircut.

Holding tension The even pressure applied to a section of hair when it is held ready for cutting.

Hood dryer An electrical item that applies dry heat to the head by sitting beneath it. The heat is adjustable and the timer can be pre-set to enable previously wet set hair to be dried.

Hot towels These towels are heated and used in barbering for shaving services.

Humectant A hygroscopic substance attracting water or locking moisture into the hair.

Humidity The level of moisture in the air.

Hydrogen peroxide An oxidizing agent used in many hairdressing processes. It readily gives off oxygen in chemical reactions, developing or processing colours, lighteners, etc.

Hydrophilic A term used in reference to the 'polar' detergent molecule. The hydrophilic end is attracted to water.

Hydrophobic Molecules that tend to be non-polar and, thus, prefer other neutral molecules and non-polar solvents. Hydrophobic molecules in water often cluster together, forming micelles. Water on hydrophobic surfaces will exhibit a high contact angle.

ICC (International Colour Chart) system A tabular system for identifying hair colours made by different manufacturers by their depth and tone.

Immersed Dipped into a liquid.

Impetigo A very contagious bacterial infection of the epidermal layers of the skin. It is usually identified as large brownish scabs around the mouth and cheeks. This contra-indication must be referred to a GP.

Incompatibility Refers to incompatible chemistry. When 'inorganic' compounds are present within the hair, for example colour restorers, 'Just for Men' or compound henna. They will be incompatible with organic-based chemicals made from carbon, hydrogen and oxygen (e.g. hydrogen peroxide).

Incompatibility test A method of testing hair to see if previous chemical treatments are compatible with those used with professional salons.

Incompatible Causing a chemical reaction on mixing; as between a chemical being added to the hair and another chemical already on the hair.

Individual learning plan (ILP) A specific programme or strategy of education or learning that takes into consideration an individual student's strengths and weaknesses.

Infection The communication of disease from one body to another. An infection is the colonization of a host organism by a parasite species.

Inflammation Inflammation is a process by which the body's white blood cells and chemicals protect us from infection and foreign substances such as bacteria and viruses.

Influencing factors Anything which could affect the hairdressing service.

Ingrown hair A painful condition where a build-up of skin occurs at the upper end of the hair follicle, causing the hair to grow under the surface of the skin.

Inversion A term used in cutting to describe a 'V' shape within a layering pattern or perimeter outline.

Irritant An agent that induces irritation.

Job description A documented set of written details pertaining to a person's specific job role, duties and responsibilities.

Jojoba (shampoo ingredient) A natural base better on normal to drier hair types.

Knots The effect produced when long hair is wound, positioned and secured to take on a tied or knotted rope-like effect.

Lacquer A fixative originally derived from shellac, now made from water soluble compounds and commonly known as hairspray.

Layering (layered cut) A cutting technique carried out on either short or long hair to produce a multi-length effect.

Legal requirements The laws affecting the way businesses are operated, how the salon or workplace is set up and maintained, people in employment and the systems of working which must be maintained.

Legislation Laws created by parliament.

Lemon (shampoo ingredient) Contains citric acid ideal for oily scalp types or for removing product build-up.

Lighteners Products that remove natural tone from the hair such as bleach or high lift colour.

Linear patterns Patterns created from either straight or curving lines, or a combination of both.

Lip-line moustache A narrow-lined moustache.

Long facial shape An outline perimeter facial shape that has proportions that are longer from the forehead to the chin than from ear to ear.

Male pattern alopecia/Male pattern baldness (MPB) A type of alopecia caused by sensitivity to androgens (male hormones).

Manual Handling Operations Regulations (1992) Legislation requiring employers to carry out a risk assessment of all activities which involve manual handling (lifting and moving objects) with the aim being to prevent injury due to poor working practice.

Manufacturer's instructions Stated guidance issued by manufacturers or suppliers of products or equipment, concerning their safe and efficient use.

Materials A variety of items other than tools and equipment for carrying out work including colouring packets, foils, wraps, meche, etc.

Medicated shampoo Helps to maintain the normal state of the hair and scalp. Medicated shampoo contains antiseptics such as juniper or tea tree oil.

Medulla The central part of the hair that is only found in coarser hair types.

Melanin The hair pigments eumelanin, pheomelanin, and trichosiderin are collectively known as melanin.

Metallic dye A hair colour containing metallic salts.

Mexican moustache A moustache following the line of the upper lip and extending around and down towards the chin.

Micro-organisms Living organisms, bacteria, etc. of microscopic size.

Mint (shampoo ingredient) A natural base suited to normal to slightly oily scalps, often used as a frequent use shampoo.

Monilethrix The technical term that describes a rare condition that under a microscope looks like the hair is 'beaded', i.e. thicker and thinner areas of hair along the hair shaft due to uneven cellular production.

Mood board A collection of ideas, themes, textures, colours, etc. that form the basis of a design plan, e.g. a competition mood board.

Moulding clay A dual purpose product for styling or finishing that bonds the hair with a firm hold. It is used on most hair lengths to give a firm textural bond.

Movement The direction that the hairs take, individually and collectively which affects the overall style.

Nape The back (posterior) part of the neck.

Nape whorls A hair growth pattern which affects shorter, cut hairstyles. The nape hair grows inwards, towards the centre of the back, rather than downwards. This is a limiting factor for some hairstyles.

National Occupational Standards (NOS) The standards defined by an industry for different levels of ability covering all the tasks and processes involved in the industrial sector.

Natural hair Hair that still has its original, natural structure.

Neck brush A small hand brush with very flexible bristles for clearing debris away from the client's face, neck, etc. during and after styling.

Neck wool A continuous 'sausage-like' length of cotton wool used during perming (and other services) to protect the client from spillages and debris.

Nine-section wind A classic technique for perming that starts by sectioning and securing the hair into nine, pre-defined workable areas.

NVQ An abbreviation for National Vocational Qualifications. These are job ready qualifications at a range of different levels.

Oblong facial shape An outline perimeter facial shape that has proportions that roughly resemble an oblong shape.

Occipital bone The protruding part at the back of the head (cranium) that provides contour and shaping to shorter cut, layered hairstyles.

Oil (shampoo ingredient) Can contain a range of natural bases such as pine, palm and almond. These are used to smooth and soften drier hair and scalps.

Oily scalp A condition caused by the over-production of natural oils, i.e. sebum, which exudes from glands within the scalp on to the surface and eventually the hair affecting its handling, maintenance and style durability.

One-length haircut A cutting technique where all the hair is cut with the natural hair fall to produce a one-length effect, i.e. the classic 'bob'.

Open or 'cut throat' style razor A razor that has a fixed, rigid blade that folds into its handle for safety. The blade is kept keen (sharp) by regular stropping and honing. The razor must be sterilized before each use.

Organic A substance that contains the chemical element carbon and relates to living (or once living) sources.

Ornamentation The term refers to the accessorizing of hair with enhancements, e.g. jewellery, beads, ribbons, tiaras, decorative pins/grips, etc.

Outlines The shapes created by the perimeter of nape and front hairlines.

Oval facial shape An outline perimeter facial shape that has proportions that roughly resemble an oval or elliptical shape.

Oxidation A chemical reaction where oxygen is added to a substance or compound during the chemical process.

Papilla The lower part of the follicle where living cells migrate upwards producing hair growth.

Para-phenylenediamine (PPD) A dye compound found in many permanent colours.

Parasite An animal or vegetable living upon or within another organism.

Parietal bone The two bones that form the sides of the cranium.

Partial colouring A term that applies to areas of the head and could include techniques such as slices, block colour, polishing/shoe shining, woven or pull through highlights and lowlights, etc.

Pediculosis capitis The trichological term for the head louse. An infestation of animal parasites. A very contagious contra-indication. See also nit.

Pencil moustache A narrow shape following the natural line of the upper lip.

Penetrating conditioner A name given to a group of deeper acting conditioners that work on the inner cortex of the hair.

Permanent colour/tint A penetrating colour product that adds synthetic pigments to natural hair until it grows out.

Perming (permanent wave) A two-part system for adding movement to hair by chemical means.

Personal development plan An ongoing action plan for self-improvement that defines personal objectives or targets set over a period of time and often reviewed during an appraisal.

Personal presentation Professional personal presentation can refer to personal health and hygiene, the use of personal protective equipment, clothing and accessories suitable for salon work.

Personal protective equipment (PPE) This health and safety term refers to all of the items of personal equipment that are supplied by the employer for employees' safety such as gloves, aprons, etc.

Personal Protective Equipment at Work Regulations (1992) Legislation requiring employers to identify, through risk assessment, those activities which require special protective equipment to be worn or used. Instruction should be provided on how the personal protective equipment should be used or worn in order to be effective.

Petrissage A slower circulatory kneading massage movement of the skin that lifts and compresses underlying structures of the skin. This movement is generally used for a scalp massage when applying conditioner.

pH The presence of positive hydrogen ions with a compound which denotes its levels of acidity or alkalinity.

pH balance The natural acid mantle of skin and hair at pH 5.5.

pH level A measurement of a solution that denotes whether it is alkaline (pH 8–14), or acid (pH 6–1). A neutral solution is pH 7.

Pharaoh A beard that projects from the base of the chin.

Pheomelanin A naturally occurring hair pigment that is yellowish or golden in colour.

Pigments The natural substances, eumelanin, pheomelanin and trichosiderin, within the hair that gives us our hair colour.

Pityriasis capitis A granular form of colouration that can be natural or artificial.

Pleat A visual description of hair that is folded, such as a French pleat.

Point cutting A cutting technique where the cutting angle is changed to remove hair bulk from the ends of each cutting section.

Porosity The speed at which hair absorbs (and retains) moisture.

Porosity test A test to indicate the condition (or damage) of the outer cuticle of the hair. This is a good indicator of the hair condition and its ability to absorb chemicals and moisture.

Porous hair Hair that has lost surface protection and therefore has a greater absorption and less resistance to chemicals and products. This affects the hair's manageability, handling and ability to hold in a style.

Portfolio A system for recording experiences, case studies, personal accounts, results from tests or assessments and the findings from projects and assignments.

Post-damping The application of perming lotion after winding in the curlers. This means that the time taken winding doesn't affect the overall processing time.

Posture The positioning of the body. Good posture is when the body is in alignment. Correct posture enables you to work longer without becoming tired. It prevents muscle fatigue (tiredness) and stiff joints.

Practise block A training head or modelling head that can be used to practise hairdressing techniques and styling effects.

Pre-damping The application of perming lotion prior to winding in the curlers.

Pre-perm treatment A product applied to the hair before perming to balance out uneven porosity.

Pre-pigmentation The preparatory process of adding warm tones to pre-lightened hair when (and before) re-introducing depth. This counteracts the unwanted effects that will often appear if this process is not carried out first, e.g. green hues.

Pre-soften A process to soften resistant white hair with hydrogen peroxide.

Prices Act (1974) The price of products has to be displayed in order to prevent a false impression to the buyer.

Professional advice Providing information based upon experience and knowledge.

Project Private study focusing upon a set topic or object. See also assignment.

Proportion The comparative relationship of one thing to another.

Provision and Use of Work Equipment Regulations (1998) (PUWER) Regulations laying down the ways in which work equipment must be used safely.

Psoriasis Non-infectious areas of thickening skin/epidermal layers usually around the elbows and knees.

Public liability insurance A compulsory insurance protecting employees, customers and visitors against the consequences of personal injury.

PW Appointment abbreviation for permanent wave (perm).

Quasi-permanent (colour) A colour that is mixed with a low-strength developer to create a longer-lasting effect. This treatment does show a regrowth and does need a skin test 24–48 hours prior to the service.

Radial brush A completely round brush. The inner body of the brush is usually metal, allowing the brush to heat up. It is used for blow-drying with volume, lift, wave and curl on short and long length hair.

Record cards Confidential cards recording the personal details of each client registered at the salon. These cards also record services a client received and retail product purchases. The information may be stored electronically on the salon's computer.

Reducing agent A product that releases hydrogen into the hair such as colour strippers, de-colour, or perm lotion.

Referral (client) The situations where you need to redirect clients to other sources of treatment or service, i.e. when there are adverse hair and skin conditions, or because of other services that your salon doesn't provide.

Regrowth The band of natural hair growing back at the root area (12.5mm per month) which will require some form of processing to match the mid-lengths and ends.

Relaxer/relaxing A chemical process (usually in two parts) which removes natural movement/curl from the hair.

Resale Prices Acts (1964 and 1976) The manufacturers can supply a recommended retail price (MRRP), but the seller is not obliged to sell at the recommended price.

Reshape/reshaping Cutting hair back into style. A six-weekly reshape cut will maintain a hairstyle.

Resources The variety of means available to a business that can be utilized or employed within any given task or project including time, money, staff, equipment, stock, etc.

Restructurant A deep acting treatment that will help to re-strengthen natural hair.

Restyle Cutting hair into a new style.

Reverse graduation A cutting technique that joins together shorter hair down to longer hair in one continuous cutting angle.

RIDDOR Reporting of Injuries, Diseases and Dangerous Occurrences Regulations. This legislation requires the employer to report certain injuries or diseases occurring in the workplace.

Ringworm A fungal disease also known as tinea capitis. It is a very contagious contra-indication and must be referred to a GP.

Risk The likelihood of harm occurring from a potential hazard.

Risk assessment A process of looking for and assessing the hazards within the workplace.

Rollers A variety of circular formers of differing diameters used for setting hair when dry (e.g. Velcro self-cling) or wet (e.g. 'Skelox').

Rooftop moustache A shape that extends from under the nose to form a straight 'chevron' or inverted 'V' shape.

Root lift mousse A mousse that has a directional nozzle allowing you to apply foam at or near to the roots. It is used on hair that needs body.

Rotary massage A quicker and firmer circular movement used during the shampooing process.

Round facial shape An outline perimeter facial shape that has proportions that roughly resemble a circular or round shape.

Safety razor A hand-held razor that is fitted with disposable blades, providing a more convenient, hygienic option, as the blades can be replaced for each client.

Sale and Supply of Goods Act (1994) The vendor must ensure that the goods they sell are of satisfactory quality and reasonably fit. The goods must be the standard that would be regarded by a reasonable person as satisfactory having taken into account the description of the goods, the price and other relevant circumstances. The vendor must ensure that the goods can meet the purpose they are claimed to do.

Salon policy The hairdressing procedures or work rules issued by the salon management.

Salon services The extent and variety of all the services offered in your workplace.

Scabies The common name of the itch mite. This animal parasite burrows beneath the surface of the skin and is very highly contagious. Referral to a GP is essential.

Scalp The skin covering the top of the head.

Scalp plaits Also known as a French plait, a cane row or cornrow.

Scissor over comb A technique of cutting hair with scissors, using the back of the comb as a guide. This technique is usually used when the hair is at a length that cannot be held between the fingers.

Scrunch drying A form of finger drying technique, where the lengths of the hair are dried (often with the aid of a diffuser) and compacted/crushed by the fingers to maximize the hair's natural movement.

Sebaceous cyst A swelling of the oil gland within the hair follicle.

Sebaceous glands Sack-like appendages on the sides of the follicle that secrete sebum onto the hair shaft.

Seborrhea An overproduction of natural oils causing a greasy scalp and hair.

Sebum A natural oil produced by the sebaceous gland.

Semi-permanent colour A semi-permanent colour is not mixed with hydrogen peroxide. It only penetrates to the lower cuticle and therefore lasts for a few washes.

Senegalese twists A twisting technique that resembles the plaited effect created by cornrows.

Serum A silicone based product that is used as a finishing product to smooth the hair and to add shine.

Shape, proportion and balance The physical and notional aspects that control hair design and hairstyling.

Shaper razor A type of razor with disposable blades that is used for cutting and styling hair, but not for shaving. It therefore has uses for both women's and men's hairstyling.

Sharps A term to describe sharp objects, e.g. razors, razor blades and scissors.

Sharps box A sharps box is a designated sealed container used for the safe disposal of sharp items, e.g. used razor blades.

Shaving cream Moisturizes the skin while providing a good lubricant for shaving. Moisturizing shaving creams can be used for all skin types, but normal to drier skins will benefit most from the creams.

Short graduations Haircuts where the inner and upper layers of a haircut are longer than the lengths of the outline, perimeter hair.

Skin tests As with hair tests, there are a number of tests that can be carried out prior to a service to help evaluate the effects of processing upon the skin. These tests could reveal contra-indications to services by providing information on how the skin reacts under certain conditions.

Slicing A texturizing technique for cutting hair using the sharp blades of scissors without opening and closing them, like using a razor or shaper.

Slicing (colouring) Sections of colour placed in the hair to bring attention to style lines or styling features.

Soya (shampoo ingredient) Helps to lock in moisture for the hair and scalp.

Sphenoid bone The bone at the base of the cranium, behind the eye sockets.

Spiral wind A perming technique of winding longer hair from root to point to create cascading curls.

Split ends A condition of the hair where a damaged cuticle exposes the inner cortex of the hair, allowing it to split along its length (fragilitas crinium).

Square facial shape An outline perimeter facial shape that has proportions that roughly resemble a square shape.

Steamer An item of salon equipment that is used for accelerating the development time of bleach lighteners. It produces a moist heat which stops the bleach drying out during the lightening process.

Sterile Free from germs.

Sterilization The complete eradication of living bacteria and germs.

Straightener (chemical) An ammonium-based lotion similar to perms that can be used to remove wave in hair.

Straightening Reducing the curl or wave in hair.

Strand test A test carried out upon hair prior to chemical services to determine the effects of processing.

Strengths and weaknesses The difference between personal skill areas that you excel in and those that you need to work on.

Style line The directions in which the hair is positioned or appears to flow.

Styling mousse A general styling aid for adding volume and providing hold when blow-drying or setting.

Stylist Another name for a qualified hairdresser or hairstylist.

Subcutaneous fatty layer/Subcutaneous tissue A fatty layer of cells at the lower dermis beneath the skin.

Surface conditioner A light conditioner that works on the outside of the hair to smooth and fill areas of damaged, missing or worn cuticle until the next shampoo.

Surfactant A surface-acting chemical detergent that cleanses the surface of the hair and skin.

Sweat A clear, salty liquid produced by glands in the skin that helps to regulate body temperature.

Sweat gland Small tubes in the skin of the dermis and epidermis which excrete sweat. Their function is to regulate body temperature through the evaporation of sweat from the skin's surface.

Sycosis An inflammatory disease affecting the follicles, particularly the beard. Appearing as pustules or papules, perforated by the hair.

Symmetrical Balanced by means of an even and equal distribution of hair on either side.

Synthetic colour Any form of colour that is not a naturally occurring pigment. A term that is often used instead of artificial colour.

T liner A type of clipper with a different blade type to standard clippers, enabling closer cut outlines around ears, necklines and facial hair shapes.

T-section highlights A partial highlighting technique around the hairline and along the parting only.

Tail or pin comb A comb that provides tension when combing through sections and helps to manage hair. It is used for sectioning hair into workable sizes, depending on the setting, plaiting or twisting technique used.

Tapered necklines Soft outlines that follow the natural hairline shape so that the nape outline appears to fade out with no harsh lines visible.

Tapering Cutting a hair section by removing thickness towards the ends of the hair to form a tapered point, i.e. a point like that of a sharpened pencil.

Tapotement A brisk tapping or slapping massage movement which is also known as percussion.

Tea tree oil (shampoo ingredient) A natural essential oil, like an antiseptic, which will fight infections on the scalp.

Telogen The period during which a hair ceases to grow before it is shed.

Temporal bones Bones which form the lower sides of the head.

Temporary bonds The hydrogen bonds within the hair that are modified and fix the style into shape.

Temporary colours Colours that do not penetrate the hair cuticle or affect the natural hair colour, but remain on the hair until washed off.

Tensile strength test A test that will determine the breaking point of a hair. This relates directly to the internal structure of the hair within the cortex.

Tension The state of being stretched.

Terminal hair The coarser type of hair that is found on the scalp and other areas of the body. There are three specific stages of terminal hair growth: anagen, telogen and catagen.

Texturizing A variety of cutting techniques that are used to achieve different effects within the cutting scheme of a hairstyle.

Thinning A way of reducing the thickness or amount of hair without having an effect on the overall (apparent) hair length. Techniques would include razoring, texturizing or using thinning scissors.

Thinning scissors Scissors which will remove uniform bulk from any point between the root area and ends.

Tinea capitis A fungal disease commonly known as ringworm. It is a very contagious contra-indication and must be referred to a GP.

Tone Refers to the tonal (the colour) properties of hair. These are grouped into reds, golds, mahogany, ash, chestnut, etc.

Toner/toning Adding pastel colours to previously lightened hair to control the final desired effect. Toning can neutralize unwanted tones or add depth or colour to hair that is too light.

Tonging A technique of styling hair with heated equipment. The tongs are cylindrical in shape and, when heated, hair is wound around and held in place for a few seconds and then released.

Total look A term that is often used to describe a visual themed effect that incorporates hair, clothes, accessories and make-up.

Traction alopecia An area of baldness that is caused by the excessive pulling of hair at the root. It is often associated with longer hair worn in plaits, twists, hair-ups and extensions.

Trade Descriptions Act (1968) Products must not be falsely or misleadingly described in relation to their quality, fitness, price or purpose, by advertisements, orally, displays or descriptions. Since 1972 it is also a requirement to label a product clearly, so that the buyer can see where the product was made.

Triangular facial shape An outline perimeter facial shape where the chin is very narrow.

Trichologist A professionally qualified person who specializes in the diagnosis and treatment of hair and scalp problems.

Trichorrhexis nodosa A condition where the hair has damaged sites of cuticle allowing the fibrous cortex to break through. This makes the hair weakened, very knotted and hard to manage.

Trichosiderin An iron-containing pigment found in human red hair.

Trim/Trimming A trim denotes a haircut where very little is taken off in order to maintain a hairstyle. Typically a six-weekly reshape is another name for a trim.

Twist A technique of styling hair, or multiple stems of hair, by twisting them together.

Ultraviolet radiation A form of sterilization carried out in salons by putting tools and equipment into a UV cabinet.

Uniform layer cut This type of haircut has sections that are equal, i.e. the same length throughout.

Velcro rollers Self-cling setting rollers for use on dry hair. They produce a softer curl effect than wet setting rollers.

Vented brush A parallel, flat brush with a double row of rigid, plastic bristles (short and long) affixed to a brush head that is not solid. It is used for general brushing and straightening of short to mid-length hair.

Virus The smallest micro-organisms that cause infection and disease.

VRQ An abbreviation for Vocationally Related Qualifications. These are job ready qualifications at a range of different levels.

W/C Appointment abbreviation for wet cutting.

Warmth A reference to hair tones that appear golden, copper or red in colour.

Wefts Long continuous strands of pre-coloured, pre-bonded hair that create a 'curtain' of hair that can be used to add to, or extend, a client's own natural hair.

Wetting agent A chemical agent that allows a liquid to spread more easily across or into a surface by lowering the liquid's surface tension.

Whorls A circular hair growth pattern that will influence or limit the styling options for a client, e.g. nape whorls.

Widow's peak A distinct point in the hairline in the centre of the forehead.

Index